MANAGEMENT OF
OCULAR INJURIES
AND
EMERGENCIES

From the second
greatest ophthalmologist,
to the first greatest.
—and the greatest
Dad!

Love,
Your Son,
John

MANAGEMENT OF
OCULAR INJURIES
AND
EMERGENCIES

Edited by

Mathew W. MacCumber, M.D., PH.D.
Assistant Professor
Retina Service
Department of Ophthalmology
Rush Medical College
Chicago, Illinois

Visiting Assistant Professor of Ophthalmology
Wilmer Eye Institute
The Johns Hopkins University School of Medicine
Baltimore, Maryland

Illustrations by
Brent A. Bauer, M.F.A., C.M.I., F.A.M.I.
Assistant Professor
Art as Applied to Medicine
The Johns Hopkins University School of Medicine
Baltimore, Maryland

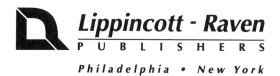

Lippincott - Raven
P U B L I S H E R S

Philadelphia • New York

Developmental Editor: David Dritsas
Manufacturing Manager: Dennis Teston
Production Manager: Lawrence Bernstein
Production Editor: Jeffrey Gruenglas
Cover Designer: Jeanette Jacobs
Indexer: Pilar Wyman
Compositor: Compset Inc.
Printer: Maple Press

Printed in the United States of America

9 8 7 6 5 4 3 2 1

Library of Congress Cataloging-in-Publication Data
The management of ocular injuries and emregencies / edited by Mathew
    W. MacCumber; illustrations by Brent A. Bauer.
        p.   cm.
    Includes bibliographical references and index.
    ISBN 0-397-51496-4 (paperback)
    1. Ophthalmologic emergencies.   2. Eye—Wounds and injuries.
    MacCumber, Mathew W.
    [DNLM: 1. Eye Injuries—therapy.   2. Eye Injuries—diagnosis.
3. Emergencies.   WW 525 M2658 1997]
    RE48.M335   1997
    617.7'025—dc21
    DNLM/DLC   97-26482
    for Library of Congress   CIP

Contents

Contributors ix

Foreword by Morton F. Goldberg xv

Foreword by Thomas A. Deutsch xvii

Preface xix

Acknowledgments xxi

1. Emergent Clinical Scenarios: Differential Diagnosis and
   Recommended Guidelines for Timing of Specialized
   Evaluation 1
   *Mathew W. MacCumber, John B. Kerrison, Dante J. Pieramici,
   and Morton F. Goldberg*

2. The Epidemiology of Ocular Trauma: A Preventable Ocular
   Emergency 9
   Nathan G. Congdon and Oliver D. Schein

3. Ocular Evaluation 29
   Nathan G. Congdon and Mathew W. MacCumber

4. Special Issues in Pediatric Ocular Trauma 39
   Arman K. Fard and Michael X. Repka

5. Radiographic and Echographic Imaging Studies 55
   Daniel P. Joseph, Cathy DiBernardo, and Neil R. Miller

6. Timing Guidelines for Emergent Surgery 79
   Sharon Fekrat and Eugene de Juan, Jr.

7. Preoperative Preparation and Anesthesia 91
   William E. Vickers and Marc A. Feldman

8. Injuries of the Lid and Lacrimal System 97
   Shannath L. Merbs and Nicholas T. Iliff

9. Orbital Trauma 107
   *John B. Kerrison, Mami Aiello Iwamoto, Shannath L. Merbs,
   and Nicholas T. Iliff*

10. Infections of the Lacrimal System, Eyelids, and Orbit 117
    Srinivas R. Sadda and Nicholas T. Iliff

11. Ocular and Periocular Inflammatory Syndromes 137
    Srinivas R. Sadda, Arman K. Fard, and Daniel A. Johnson

12. Ocular Burns 163
    Julie S. Yu, Robert A. Ralph, and Jonathan B. Rubenstein

13. Noninfectious Disorders of the Conjunctiva and Cornea 173
    *Laura L. Harris, Jonathan B. Rubenstein, Walter J. Stark, and
    Dimitri Azar*

14. Infectious Conjunctivitis and Keratitis 185
    Laura L. Harris and Terrance P. O'Brien

15. Corneoscleral Lacerations and Ruptures 207
    *Martin G. Edwards, Dante J. Pieramici, Sharon Fekrat,
    Dimitri T. Azar, Walter J. Stark, and Mathew W. MacCumber*

16. Injuries of the Anterior Segment 227
    Sharath C. Raja and Morton F. Goldberg

17. Glaucomatous Emergencies 235
    Michael J. Cooney and Harry A. Quigley

18. Management of the Injured Lens: Anterior Segment
    Reconstruction 257
    *Dante J. Pieramici, Mathew W. MacCumber, Dimitri T. Azar,
    and Walter J. Stark*

19. Endophthalmitis 275
    *Shannath L. Merbs, Lisa S. Abrams, and
    Peter A. Campochiaro*

20. Acute Management of Posterior Segment Injuries and
    Emergencies 285
    *Sharon Fekrat, Mathew W. MacCumber, and
    Eugene de Juan, Jr.*

21. Management of Intraocular Foreign Bodies 309
    Michael U. Humayun, Arturo Santos, and Eugene de Juan, Jr.

22. Traumatic Maculopathies 319
    *Mathew W. MacCumber, Thomas B. Connor, Jr., and
    Neil M. Bressler*

23. Sudden Nontraumatic Visual Loss and Visual Disturbances . . . 333
    *Mark J. Rivellese, Mathew W. MacCumber, and
    Andrew P. Schachat*

24. Disorders of the Optic Nerve and Afferent Visual System   351
    John B. Kerrison and Neil R. Miller

25. Traumatic and Other Acute Disorders of Eye Movements and
    Pupils   369
    John B. Kerrison and Neil R. Miller

26. Neurovascular Disorders: Carotid Cavernous Sinus Fistula,
    Cavernous Sinus Thrombosis, and Aneurysm   387
    John B. Kerrison and Neil R. Miller

27. Selected Intraoperative and Postoperative Emergencies   393
    Michael A. Johnson and John D. Gottsch

28. Sympathetic Ophthalmia and Enucleation   407
    Angelo P. Tanna and Nicholas T. Iliff

29. Nonorganic Visual Loss and Medical/Legal Considerations . . .   417
    J. B. Harlan, Jr., and Neil R. Miller

Appendix A: Pediatric Dosing of Commonly Used Medications . .   427
    Sharon Fekrat

Appendix B: Preparation of Antibiotics   429
    Shannath L. Merbs and Peter A. Campochiaro

Appendix C: Evaluation of Visual Disability   433
    J. B. Harlan, Jr., and Neil R. Miller

Subject Index   457

Contributors

ASSISTANT EDITORS

John Barnwell Kerrison, Capt., U.S.A.F., M.D.
Ophthalmologist
89 MDOS/SGOSE
Malcolm-Grow Medical Center
1050 West Perimeter Road
Andrews Air Force Base, Maryland 20762–6600,
Instructor
Department of Surgery
Uniformed Services Health Sciences University,
Clinical Assistant Professor
Department of Ophthalmology
Georgetown University School of Medicine, and
Post-Doctoral Fellow
Wilmer Eye Institute
The Johns Hopkins University School of Medicine
600 North Wolfe Street
Baltimore, Maryland 21287

Dante J. Pieramici, M.D.
Assistant Professor
Department of Ophthalmology and Visual Science
Vitreoretinal Section
Yale University School of Medicine
330 Cedar Street
New Haven, Connecticut 06520–8061

Lisa S. Abrams, M.D.
Assistant Professor of Ophthalmology
Department of Ophthalmology
Wilmer Eye Institute
600 North Wolfe Street
Baltimore, Maryland 21287

Dimitri T. Azar, M.D.
Associate Professor and Director of Corneal Service
Department of Ophthalmology
Massachusetts Eye and Ear Infirmary
Harvard Medical School
243 Charles Street
Boston, Massachusetts 02114

Brent A. Bauer, M.F.A., C.M.I., F.A.M.I.
Assistant Professor
Art as Applied to Medicine
The Johns Hopkins University School of Medicine
1830 East Monument Street, Suite 7000
Baltimore, Maryland 21205

Neil M. Bressler, M.D.
Associate Professor of Ophthalmology
Department of Ophthalmology
Wilmer Eye Institute
The Johns Hopkins University School of Medicine
550 North Broadway, Suite 902
Baltimore, Maryland 21205

Peter A. Campochiaro, M.D.
Professor of Ophthalmology and Neuroscience
Department of Ophthalmology
Wilmer Eye Institute
The Johns Hopkins University School of Medicine
600 North Wolfe Street
Baltimore, Maryland 21287–9277

Nathan G. Congdon, M.D., M.P.H.
Fellow in Glaucoma
Glaucoma Service
Wills Eye Hospital
900 Walnut Street
Philadelphia, Pennsylvania 19107–5599

Thomas B. Connor, Jr., M.D.
Assistant Professor, Ophthalmology
Vitreoretinal Section
Retina Service
Medical College of Wisconsin
925 North 87th Street
Milwaukee, Wisconsin 53226

Michael J. Cooney, M.D.
Resident in Ophthalmology
Department of Ophthalmology
Wilmer Eye Institute
The Johns Hopkins University School of
* Medicine*
600 North Wolfe Street, Wilmer B-20
Baltimore, Maryland 21287

Eugene de Juan, Jr., M.D.
Professor of Ophthalmology
Department of Ophthalmology
Wilmer Eye Institute
The Johns Hopkins University School of
* Medicine*
600 North Wolfe Street, Maumenee 721
Baltimore, Maryland 21287

Thomas A. Deutsch, M.D., F.A.C.S.
Professor and Chairman
Department of Ophthalmology
Rush Medical College
Chicago, Illinois 60612

Cathy W. DiBernardo, R.N.,
R.D.M.S., R.O.U.B.
Assistant Professor of Ophthalmology,
* and Director of Echography*
Department of Ophthalmology
Wilmer Eye Institute
The Johns Hopkins University School of
* Medicine*
600 North Wolfe Street
Baltimore, Maryland 21287–9275

Martin G. Edwards, Maj., M.D.
Chief of Ophthalmology
Department of Ophthalmology
Walson Airforce Hospital
McGuire Air Force Base, New Jersey
* 08641*

Arman K. Fard, M.D.
Resident in Ophthalmology
Department of Ophthalmology
Wilmer Eye Institute
The Johns Hopkins University School of
* Medicine*
600 North Wolfe Street, Wilmer B-20
Baltimore, Maryland 21287–5001

Sharon Fekrat, M.D.
Assistant Chief of Service, Instructor, and
* Director of Ocular Trauma*
Department of Ophthalmology
Wilmer Eye Institute
The Johns Hopkins University School of
* Medicine*
600 North Wolfe Street, Wilmer B-20
Baltimore, Maryland 21287

Marc A. Feldman, M.D., M.H.S.
Assistant Professor
Department of Anesthesiology and
* Critical Care Medicine, and Division*
* Chief of Anesthesiology*
Wilmer Eye Institute
The Johns Hopkins University School of
* Medicine*
600 North Wolfe Street
Baltimore, Maryland 21287

Morton F. Goldberg, M.D.,
F.R.A.C.O. (Honorary), M.D.
(Honorary, University of
Coimbra)
William Holland Wilmer Professor, and
* Director*
Wilmer Eye Institute
The Johns Hopkins University School of
* Medicine*
600 North Wolfe Street
Baltimore, Maryland 21287

John D. Gottsch, M.D.
Associate Professor of Ophthalmology
Department of Ophthalmology
Wilmer Eye Institute
The Johns Hopkins University School of
    Medicine
600 North Wolfe Street, Maumenee 321
Baltimore, Maryland 21287

J. B. Harlan, Jr., M.D.
Resident in Ophthalmology
Wilmer Eye Institute
The Johns Hopkins University School of
    Medicine
600 North Wolfe Street, Wilmer 320
Baltimore, Maryland 21287

Laura L. Harris, M.D.
Fellow in Cornea
Wilmer Eye Institute
The Johns Hopkins University School of
    Medicine
600 North Wolfe Street, Wilmer 320
Baltimore, Maryland 21287

Michael U. Humayun, M.D.
Ophthalmologist
5615 April Journey
Columbia, Maryland 21044

Nicholas T. Iliff, M.D.
Associate Professor of Ophthalmology
    and Plastic Surgery
Department of Ophthalmology
Wilmer Eye Institute
The Johns Hopkins University School of
    Medicine
600 North Wolfe Street
Baltimore, Maryland 21287–9218

Mami Aiello Iwamoto, M.D.
Department of Ophthalmology
Brigham and Women's Hospital
75 Francis Street
Boston, Massachusetts 02115

Daniel A. Johnson, M.D.
Wilmer Eye Institute
The Johns Hopkins University School of
    Medicine
600 North Wolfe Street
Baltimore, Maryland 21287

Michael A. Johnson, M.D.
Scheie Eye Institute
51 North 39th Street
Philadelphia, Pennsylvania 19104

Daniel P. Joseph, M.D., Ph.D.
Department of Ophthalmology
Washington University at Barnes
1 Barnes Plaza, Suite 17413
St. Louis, Missouri 63110

Mathew W. MacCumber, M.D.,
    Ph.D.
Assistant Professor
Retina Service
Department of Ophthalmology
Rush Medical College
1725 West Harrison Street
Chicago, Illinois 60612, and
Visiting Assistant Professor of
    Ophthalmology
Wilmer Eye Institute
The Johns Hopkins University School of
    Medicine
600 North Wolfe Street
Baltimore, Maryland 21287

Shannath L. Merbs, M.D., Ph.D.
Resident in Ophthalmology
Department of Ophthalmology
Wilmer Eye Institute
The Johns Hopkins University School of
    Medicine
600 North Wolfe Street, Wilmer B-20
Baltimore, Maryland 21287

Neil R. Miller, M.D.
*Professor of Ophthalmology, Neurology,
Neurosurgery, and Neuro-
Ophthalmology
Departments of Ophthalmology,
Neurology, and Neurosurgery
Wilmer Eye Institute
The Johns Hopkins University School of
Medicine
600 North Wolfe Street
Baltimore, Maryland 21287*

Terrence Patrick O'Brien, M.D.
*Assistant Professor of Ophthalmology
Department of Ophthalmology
Wilmer Eye Institute
The Johns Hopkins University School of
Medicine
600 North Wolfe Street
Baltimore, Maryland 21287–9121*

Harry A. Quigley, M.D.
*Professor of Ophthalmology
Department of Ophthalmology
Wilmer Eye Institute
The Johns Hopkins University School of
Medicine
600 North Wolfe Street, Wilmer 120
Baltimore, Maryland 21287*

Sharath C. Raja, Capt., M.D.
*Ophthalmologist
Department of Ophthalmology
Walson Airforce Hospital
McGuire Air Force Base, New Jersey
08641*

Robert A. Ralph, M.D.
*Clinical Professor of Ophthalmology
Georgetown University
6212 Montrose Road
Rockville, Maryland 20852, and
Assistant Professor of Ophthalmology
Wilmer Eye Institute
The Johns Hopkins University School of
Medicine
600 North Wolfe Street
Baltimore, Maryland 21287*

Michael X. Repka, M.D.
*Assistant Professor of Ophthalmology
and Pediatrics
Wilmer Eye Institute
The Johns Hopkins University School of
Medicine
600 North Wolfe Street
Baltimore, Maryland 21287–9009*

Mark J. Rivellese, M.D.
*Resident in Ophthalmology
Department of Ophthalmology
Rush-Presbyterian St. Luke's Hospital
Rush Medical College
1725 West Harrison Street, Suite 906
Chicago, Illinois 60612*

Jonathan B. Rubenstein, M.D.
*Associate Professor of Ophthalmology
Department of Ophthalmology
Rush Medical College
1725 West Harrison Street
Chicago, Illinois 60612*

Srinivas R. Sadda, M.D.
*Resident in Ophthalmology
Department of Ophthalmology
Wilmer Eye Institute
The Johns Hopkins University School of
Medicine
600 North Wolfe Street
Baltimore, Maryland 21287*

Arturo Santos, M.D.
*Professor of Ophthalmology
Department of Health Science
University of Guadalajara
P.O. Box 5–902
Guadalajara, Jalisco 45042
Mexico*

Andrew P. Schachat, M.D.
Professor of Ophthalmology
Department of Ophthalmology
Wilmer Eye Institute
The Johns Hopkins University School of
*   Medicine*
600 North Wolfe Street, Maumenee 713
Baltimore, Maryland 21287–9275

Oliver D. Schein, M.D., M.P.H.
Associate Professor
Departments of Ophthalmology and
*   Epidemiology*
Wilmer Eye Institute
The Johns Hopkins University School of
*   Medicine*
600 North Wolfe Street, Wilmer 116
Baltimore, Maryland 21287–9019

Walter J. Stark, M.D.
Professor of Ophthalmology
Department of Ophthalmology
Wilmer Eye Institute
The Johns Hopkins University School of
*   Medicine*
600 North Wolfe Street, Maumenee 327
Baltimore, Maryland 21287–9238

Angelo P. Tanna, M.D.
Resident in Ophthalmology
Department of Ophthalmology
Wilmer Eye Institute
The Johns Hopkins University School of
*   Medicine*
600 North Wolfe Street
Baltimore, Maryland 21287

William E. Vickers, M.D.
Resident Physician
Department of Anesthesiology and
*   Critical Care Medicine*
Wilmer Eye Institute
The Johns Hopkins University School of
*   Medicine*
600 North Wolfe Street
Baltimore, Maryland 21287

Julie S. Yu, M.D.
Resident in Ophthalmology
Department of Ophthalmology
Rush-Presbyterian St. Luke's Medical
*   Center*
1753 West Congress Parkway
Chicago, Illinois 60612

Foreword by Morton F. Goldberg

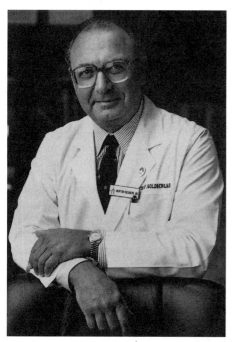

Morton F. Goldberg, M.D.

If a physician understands the diagnosis and management of ophthalmic emergencies, there need not be irrational anxiety when such events occur. And occur they do, despite some efforts at prevention, both personal and public. Indeed, the sad observation offered in the first volume in this series of books (1–3) related to ophthalmic trauma and emergencies is still valid: "Modernization of society has clearly not lessened the occurrence of accidental and intentional assaults on the human body; in many respects it has increased them."

In the three decades since our first book appeared, there has been definite progress in the technical management of ocular trauma and emergencies. Clearly, there are better diagnostic and therapeutic methods and machines; such as radiologic and ultrasonic scanning technologies, vitrectors and phacoemulsifiers, more effective intraocular lenses, and so on. It is not clear, however, that the visual prognosis for the most serious injuries and emergencies has improved substantially (4). Furthermore, it is obvious that much ocular trauma could and should be prevented. Why, for example, are some popular sports with balls, sticks, and racquets permitted without contemporary eye protection with sport goggles or other devices? (5) Racquetball and other sports are not quite as genteel as their advocates might wish to believe. Why can administrators of amateur sporting groups not understand the implications of eye trauma and blindness and take effective action? Why does society not regulate the use of BB-guns, unprotected boxing, and other violent activities, when it is our society that bears the brunt of the health costs which are incurred? Why should $200 million per year still be required to pay for eye injuries in the United States? Why are there close to 1 million occupational eye injuries in this country per year? Why is eye trauma the leading cause of unilateral blindness in the world today? We must hope that the content of this book will awaken parents, teachers, legislators, manufacturers, sports authorities, other physicians, and of course, individual citizens to the importance of preventable eye injuries.

This book, as reflected in the Contents, is much more comprehensive than its predecessors. Chapters are included on epidemiology, diagnostic devices, therapeutic strategy, pharmacologic and surgical choices, and legal/administrative issues. This book now makes available the remarkably extensive knowledge and experience of the residents and senior staffs of the Wilmer Eye Institute. Busily functioning 24 hours a day, Wilmer's Emergency Department provides an expert, specialized environment where patients and physicians together strive to remedy both purposeful and inadvertent damage to the eye and its surrounding tissues. The advice of our residents and staff, presented for the benefit of our colleagues and their patients, represents poignant testimony to the traumatic and urgent sides of our modern existence, as well as our frequently, but not universally, successful efforts to cope with these unfortunate events.

REFERENCES

1. Paton D, Goldberg MF. *Injuries of the Eye, the Lids, and the Orbit. Diagnosis and Management.* Philadelphia: WB Saunders, 1968
2. Paton D, Goldberg MF. *Management of Ocular Injuries.* Philadelphia: WB Saunders, 1976.
3. Deutsch TA, Feller DB. In Paton D, Goldberg MF, eds. *Management of Ocular Injuries.* 2nd ed. Philadelphia: WB Saunders, 1985.
4. Pieramici DJ, MacCumber MW, Humayun MV, Marsh MJ, de Juan E. Open globe injury. Update on types of injuries and visual reports. *Ophthalmology* 1996;103:1798–1803.
5. Napier SM, Baker RS, Sanford DG, Easterbrook M. Eye Injuries in Athletes and Recreation. *Surv Ophthalmol* 1996;41:229–244 (Philadelphia: WB Saunders, 1996).

Foreword by Thomas A. Deutsch

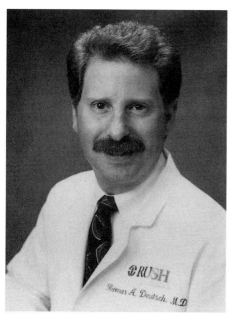

Thomas A. Deutsch, M.D.

Despite attempts to reduce the number of eye injuries through the education of workers and athletes, ocular injuries and emergencies continue to constitute a significant number of emergency room visits. The previous editions of this book have attempted to condense the best information available at the time for the benefit of those who care for eye injuries. Unfortunately, the former editions are hopelessly out of date in terms of the techniques and knowledge now available. Fortunately, Mathew W. MacCumber, M.D., has harnessed the talents and experience of a great many ophthalmologists to bring this new edition together.

This edition greatly transcends the former works, completely rearranging the topics, providing all new figures, and adding important new areas, including ocular emergencies. This book will provide another generation of physicians with the basis of theory and practice in the eye emergency room.

The original edition was authored by two of the outstanding former chief residents of the Wilmer Ophthalmological Institute: David Paton, M.D., and Morton F. Goldberg, M.D. The second edition was authored by two chief residents in Dr. Goldberg's department of almost 20 years at The University of Illinois Eye and Ear Infirmary, Daniel B. Feller, M.D., and myself. This edition is edited by Dr. Goldberg's chief resident at the Wilmer Eye Institute, Mathew W. MacCumber, M.D. I am particularly pleased that Dr. MacCumber is now in my department at Rush Medical College.

It is certain that the eye will continue to be vulnerable to injury. As practitioners, we should all be grateful to this editor and to these authors for guiding us towards the best practices for these challenging patients.

Preface

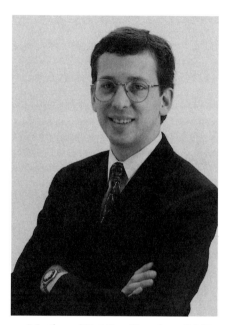

Mathew W. MacCumber, M.D.

This book follows in a tradition established by Morton F. Goldberg, M.D., when, as Chief Resident and Assistant Chief of Service at the Wilmer Eye Institute at Johns Hopkins, he wrote with David Paton, M.D., the first edition to *Management of Ocular Injuries.* During my year as Chief Resident, Assistant Chief of Service and Director of Ocular Trauma Service, I not only had the honor of working closely with Dr. Goldberg, but with an outstanding group of resident ophthalmologists as well. The residents and I organized an ocular emergencies conference at Wilmer on a snowy February day in 1996 which provided the basis for this expanded edition. The final product, however, could have not been completed without the expert supervision of the Wilmer Eye Institute and Rush Medical College faculty members, who worked closely with the resident authors at both institutions.

This book is designed to be a resource "of everything one needs to know" for the management of an ocular injury or other ocular emergency within the first 48 hours. In our experience, this provides sufficient time for the treating physician to read more detailed texts or to search the medical literature for the most up-to-date therapy. For an emergency room, it can stand alone as the one book on ophthalmology.

Chapter One gives guidelines to primary care physicians, regarding when patients should receive consultation by an ophthalmologist or other specialty physician. The following six chapters provide information for the thorough evaluation of the patient and preparation for surgery, if necessary. The remaining bulk of the work then outlines in detail the medical and surgical steps that should be taken for each disorder. Although useful for resident ophthalmologists, the surgical chapters are not intended to teach a novice a new surgical procedure, but rather to provide suggestions and reminders to ensure that patients will have the best overall outcome. The book provides suggestions for the follow-up care of many ophthalmic injuries and emergencies. Finally, the appendices contain information that treating physicians may find helpful when they do not have other resources readily available (such as *AMA Guides to the Evaluation of Permanent Impairment*).

Mathew W. MacCumber, M.D., Ph.D.

Acknowledgments

I am indebted to several individuals who went well beyond the call of duty during the process of completing this book. First, I thank Morton F. Goldberg, M.D., Director of the Wilmer Eye Institute at Johns Hopkins, for the inspiration and guidance he provided during my year as Chief Resident, Assistant Chief of Service and Director of Ocular Trauma Service. I never cease to be impressed by the stellar group of residents both at Wilmer and in the Department of Ophthalmology at Rush Medical College. In particular, I want to thank John B. Kerrison, M.D., Dante J. Pieramici, M.D., Shannath L. Merbs, M.D., Ph.D., Nicholas T. Iliff, M.D., and all of "The First Years" for their commitment to this project. I have been extremely lucky to have been associated with Brent Bauer, one of the finest medical illustrators in the world. I thank my fellow associates at Illinois Retina Associates for their support, and my current chairman in the Department of Ophthalmology at Rush Medical College, Thomas A. Deutsch, M.D. (also a past author of a book in this series). Special thanks to Kirk Packo, M.D., for donating several critical color photographs. I am grateful to Stuart Freeman and the editors at Lippincott–Raven Publishers for skillfully guiding the book through the publication process. I had expert technical assistance by Ruth Shea and Sharon Welling. Finally, this book is dedicated to Judith and Abigail, who provide immeasurable joy in my life and from whom precious time was taken for the book's completion.

MANAGEMENT OF

OCULAR INJURIES

AND

EMERGENCIES

Management of Ocular Injuries and Emergencies,
edited by Mathew W. MacCumber.
Lippincott–Raven Publishers, Philadelphia ©1998.

1

Emergent Clinical Scenarios: Differential Diagnosis and Recommended Guidelines for Timing of Specialized Evaluation

Mathew W. MacCumber, John B. Kerrison, Dante J. Pieramici, and Morton F. Goldberg

Retina Service, Department of Ophthalmology, Rush Medical College, Chicago, Illinois 60612; Department of Ophthalmology, Wilmer Eye Institute, The Johns Hopkins University School of Medicine, Baltimore, Maryland 21218; and Department of Ophthalmology and Visual Science, Vitreoretinal Section, Yale University School of Medicine, New Haven, Connecticut 06520–8061

Of the variety of ophthalmic conditions that cause affected individuals to present for emergent evaluation, only two, chemical burns and retinal artery occlusion, require immediate therapy (within minutes). A variety of other conditions require attention within hours, such as endophthalmitis, intraocular foreign bodies, and orbital cellulitis. Thus, in general there is adequate time for examination, unhurried decision making, and optimal preparation for the initiation of therapy. However, it is critical that a few hours do not become several hours or days because of incorrect or incomplete diagnosis (e.g., a missed intraocular foreign body with early endophthalmitis). Proper evaluation often requires consultation by an experienced ophthalmologist and, for some conditions, other health-care professionals, such as a radiologist, otolaryngologist, neurologist, or neurosurgeon.

Below are several clinical scenarios occurring in emergency rooms and clinicians' offices on an emergent basis. To ensure that important diagnoses are not missed, the most serious conditions are listed for differential diagnosis. For general and emergency room physicians, guidelines are presented for the timing of referral to an ophthalmologist or other key specialists so harmful delays in instituting necessary therapy can be avoided.

If ophthalmologic or other specialized evaluation requiring anesthesia is indicated within a few hours, the patient should be maintained NPO (nothing by mouth). All traumatically injured eyes should be properly shielded (Fig. 1–1) and consideration should be given to bilaterally shielding the patient if there is risk of binocular traumatic injury. Dilating drops or ointments of any kind should be avoided until evaluation by the ophthalmologist or other specialist is performed.

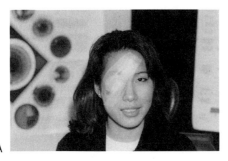 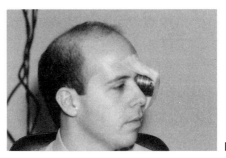

A   B

FIG. 1–1. A: Patching of injured eye with a metal shield. **B:** Patching of injured eye with a stiff paper cup when metal shield is unavailable.

Splash Injury (see Chapter 12)
Differential diagnosis
  Chemical burn until proven otherwise
Initial management
  Therapy (irrigation) should begin immediately at scene of accident if possible.
  Arrange evaluation by an experienced physician within minutes if possible and
    then by an ophthalmologist within a few hours.
Sudden Painless Atraumatic Loss of Vision (see Chapters 23 and 24)
Differential diagnosis
  Retinal artery occlusion
  Retinal vein occlusion
  Giant cell arteritis
  Nonarteritic ischemic optic neuropathy
  Cerebrovascular accident (stroke)
  Retinal detachment
  Vitreous hemorrhage
  Choroidal neovascularization ± subretinal hemorrhage
  Malingering (see Chapter 29)
Initial management
  If no other neurologic findings, arrange evaluation by an ophthalmologist
    within 30 to 60 minutes if central retinal artery occlusion is possible and
    within a few hours otherwise.
If other neurologic findings are present, stabilize patient, arrange head and optic
  nerve CT scanning, and arrange evaluation by a neurologist/neurosurgeon and
  by an ophthalmologist within a few hours (within minutes, if possible, if patient
  could qualify for thrombolytic protocol).
Transient Atraumatic Loss of Vision (see Chapter 23)
Differential diagnosis
  Amaurosis fugax

Migraine headache

Corneal or tear film abnormality

Initial management

Arrange evaluation by an ophthalmologist or neurologist/neurosurgeon within 24 hours

Sudden Painful Atraumatic Loss of Vision

Differential diagnosis

Angle-closure glaucoma (see Chapter 17)

Endophthalmitis (see Chapter 19)

Anterior uveitis (see Chapter 11)

Giant cell arteritis (see Chapter 24)

Optic neuritis (see Chapter 24)

Keratitis (see Chapter 14)

Initial management

Arrange evaluation by an ophthalmologist within a few hours.

Blunt Injury

Differential diagnosis (there may be multiple diagnoses)

Globe rupture (see Chapter 15)

Corneal abrasion (see Chapter 13)

Hyphema and/or other anterior segment injuries (see Chapter 16)

Retinal tear or detachment (see Chapter 20)

Traumatic maculopathy (see Chapter 22)

Lid laceration (see Chapter 8)

Orbital fracture (see Chapter 9)

Initial management

Arrange evaluation by an ophthalmologist within a few hours.

Penetrating Injury

Differential diagnosis (there may be multiple)

Globe laceration (see Chapter 15)

Endophthalmitis (see Chapter 19)

Intraocular foreign body (see Chapter 21)

Lid laceration (see Chapter 8)

Orbital fracture (see Chapter 9)

Orbital cellulitis (see Chapter 10)

Initial management

Arrange evaluation by an ophthalmologist within a few hours.

Atraumatic Double Vision (see Chapter 25)

Differential diagnosis

Monocular (double vision persists when unaffected eye is covered, rarely acute)

Refractive error

Corneal or lenticular opacity

Binocular vision (no double vision when either eye covered)

Cranial nerve III, IV, or VI palsy (see Chapter 25 for differential diagnosis which includes intracranial aneurysm)

Myasthenia gravis (often intermittent double vision)
Orbital pseudotumor
Thyroid eye disease (orbitopathy)
Cavernous sinus/superior orbital fissure syndrome
Cerebrovascular disease
Demyelinating disease
Decompensated phoria
Decentered spectacles
Initial management
Arrange evaluation by an ophthalmologist and/or neurologist/neurosurgeon within a few hours if acute, otherwise within one to a few days.

Traumatic Double Vision (see Chapter 25)
Differential diagnosis
Orbital fracture with extraocular muscle involvement
Orbital hemorrhage
Trochlear injury
Cranial nerve III, IV, or VI palsy (see Chapter 25 for further differential diagnosis)
Initial management
If evidence of central nervous system trauma, arrange evaluation by a neurosurgeon within minutes if possible. If isolated to the orbit, arrange evaluation by an ophthalmologist within a few hours.

Acute Visual Distortion (see Chapter 23)
Differential diagnosis
Choroidal neovascularization
Retinal detachment
Central serous chorioretinopathy
Corneal, lenticular, or spectacle abnormality (less common)
Initial management
If central vision is not affected, arrange evaluation by an ophthalmologist within a few hours (for diagnosis of a macular-on retinal detachment).
If central vision is affected, arrange evaluation by an ophthalmologist within 24 hours.

Acute Visual Disturbance in the Immunocompromised Individual (see Chapter 11)
Differential diagnosis
Endogenous endophthalmitis
Cytomegalovirus retinitis
Toxoplasmosis retinochoroiditis
Herpes necrotizing retinitis
Syphilitic retinitis/neuritis
Retinal detachment
Other causes unrelated to the immunocompromised state
Initial management
Arrange evaluation by an ophthalmologist within a few hours if marked and within 24 hours if mild (e.g., limited to floaters).

Acute Visual Disturbance in the Postoperative Patient
Differential diagnosis
   Endophthalmitis (see Chapter 19)
   Retinal detachment (see Chapter 20)
   Postoperative inflammation
   Ocular nerve or muscle injury (double vision)
   Other causes possibly unrelated to the surgery
Initial management
   Arrange evaluation by an ophthalmologist (preferably the operating surgeon)
      within a few hours.
Floaters (see Chapters 11 and 23)
Differential diagnosis
   Posterior vitreous detachment ($\pm$ retinal tear/detachment)
   Vitreous hemorrhage
   Retinitis in the immunocompromised individual
   Intermediate or posterior uveitis
Initial management
   Arrange evaluation by an ophthalmologist within 24 hours.
Flashes of Light (Photopsia) (see Chapter 23)
Differential diagnosis
   Posterior vitreous detachment
   Retinal tear
   Migraine
   Retinitis (infectious or inflammatory)
   Ocular tumor
Initial management
   Arrange evaluation by an ophthalmologist within 24 hours.
Acute Proptosis (see Chapters 11, 25, and 26)
Differential diagnosis
   Orbital pseudotumor
   Thyroid eye disease (orbitopathy)
   Traumatic orbital hemorrhage or foreign body
   Orbital cellulitis
   Carotid-cavernous sinus fistula (typically bilateral)
   Cavernous sinus thrombosis (typically bilateral)
   Leukemia or lymphoma
   Rhabdomyosarcoma or metastatic neuroblastoma (in children)
   Hemorrhage into lymphangioma (in children)
Initial management
   Arrange evaluation by an ophthalmologist within a few hours, particularly if se-
      vere or in a child.
Acute Red Eye (see Chapters 13 and 14)
Differential diagnosis
   Conjunctivitis
   Allergic

Infectious

Toxic

Corneal abrasion or foreign body

Episcleritis

Kerititis

Scleritis

Uveitis

Endophthalmitis

Blepharitis

Initial management

Arrange evaluation by an experienced physician within a few hours; arrange consultation with or evaluation by an ophthalmologist at this time.

Sudden Corneal Foreign Body Sensation (see Chapters 13 and 14)

Differential diagnosis

Corneal abrasion; recurrent erosion

Corneal foreign body

Keratitis

Spontaneous perforation/ruptured descemetocele

Conjunctivitis

Dry eye

Initial management

Arrange evaluation by experienced physician within a few hours.

Therapy (e.g., removal of a corneal foreign body) should be initiated by or in consultation with an ophthalmologist.

Acute Periocular Itchiness (see Chapter 13)

Differential diagnosis

Blepharitis

Conjunctivitis (e.g., viral, allergic, or vernal)

Topical drug allergy (e.g., atropine)

Dermatitis

Initial management

Arrange evaluation by an ophthalmologist within a few days, sooner if severe.

Acute Tearing (see Chapters 13 and 14)

Differential diagnosis

Painful

Corneal abrasion or recurrent erosion

Corneal foreign body

Keratitis

Trichiasis (aberrant eyelash)

Anterior uveitis

Minimal or no pain

Dry eye syndrome

Conjunctivitis

Punctal, cannalicular, or lacrimal sac obstruction

Nasolacrimal duct obstruction (particularly in infant)

Congenital glaucoma (in infant)
Initial management
   If painful, arrange evaluation by an experienced physician in consultation with
      an ophthalmologist within a few hours. If minimally painful, arrange evalua-
      tion by an ophthalmologist within a few days.
Acute Atraumatic Periocular Pain (see Chapter 11 and as indicated)
Differential diagnosis
   Angle-closure glaucoma (see Chapter 17)
   Headache/migraine
   Sinusitis
   Scleritis/episcleritis
   Orbital pseudotumor
   Preseptal/orbital cellulitis
   Herpes zoster ophthalmicus/postherpetic neuralgia
   Anterior uveitis
   Endophthalmitis (see Chapter 19)
   Corneal abrasion or recurrent erosion (see Chapter 13)
   Corneal foreign body (see Chapter 13)
   Kerititis (see Chapter 14)
Initial management
   Arrange evaluation by an ophthalmologist within a few hours.
Atraumatic Periocular Swelling (see Chapter 11)
Differential diagnosis
   Chalazion/hordeolum
   Conjunctivitis (viral, allergic)
   Preseptal/orbital cellulitis
   Dermatitis (contact, allergic)
   Dacryoadenitis (upper lid, temporally)
   Dacryocystitis (lower lid, nasally)
   Prolapsed fat (noninflammatory)
   Fluid retention/head-dependent positioning (noninflammatory)
Initial management
   Arrange evaluation by an ophthalmologist within a few hours if severe or if or-
      bital or preseptal inflammatory signs are present. Otherwise, arrange evalua-
      tion by an experienced physician or ophthalmologist within 24 hours.
Acute Eyelid Twitching
Differential diagnosis
   Corneal abrasion, dryness or foreign body
   Blepharospasm
   Hemifacial spasm
   Fatigue
   Excess caffeine
Initial management
   Arrange evaluation by an experienced physician within a few hours if severe;
      arrange evaluation by an ophthalmologist within a few days if mild.

Acute Eyelid Droop (Ptosis) (see Chapter 25)

Differential diagnosis

    Traumatic or after intraocular surgery

    Myasthenia gravis

    Horner's syndrome

    Cranial nerve III palsy

    Reflexive secondary to corneal or anterior segment disorder

Initial management

    Arrange evaluation by an ophthalmologist within a few hours, particularly if associated with other neurologic signs or symptoms.

Anisocoria (see Chapter 25)

Differential diagnosis

    Intracranial third nerve palsy (if painful includes possibility of aneurysm)

    Horner's syndrome

    Adie's pupil

    Ophthalmoplegic migraine

    Trauma to ciliary nerves or ganglia

    Traumatic mydriasis or miosis/iris sphincter tear

    Pharmacologic

    Benign physiologic anisocoria

Initial management

    If painful and atraumatic, consider the possibility of intracranial aneurysm and arrange evaluation by ophthalmologist, neurologist, or neurosurgeon within a few hours.

    If traumatic, arrange evaluation by an ophthalmologist within a few hours. Otherwise, arrange evaluation by an ophthalmologist within a few days.

"Blurred" Optic Nerve Head (see Chapter 24)

Differential diagnosis

    Elevated intracranial pressure (e.g., pseudotumor cerebri, true mass lesions)

    Accelerated hypertension

    Giant cell arteritis

    Nonarteritic ischemic optic neuropathy

    Traumatic optic neuropathy

    Optic neuritis

    Optic nerve head drusen

    Hypotony

    Hyperopia and physiologic variants

    Diabetic papillopathy

Initial management

    Measure blood pressure.

    If systemic or neurologic findings are present, arrange evaluation by a neurologist within a few hours.

    If ocular symptoms are present, arrange evaluation by an ophthalmologist within a few hours. Otherwise, arrange evaluation by an ophthalmologist within a few days.

Management of Ocular Injuries and Emergencies,
edited by Mathew W. MacCumber.
Lippincott–Raven Publishers, Philadelphia ©1998.

2

The Epidemiology of Ocular Trauma: A Preventable Ocular Emergency

Nathan G. Congdon and Oliver D. Schein

Glaucoma Service, Wills Eye Hospital, Philadelphia, Pennsylvania 19107–5599 and Departments of Ophthalmology and Epidemiology, Wilmer Eye Institute, The Johns Hopkins University School of Medicine, Baltimore, Maryland 21287

Incidence and Risk Factors   10
   Gender   10 · Race   11 · Socioeconomic Status   11 · Age   11
Etiology   13
   Occupational Injuries   13 · Sports   18 · Airguns/BB Guns   20 · Assault   21
   War   22 · Motor Vehicle Accidents   24
Direct and Indirect Costs of Ocular Trauma   24
Prevention of Ocular Trauma   24

Over the past 10 years, there has arisen a significant body of research regarding the epidemiology of ocular trauma (1). This awakening interest in ocular trauma has been accompanied by a growing awareness of the financial and visual impact of eye injuries, which are estimated to have cost $175 to 200 million for 227,000 days of hospital care in 1986 (2). Statistics from the National Institute for Occupational Safety and Health (NIOSH) indicate that the 900,000 on-the-job eye injuries reported in 1982 were second only to dermatologic complaints (3). From the international perspective, an estimated 500,000 blinding eye injuries occur annually worldwide, making ocular trauma the principal cause of unilateral blindness in the world today (4,5) and the second-leading cause of blind eyes in at least one recent major study from the developing world (6).

Epidemiologic study of ocular trauma in the United States has benefited from the relatively recent proliferation of data bases recording eye injuries on a local or national basis. These include the National Eye Trauma System (NETS) Registry (7), which records penetrating trauma at 52 centers throughout the United States; the United States Eye Injury Registry (USEIR), started in 1982 in Alabama (8) and now a federation consisting of 22 state registries involving 117 million persons; the National Electronic Injury Surveillance System (NEISS) (9), a consumer safety survey established in 1973 by the same legislation that created the Consumer Products Safety Commission, and which records all emergency room visits related to unsafe products; the National Athletic Injury/Illness Reporting System (10), which follows injury rates in participating schools; and larger health data bases providing useful information on eye injuries, such as the National Hospital Discharge Survey (11), and similar state records of hospital discharges, such as the Maryland State Health Services Cost Review Commission (2).

Each of these data bases has its weaknesses, however, and none satisfies ideal epidemiologic criteria of unbiased inclusiveness and broad geographic representation. NETS is in fact only a large case series with no claims as to random sampling. In fact, there is reason to doubt that the large trauma centers that comprise NETS are representative of all hospitals. The lack of accurate catchment area figures for these centers mean that population rates cannot be calculated. Finally, a low proportion of cases in NETS involve any clinical follow-up with regards to final outcome (7).

A significant limitation of the National Hospital Discharge survey is lack of incentive to use E codes in documenting ocular trauma: between 24 and 26% of discharges studied by Klopfer had full E-code information (12). The NEISS only reports emergency room visits related to injuries caused by products, a minority of severe ocular trauma (9). Finally, USEIR provides a unique advantage in that it records office visits, which many other data bases omit; however, coverage is limited to only 22 states, and the records are not comprehensive (8).

INCIDENCE AND RISK FACTORS

Traditional studies of ocular trauma have taken the form of clinic-based case series, with their attendant limitations as to selection and representation. More recently, an increasing number of population-based surveys have become available, providing incidence rates for medically treated ocular injuries ranging from 1.8 to 5.6 per thousand per year for urban Americans 40 years of age and above in Baltimore (13), 4.23 per thousand per year for rural Americans in Wisconsin (14), and 9.75 per thousand per year for individuals over 18 in New England (15). The annual incidence of ocular trauma requiring in-patient hospital treatment was roughly one tenth this rate, or 13.2 per 100,000 per year in Maryland (16). Between 10% and 20% of persons 40 years of age and above reported ever having had an eye injury in the Baltimore Eye Survey (13).

Gender

Hospital-based studies of all ocular injuries (17–19), injuries requiring hospitalization (10), and open globe injuries (20–22) all indicate that 70% to 85% of those with a spectrum of superficial to severe ocular injuries are male. Population-based studies (13,15,23) give comparable results, although there is some suggestion that the gender difference is less pronounced among Blacks (13).

Race

Although the number of studies estimating population rates of ocular injury by race is small, available reports all indicate that blacks are at greater risk than whites (15). Black men had a 25% greater incidence of ocular injury than did white men, whereas black women had nearly three times the rate of eye trauma compared with white women in Baltimore (13). The incidence of open globe injury among blacks in Allegheny County was 2.2 times that among whites (21). Even more disturbingly, the prevalence of visual impairment and blindness due to trauma among black men in the Baltimore Eye Survey was three to four times higher than among white men, a difference that could not be explained entirely by differential access to eye care (13).

Socioeconomic Status

A related risk factor of international importance in ocular trauma is socioeconomic status. Studies among children in Brazil (24) and Australia (25) have found eye injuries to be more common and severe among children of poorer families. The Nepal Eye Study (6) similarly found that individuals in the socioeconomically higher classes had both fewer ocular injuries and less trauma-related blindness.

Age

At least two large studies (10,15) have suggested a bimodal age distribution, with the maximum risk occurring among young adults and individuals 70 years of age and above. The excess risk of severe trauma among very young individuals has been reported in many studies: Schein's study at the Massachusetts Eye and Ear Infirmary (18) found that although subjects under 15 years of age made up only 8% of the study population, they incurred one third of severe injuries, including 36% of hyphemas and 25% of all open globes. A large national study in Israel reported that 47% of nearly 2,500 ocular injuries occurred in children 17 years of age or under (26). Recent studies from as far afield as Finland and Malawi have generally reported one to two thirds of ocular injuries occurring among children (Table 2–1).

Because of difficulties in managing pediatric cataracts and the potential for amblyopia, the outcome of pediatric ocular injury may be particularly severe: Takvam (27) reports some visual deficit on follow-up in fully 49% of children admitted to hospital for ocular injuries. Among children with open globe injuries, Baxter (28) noted that good prognostic indicators include age greater than 8 years, good preoperative visual acuity, injury outside the visual axis, and low postoperative astigmatism. Alfaro (29) and most other investigators concur that involvement of the lens and need for lensectomy carries a relatively grave prognosis.

The type and mechanism of ocular injury tends to vary with age as well. Various investigators report falls as a leading cause of open globe trauma in the elderly

TABLE 2-1. Eye injuries in children

Source	Place	Year[a]	Type of survey	Total no. of cases	Percentage of children	Sex M	Sex F	Circumstance of occurrence
Werner	Finland	1946–1950	Children	Total, 1,166 Children, 215	18.4	170	45	...
Niiranen and Raivio	Finland	1977	Children	Total, 319 Children, 110	34.5	90	20	Sport and play, 82% Accident in home, 17%
Ilsar et al.	Malawi	1976–1977	General	Total, 205 Children, 71	34.6	53	18	Sport, 2.8% Domestic activity, 56.4%
Canavan et al.	Ireland	1967–1976	General	Total, 2,032 Children, 1,437	71	1,199	238	Sport and play, 82.1% Accident in home, 7.7%
Thordarson et al.	Iceland	1965–1976	General	Total, 105 Children, 39	37	33	6	Sport, 10% Accident in home, 26%
Savir et al.	Israel	1965–1975	Children	Children, 658	...	520	138	Accident in street, 50% Accident in home, 25%
Gordon and Mokete	Maseru, Lesotho, South Africa	1982 (published)	Children	Children, 110	...	81	29	Outdoor setting, 93.6% Indoor setting, 6.4%
Present study	Israel	1980–1983	Children	Total, 2,276 Children, 1,127	47	894	233	Play and sport, 65.1% Accident in home, 16.9%

[a]Year represents time span between research study and publication of data.
Courtesy of *Arch Ophthalmol* 1990;108:376–379. Copyright 1990, American Medical Association.

(13,16,30), whereas Klopfer adds complications of surgery (presumably trauma to old surgical wounds) (13). For young adults, motor vehicle accidents (13,31), occupational trauma (see related section below), and assault (17) are important etiologies of serious ocular injury. Among children, domestic accidents, play, and organized sports accounted for greater than 70% of open globe injuries in one recently reported series (28).

ETIOLOGY

Trauma research has usually divided ocular trauma according either to the mechanism of injury (e.g., blunt versus penetrating) or the activity or context within which the injury occurred (e.g., occupational, sports, assault). This second mode of treating ocular injuries offers the potential advantage of aiding in the formulation of specific prevention strategies. For this reason, we choose to characterize trauma according to etiology, and discuss potential preventive strategies specific to each etiology below.

Occupational Injuries

Occupational ocular injuries have been studied extensively since Garrow's ground-breaking work in 1923 (32). Differences in sampling method and populations and type of injury studied make comparisons difficult, but certain themes are apparent. Studies conducted in the west before modern workplace regulations were enacted show occupational eye injuries comprising as much as 70% (32) of all ocular injuries. Reports from the developing world where workplaces are often still comparatively unregulated also show occupational injuries to be the leading cause of ocular trauma (5), comprising up to two thirds of all serious trauma in one series (33). Comprehensive, modern-day studies of ocular trauma in western settings tend to report that workplace eye injuries make up 15% to 40% of all ocular injuries (Table 2–2).

Occupations at particular risk for ocular injury are identified differently as various schemes are used to parcel out different job types. Schein (18), Punnonen (34), and Hassett (35), among many others, cite construction as the single industry most prone to ocular injuries. Others have noted a high incidence of ocular injuries in the metal (18,36,37), chemical (34,38), and automotive (18) industries. In the developing world and other agrarian areas, agricultural injuries, particularly fungal and other microbial corneal infections caused by vegetable matter, are of great importance (5,39) (Table 2).

As an index of the impact of occupational injuries, NIOSH statistics indicate that of 900,000 occupational injuries occurring in the United States in 1982, 16% were thought to involve serious damage to the eye (40). One report from Ireland (32) indicates that over 25% of subjects with ocular injuries became unemployed as a result of the injury, whereas a permanent disability rate after ocular injury of 5% is reported from Finland (34).

TABLE 2–2. *Key findings of published reports on work-related eye injuries*

Source, yr	Type of report	Type of injuries	Location	Total no. of injuries	No. (%) of occupational injuries	Major occupations	Agents of injuries	Outcomes
Belfort et al., 1972	Review of clinic records	Conjunctivitis, foreign bodies, and corneal ulcers	Sãu Paulo, Brazil	500	500 (100)	Grinders, welders, and machine operators	Not reported	Visual acuity improved during treatment in 58% of the cases
Blomdahl and Norell, 1984	Population-based registry of hospitalized patients	Perforating eye injuries	Stockholm County (Sweden)	320	87 (27)	Construction workers, building metal workers, carpenters, and technical workers	Occupational perforating injuries only: 43% metal fragments; and 14% nails	Not reported
Bureau of Labor Statistics, 1980	OSHA survey of worker's compensation claims	Abrasions, chemical burns, lacerations, and others	19 states in United States	1,052	1,052 (100)	Craft workers, operatives, and laborers	52% metal items, and 18% chemicals	Not reported
Cole et al., 1987	Review of hospital records	Perforating eye injuries	England	381	107 (28)	Machine operators and others	Hammer with or without chisel and operating machines	Not reported
Glynn et al. 1988	Population-based telephone survey	Any eye injury needing medical attention	6 states in New England	27	16 (59)	Not reported	Not reported	10 of 16 injured workers lost at least 1 day of work
Karlson and Klein, 1986	Population-based hospital records	Hospital-treated eye injuries	Dane County (Wisconsin)	1,347 total: 13 severe	188 Total (14): 4 severe (31)	Miscellaneous	2 chemical burns, 2 wire foreign bodies	Not reported

Kaufmann, 1956	Industrial medical log books	Foreign bodies, corneal abrasions, burns, and others	Montreal, Quebec	1,107	1,107 (100)	Heavy industry, construction, and garment industry	Metal foreign bodies and chemical burns	26 cases required prolonged treatment
Lambah, 1969	Review of hospital records	Corneal, eyelid and conjunctival injuries, penetrating injuries, and others	Wolverhampton, United Kingdom	1,017	Approximately 800 (80)	Heavy industry, light industry, and mining	Hammering hot metal	44% with perforating injuries were blind
Landen et al., 1990	Review of hospital records	Perforating eye injuries	Allegheny County (Pennsylvania)	345	36 (10)	Not reported	Metal and wood foreign bodies	Not reported
Liggett et al., 1990	Review of urban trauma center records	Blunt trauma, penetrating injuries, chemical and thermal burns, and others	Los Angeles, Calif	1,132	Approximately 90 (80)	Not reported	Blunt objects and sharp objects (total group)	Not reported
Macewen, 1989	Review of ER records	Extraocular foreign bodies, corneal abrasions, flash burns, and others	Scotland	5,671	3,963 (70)	Light industry, grinding/buffing, and welding	67% extraocular foreign bodies	14 of 3,963 (0.4%) hospitalized; 12 of 14 hospitalized had good visual outcomes
Maltzman et al., 1976	Review of hospital records	Hyphema, traumatic cataract, perforating trauma, eyelid trauma and others	New Jersey	468	Approximately 40%	Not reported	Metal foreign bodies and other projectiles	Good outcomes reported for hyphemas (total group)

continued

TABLE 2-2. Continued.

Source, yr	Type of report	Type of injuries	Location	Total no. of injuries	No. (%) of occupational injuries	Major occupations	Agents of injuries	Outcomes
Mencia-Gutiérrez et al., 1988	Review of records at one hospital	Perforating eye injuries only	Madrid, Spain	77	77 (100)	Industry, agriculture, and service trades	43% metal foreign bodies and 21% metal sharp objects	47% had acuity 5/10 or better, 49% corneal scars
Morris et al., 1987	Statewide eye trauma registry	All serious eye injuries	Alabama	736	196 (27)	Not reported	32% blunt injury; 23% sharp injury (total group)	Almost 90% of initial acuity 20/100 or better had outcomes at least as good as initially
Niranen, 1978	Review of hospital records	Perforating eye injuries	Helsinki, Finland	2,015	1,160 (58)	Metal workers, agriculture, and construction	Metal foreign bodies, sharp objects, and explosions	Prognosis improved from 1930s to 1950s
Punnonen, 1989	Review of records at one hospital	Perforating eye injuries	Helsinki, Finland	387	139 (36)	Construction work (42%); industry (30%); and transport commerce, and storage (15%)	Not reported	22% of injured eyes remained blind; 15% could not work or changed jobs because of injury
Saari and Aine, 1984	Review of hospital records	Blunt trauma, perforating eye injuries, chemical burns, and others	Tampere, Finland	662	278 (42); 96 agricultural workers (only 70 at work)	Agriculture and construction industry	Cow horn, wood chips, metal foreign bodies, and chemical burns	Better in farming and lumbering, worse in dairying

Study	Method	Type of injuries	Location	Total number	Number (%)	Setting	Cause/Object	Comments
Saari and Parvi, 1984	Review of workers compensation records	Superficial injuries, radiation, burns, wounds, contusions, and others	Finland	25,380	25,380 (100); 20,102 (79) superficial; and 602 (2) wounds	Manufacturing, construction, and agriculture	Foreign bodies, machines and equipment, and chemicals	18% of all industrial injuries with 1–2 days of lost work time were due to eye injuries
Schein et al., 1988	Review of ER records at one major eye hospital	Major and minor eye injuries	Massachusetts	3,184 total; 161 severe	Approximately 1,530 (48)	Construction (63%); and automotive repair (18%)	Not reported	Ruptured globes (total group); median workdays lost, 70 days
Scherf and Zonis, 1976	Review of hospital records	Perforating eye injuries	Israel	207	142 (69) includes military war injuries	Military injuries, work injuries, and agricultural injuries	Hammering, military activity	For intraocular foreign bodies 37% had good or fair vision; and the rest were worse
Thordarson et al., 1979	Review of records at one hospital	Primarily severe eye injuries	Iceland	105	43 (41)	Construction, auto repair, agriculture, and fishing	Wire, metal or wood splints, and screwdriver	Approx 2/3 of the total group had a good outcome
Vernon 1983	Review of ER records at one hospital	Nonperforating trauma	Bristol, England	3,210	971 (30)	Not reported	Foreign bodies and abrasions high in total group	13% of eye injuries in total group required hospital admission
White et al., 1989	Statewide eye trauma registry	All serious eye trauma	Alabama	514	144 (28)	Not reported	34% sharp object; 23% blunt object; 3% gunshot	4% enucleations; 69% return to work after rehabilitation
Present study	NETS registry	Penetrating eye injuries	48 centers in United States	2,939	635 (22)	Not reported	72% projectiles; metal objects, nails, wire, and various tools	Not reported

OSHA, Occupational Safety and Health Administration: ER, emergency room: NETS, National Eye Trauma System. Courtesy of *Ophthalmology* 1993;201–207:100. (*Arch Opthalmol* 1992;843–848:110)

Legislative regulation of the workplace has been the major strategy to control on-the-job ocular injuries for over a century. Legislation protecting workers against eye injury was first introduced in the United Kingdom in 1891 to safeguard workers from bursting soda bottles, and similar laws requiring protective lenses have been in place in the United States since 1912.

However, most studies clearly show that noncompliance either by the worker or the employer with available or even mandated protective eyewear is the single greatest risk factor for ocular injury in the workplace. One report of over 600 penetrating injuries based on the National Eye Trauma Registry System indicates that only 6% of those injured were wearing safety glasses, whereas an additional 3% had on nonsafety glasses (41). As might be expected, other studies show that rates of protective eyewear use are higher (up to 20%) for cases of superficial injury (38), whereas such eyewear was only rarely worn when penetrating injury resulted. Patel reported that only one of 69 subjects who sustained penetrating ocular injury in the workplace had protective eyewear in place at the time of the accident. Patel went on to estimate that fully 90% of these injuries might have been prevented (42).

Sports

Surveys of ocular trauma indicate that sports-related injuries are both common and severe, accounting for 23% to 34% of open globe (18,43); 50% to 70% of hyphemas (8,44); 25% of all severe ocular injuries (8); and 23% of ocular trauma admissions (44) in various studies. Among patients with sports-related trauma presenting to a major eye center, nearly 14% were admitted and 13% had permanent ocular sequelae (45).

Perhaps more importantly, sports injuries are uniquely prone to preventive strategies, in that participation in team sports often occurs in the context of organized leagues bound by specific rules and under the auspices of sanctioned governing bodies. A notable success story in the prevention of sports injury is that of Canadian amateur ice hockey. In the 1972–1973 season, 287 ocular injuries resulting in 20 blind eyes occurred, and in the following year there were 258 injuries and 43 blind eyes. In 1979, the Canadian Amateur Hockey Association ruled that all players must use face protectors, whereas the professional leagues made no such changes. The age of average ocular injury in ice hockey rose from 14 to 26 (46,47). By the 1991–1992 season, the number of ocular injuries in Canadian amateur hockey had decreased to 28, with seven blind eyes (48). In 1990, similar standards for face protection were adopted by the professional hockey leagues.

The relative importance of different sports as a cause of ocular injury varies from country to country. In both the United States (49) (Table 2–3) and Japan (50), baseball has been the number one cause of recreational ocular injuries, accounting for one fifth of such injuries in the United States and nearly one half in Japan. Of the nearly 10,000 baseball-related eye injuries recorded in the United States annually, the majority occur in young, amateur players: one study in Massachusetts found that one of 238 children 5 to 19 years of age are treated at hospitals for

TABLE 2–3. *Estimated number of product-related eye injuries treated in hospital emergency departments for selected sports: United States, 1991–1992*

Sport	1991	1992
Racket sports	3,688	4,161
Badminton	156	51
Tennis	1,951	2,413
Racquetball, squash, paddleball	1,521	1,646
Handball	60	51
Hockey (all types)	1,053	971
Basketball	6,842	8,304
Baseball	6,950	8,083
Soccer	1,108	1,469
Volleyball	660	785
Football	2,930	1,745
Skiing, snow	490	604
Skiing, water	277	205
Swimming and pool sports	3,329	2,338
Wrestling	236	286
Boxing	86	112
Fishing	1,017	856
Golf	927	1,320
Horseback riding	301	308
Bicycling	2,003	2,460
Gas-, air-, spring-operated guns	1,984	2,576

NEISS data and estimates are based on injuries treated in hospital emergency departments that patients say are *related* to products. Therefore it is *incorrect,* when using NEISS data, to say the injuries were *caused* by the product.
Courtesy of *Duane's Clinical Ophthalmology.* Vol. 5. Philadelphia: Lippincott–Raven, 1993.

injuries sustained while playing baseball (51). Although other sports may be more dangerous, the large number of children playing baseball accounts for its importance. By comparison, one study of professional baseball conducted between July 1991 and July 1992 reported only 24 eye injuries among 21 players, accounting for only five missed games, and no incidence of final vision less than 20/20 (49). Suggestions to make baseball safer from an ocular standpoint have included the use of lighter, softer balls among young amateurs and requiring face shield protection while at bat or in the on-deck circle (52).

Basketball has recently surpassed baseball in the United States as the leading cause of ocular injuries (52). Ten percent of college basketball players sustain ocular injuries each season (53). Although the majority of these injuries are limited to corneal abrasions, mostly caused by the fingers and limbs of opponents, avulsion of the optic nerve has been reported from an extended finger in basketball (54). The number of ocular injuries in basketball continues to increase as the modern game evolves to allow more physical contact (55). Sports goggles have been shown to prevent ocular injury in basketball: only one of 50 eye injuries recorded in professional basketball over a 1-year period was incurred by a player wearing protective eyewear (52).

The third significant cause of ocular sports injuries in America is racket sports, now the leading cause of sports-related ocular injury in Canada (52). The risk of participating in sports such as tennis, handball, and squash without adequate eye protection to prevent small, deformable balls from making contact with the globe is significant. Of all racquetball injuries tabulated in one study, 29% were to the eye (56). The likelihood that a squash player playing without ocular protection for 25 years will sustain a serious eye injury has been estimated to be in excess of 25% (57,58). Racket sports were implicated in 51.9% of all admissions for eye trauma to the Manchester Royal Hospital (59). One study reports tennis as the leading cause of eye injuries among working-age women in Massachusetts (52). The recommendation to avoid ocular injury in racket sports is regular use of polycarbonate sports eye protectors meeting the racket sport protector standard (ASTM F 803). Various editorials have called for all tennis clubs to make the wearing of such protection mandatory for their members (44); as their use has gradually replaced unsafe street eyewear and open eye protectors, the volume of racket sport eye injuries has decreased by nearly two thirds (48).

Although the sport of boxing accounts for one tenth to one hundredth of the number of ocular injuries associated with more popular sports such as basketball (Table 2–3), it is associated with a high risk of significant ocular injury. Common ocular injuries in boxing include hyphema, angle recession, posterior subcapsular cataract, ptosis, retinal detachment, orbital fracture, and diplopia from damage to the muscles, nerves, or, most commonly, trochlea (52). One study examined 74 asymptomatic boxers who had averaged 61 bouts over 9 years. Vision-threatening injuries (significant damage to the angle, lens, macula, or peripheral retina) were found in 43 boxers (58%), and retinal tears were found in 24% (60). It does not appear that changes in equipment will be adequate to control the problem: among 13 asymptomatic Olympic boxers (who are required to wear headgear) examined in 1984, three had retinal holes or tears apparently resulting from boxing (52). Currently the most favored approach, and the one recommended by the Academy of Ophthalmology, is to require annual eye examinations as a condition for licensure to box so that injuries can be detected and treated early (61).

Airguns/BB Guns

The importance of nonpowder firearms as a cause of ocular trauma cannot be overstated. Of 50,000 nonpowder firearm injuries evaluated annually in U.S. emergency rooms (62), some 1,200 involve the eye (63). Among penetrating ocular injuries occurring in a recreational setting reported to the National Eye Trauma System, 63% were related to the use of nonpowder firearms (7). The mean muzzle velocity reported for BB guns (64) is three times the minimum velocity required to achieve ocular penetration (65). It is thus not surprising that rates of enucleation for penetrating trauma in cases of BB injury are as high as 86% (66,67), whereas nearly one fifth of all eyes involved in BB injuries are ultimately lost (66,68). Several studies report final visual acuity after BB injury in the legally blind range in nearly one half of all affected eyes (67–69).

Schein has attempted to place ocular injuries from nonpowder firearms in their social context. Of 140 shooting victims identified through the National Eye Trauma System and interviewed by telephone, 91% were male and 95% were injured by persons known to them, 40% by relatives. People were the intended targets in 45% of cases, and adults were present during only 11% of incidents. In fewer than half of cases was the weapon used in the shooting reported to have been destroyed or confiscated by parents or authorities (70). Although engineering improvements in the trigger safeties of guns might impact on the one third of cases resulting from unintentional firing, it seems clear that significant progress in this area will be difficult while "non-powder firearms are not regarded by the public as sufficiently hazardous to proscribe their routine use by young children without supervision" (70).

Assault

This category of ocular injury accounts for a steadily growing proportion of ocular trauma, particularly in American urban centers and among African Americans (Table 2–4). Assault was the single most common cause of ocular trauma in a recent series in Los Angeles (17). Examination of the National Eye Trauma System

TABLE 2–4. *Assault-related eye injury as a percentage of reported cases of ocular trauma*

Source, yr	Total no. of eye injuries	No. (%) of assault-related eye injuries	Location
Roper-Hall, 1959	267	2 (1)	England
Lambah, 1969	1,017	75 (7)	England
Johnston, 1971	295	28 (9)	Northern Ireland
Eagling, 1976	237	19 (8)	England
Scherf and Zonis, 1976	207	71 (34)[a]	Israel
Gordon and Mokete, 1981	252[b]	134 (53)	Lesotho
Niiranen, 1981	139[c]	37 (27)	Finland
Vernon, 1983	3,210	53 (2)	England
Blomdahl and Norell, 1984	318	33 (10)	Sweden
Karlson and Klein, 1986	1,347	201 (15)	Wisconsin
Cole et al., 1987	378	42 (11)	England
Morris et al., 1987	735	73 (10)	Alabama
Gilbert et al., 1987	91	27 (30)	Baltimore, Md
Macewen, 1989			
Total	5,671	113 (2)	United Kingdom
Hospitalized	102	19 (19)	United Kingdom
Punnonen, 1989	387	47 (12)	Finland
Tielsch et al., 1989	2,373	436 (18)	Maryland
Landen et al., 1990	345	47 (14)	Pittsburgh, Pa
Liggett et al., 1990	1,260	511 (41)	Los Angeles, Calif
Present study	2,939	648 (22)	United States

[a]Includes 69 military injuries.
[b]Excludes children.
[c]Excludes children and occupational injuries.
Courtesy of *Arch Ophthalmol* 1992;110:852. Copyright 1992, American Medical Association.

Registry shows 648 cases of penetrating ocular trauma due to assault occurring between 1985 and 1991, accounting for some 22% of penetrating ocular trauma reported during that time (71). As for other traumatic eye injuries, more than 80% of victims of ocular trauma related to assault are male, the majority under the age of 35 years (71,72). Alcohol is implicated in 48% to 70% of assault-related ocular injuries (68,69). Such injuries tend to be severe, involving posterior segment trauma in 70% of cases and resulting in a presenting vision of hand motions or less in 74% (71); they have a commensurately guarded prognosis, with 63% of eyes in one study having a final vision of 5/200 or less (72). As several investigators have noted, devising strategies to prevent assault-related ocular trauma is extremely difficult when compared with similar efforts in the more tightly regulated workplace or playing field.

War

At least two studies have appeared recently reporting on the experience of ocular trauma during the Desert Storm and Desert Shield campaigns in the Middle East (73,74). The more comprehensive of the two reports details serious injuries to 221 eyes of 180 patients, of which 98 involved penetrating injury. The most common cause of injury was blast fragments, accounting for 78% of all serious injuries and 94% of 35 enucleations. Interestingly, among nonmunitions injuries involving the eye, motor vehicle accidents were most common (73). Heier reported on a less serious group of ocular injuries, all of those reporting to the emergency room at one of four field hospitals supporting the campaigns. Although all troops were issued safety goggles, only 4% of those injured were wearing them at the time of injury. Heier also tabulated an increasing proportion of U.S. casualties due to ocular injuries, from 0.57% during the Civil War to 13% in the current study, presumably as a result of increasing rates of survival among individuals with severe cranial and facial injuries (Table 2–5) (74).

TABLE 2–5. *Ocular injuries as percentage of total war injuries*

War	Years	% of all war injuries	Source
American Civil War[a]	1861–1865	0.57	Steindorf, 1914
World War I[a]	1914–1918	2.0	Stone, 1950
World War II[a]	1941–1945	2.0	Reister, 1975
World War II[b]	1939–1945	2.0	Polyak, 1957
Korean conflict[a]	1950–1953	2.8	Reister, 1973
6-Day War[c]	1967	5.6	Treister, 1969
October 1973 War[c]	1973	6.7	Belkin et al., 1984
Lebanon War[c]	1982	6.8	Belkin et al., 1984
Vietnam conflict[a]	1962–1972	5-9	Hornblass, 1981
Gulf conflict[a]	1990–1991	13	Present study

[a]Forces reported were American.
[b]Forces reported were Soviet.
[c]Forces reported were Israeli Defense Forces.
Courtesy of *Arch Ophthalmol* 1993;111:745–798. Copyright 1993, American Medical Association.

TABLE 2–6. Ocular trauma secondary to motor vehicle accidents

Report	Year	No. of cases	Type of injury (%)			Uveal prolapse (%)	Lens dislocation (%)	Traumatic cataract (%)	Hyphema (%)	Vitreous prolapse (%)	Retinal incarceration (%)	Loss of ambulatory Vision (VA <20/400) (%)	Enucleation rate (%)
			C	S	CS								
Current	1992	10	20	20	60	80	10	10	40	10	10	10	0
Punnonen (Finland)	1989	21	—	—	—	—	—	—	—	—	—	25	5
Wykes (United Kingdom)	1988	27	—	—	—	—	—	—	—	—	—	—	15
Patel and Morgan (United Kingdom)	1988	16	—	—	—	—	—	—	—	—	—	50	13
Johnston and Armstrong (N. Ireland)	1986	63	—	—	—	—	—	—	—	—	—	33	13
Blake et al. (Ireland)	1983	276	30	14	56	97	17	25	—	—	—	40	23
Peter 1981 (Switzerland)	107	22	22	54	—	—	—	—	—	—	33	—	—
Canavan et al. (N. Ireland)	1980	311	—	—	—	—	—	—	—	—	—	—	19
Merté and Sipp (Germany)	1977	212	28	21	51	—	—	—	—	—	—	33	22
Briner (Australia)	1976	24	—	—	—	71	—	—	—	—	—	—	—
Mackay (United Kingdom)	1975	30	—	—	—	—	—	—	—	—	—	40	—
Soni (United Kingdom)	1973	64	29	3	69	83	34	23	6	54	3	20	17
Lavergne and Dereume-de Corte (France)	1972	97	—	—	—	—	—	—	—	—	—	29	—

C, corneal; S, scleral; CS, corneoscleral; VA, visual acuity.
Courtesy of *Ophthalmology* 1993;100:201–207.

Motor Vehicle Accidents

The reported proportion of ocular trauma due to motor vehicle accidents in the United States has ranged from 3% to 12% (17,75), whereas reports from the United Kingdom give a somewhat higher range, 23% to 30% (31,76) (Table 2–6). It is theorized that the main reasons for lower rates of eye injuries in American road accidents are the existence of compulsory seat-belt laws (not yet in place in the United Kingdom at the time of the studies cited) and the use of laminated as opposed to tempered glass windshields (75). Mackay reported a 50% reduction in the rate of ocular injury with the use of laminated glass (77), whereas Hall noted a 73% reduction in motor vehicle-related penetrating ocular injury after the adoption of mandatory seatbelt legislation in the United Kingdom in 1983 (78). Most reported cases of ocular trauma involve isolated trauma to the anterior segment with sparing of the posterior segment (75). It seems likely that the advent of the airbag may promise a further reduction in automobile-related ocular trauma, although recently reports of ocular trauma including corneal abrasion and hyphema from airbags themselves have begun to appear (79,80).

DIRECT AND INDIRECT COSTS OF OCULAR TRAUMA

As with other medical costs, those related to ocular trauma have proven difficult to control. Tielsch has reported, based on data from the state of Maryland, that although the average length of stay for hospitalized patients with ocular trauma decreased from 6.0 days in 1979 to 3.8 days in 1986, the direct cost per hospital discharge actually increased from $1,531 to $2,615 during the same period (2). The total annual direct cost for hospitalized cases of ocular trauma in the United States was estimated at $150 million (2). A recent study from Sweden found that of total direct and indirect costs for cases of ocular trauma treated at a university hospital, direct cost of hospitalization comprised only 22.9%, greatly exceeded by the 65.6% direct cost of out-patient treatment. Indirect costs for lost days of work comprised 11.1% (81). If similar proportions applied to the United States, the $150 million figure may in fact represent only a small part of the total cost of ocular trauma.

PREVENTION OF OCULAR TRAUMA

Schein and Vinger (82) recommend a simple, three-part strategy that can be used in the ophthalmologist's office to prevent loss of vision from ocular trauma:

1. Determine the patient's injury potential. This might include asking about participation in racquet sports, obtaining a history of prior ocular surgery (which might weaken the eye in the event of trauma), and identifying functionally one-eyed patients (e.g., those whose vision is less than 20/40 in the worse-seeing eye; Fig. 2–1).

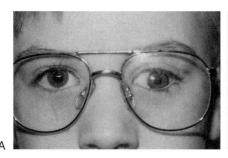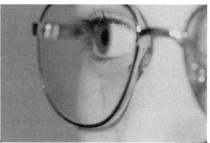

A B

FIG. 2–1. A: This 8-year-old boy has a prosthetic left eye after a penetrating BB injury. He returned on a postoperative visit, relating how he had run into a tree branch while playing in a wooded area. Note the deep scratch in his right polycarbonate lens. **B:** Close-up view of the scratch.

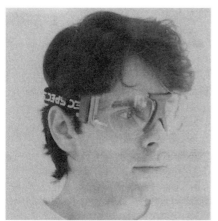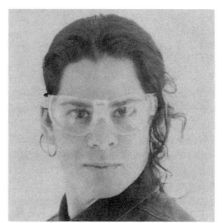

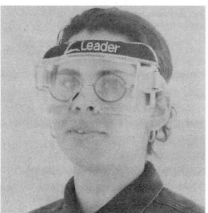

FIG. 2–2. Frames meeting F803 standards for raquet and ball sports. (From Vinger PF (52), reprinted with permission.)

2. Prescribe appropriate protective devices. The example is given of a regular squash player, whose risk for loss of vision over a lifetime is higher than that for the average glaucoma patient (54,55). Polycarbonate lenses are recommended for both streetwear and protection. Although proper protective eyewear is often mandated for individuals engaged in welding and drilling on the job, the home hobbyist may go unprotected if not identified and counseled appropriately by an eye-care professional taking a thorough history. The appropriate frame also should be specified: frames meeting American National Standards Institute Z87 specifications for work and hobby use (83) and those meeting American Society for Testing and Materials F803 standards for racquet and ball sports (Fig. 2–2, photographic example) (84).

3. Finally, recommend a supplier who is known to provide the prescribed eyewear at a reasonable price and without undue delay. Patients are unlikely to comply with suggested protective eyewear if they must pay an unwarranted premium or cope with unnecessary delays to obtain it.

REFERENCES

1. Parver L. Eye trauma: the neglected disorder. *Arch Ophthalmol* 1986;104:1452.
2. Tielsch JM, Parver LM. Determinants of hospital charges and length of stay for ocular trauma. *Ophthalmology* 1990;97:231–237.
3. Leads from the *MMWR:* Leading work-related diseases and injuries—United States. *JAMA* 1990; 251: 2503–2504.
4. Thylefors B. Present challenges in the global prevention of blindness. *Aust N Z J Ophthalmol* 1992; 20:89–94.
5. Thylefors B. Epidemiologic patterns of ocular trauma. *Aust N Z J Ophthalmol* 1992;20:95–98.
6. Brilliant LB, Pokhrel RP, Grasset NC, et al. Epidemiology of blindness in Nepal. *Bull WHO* 1985; 63:375–386.
7. Parver LM. The National Eye Trauma System. *Int Ophthalmol Clin* 1988;28:263.
8. Morris RE, Witherspoon CD, Helms HA, Feist RM, Byrne JB. Eye Injury Registry of Alabama (a preliminary report): Demographics and prognosis of severe injury. *South Med J* 1987;80:810.
9. National Electronic Injury Surveillance System. US Consumer Product Safety Commission/Directorate for Epidemiology. National Injury Information Clearinghouse, Washington, DC, 1991, 1992.
10. Damron CF, Hoerner EF, Shaw J. Injury surveillance systems for sports. In: Vinger PF, Hoerner EF, eds. *Sports Injuries: The Unthwarted Epidemic.* 2nd ed. Littleton, MA: Publishing Sciences Group, 1986:1–23.
11. Graves FJ. Detailed diagnoses and procedures, National Hospital Discharge Survey, 1987, *Vital Health Stat* 13. 1989;100:1–304.
12. Klopfer J, Tielsch JM, Vitale S, See LC, Canner JK. Ocular trauma in the United States. Eye injuries resulting in hospitalization, 1984 through 1987. *Arch Ophthalmol* 1992;110:838–842.
13. Katz J, Tielsch JM. Lifetime prevalence of ocular injuries from the Baltimore Eye Survey. *Arch Ophthalmol* 1993;111:1564–1568.
14. Karlson TA, Klein BEK. The incidence of acute, hospital-treated eye injuries. *Arch Ophthalmol* 1983;104:1473–1476.
15. Glynn RJ, Seddon JM, Berlin BM. The incidence of eye injuries in New England. *Arch Ophthalmol* 1988;106:785–789.
16. Tielsch JM, Parver L, Shankar B. Time trends in the incidence of hospitalized ocular trauma. *Arch Ophthalmol* 1989;107:519–523.
17. Liggett PE, Pince KJ, Barlow W, Ragen M, Ryan SJ. Ocular trauma in an urban population. *Ophthalmology* 1990;97:581–584.
18. Schein OD, Hibberd PL, Shingleton BJ, et al. The spectrum and burden of ocular injury. *Ophthalmology* 1988;95:300–305.
19. Zagelbaum BM, Tostanoski JR, Kerner DJ, Hersh PS. Urban eye trauma: a one-year prospective study. *Ophthalmology* 1993;100:851–856.

20. Dunn ES, Jaeger EA, Jeffers JB, Freitag SK. The epidemiology of ruptured globes. *Ann Ophthalmol* 1992;24:405–410.
21. Landen D, Baker D, LaPorte R, Thoft RA. Perforating eye injury in Allegheny County, Pennsylvania. *Am J Pub Health* 1990;80:1120–1122.
22. Parver LM, Dannenberg AL, Blacklow B, Fowler CJ, Brechner RJ, Tielsch JM. Characteristics and causes of penetrating eye injuries reported to the National Eye Trauma System Registry. *Public Health Rep* 1993;108:625–632.
23. Koval R, Teller J, Belkin M, Romem Y, Yanko L, Savir H. The Israeli Ocular Injuries Study: a nationwide collaborative study. *Arch Ophthalmol* 1988;106:776–780.
24. Moreira CA. Epidemiological study of eye injuries in Brazilian children. *Arch Ophthalmol* 1988; 106:781–786.
25. Waddy PM. The causes and effects of eye injuries in children. *Aust J Ophthalmol* 1984;12: 245–251.
26. Rapoport I, Romem M, Kinek E, et al. Eye injuries in children in Israel. *Arch Ophthalmol* 1990; 108:376–379.
27. Takvam JA, Midelfart A. Survey of eye injuries in Norwegian children. *Acta Ophthalmol* 1993;71: 500–505.
28. Baxter RJ, Hodgkins PR, Calder I, Morrell AJ, Vardy S, Elkington AR. Visual outcome of childhood anterior perforating eye injuries: prognostic indicators. *Eye* 1994;8:349–352.
29. Alfaro DV, Chaudhry NA, Walonker AF, Runyan T, Saito Y, Liggett PE. Penetrating eye injuries in young children. *Retina* 1994;14:201–205.
30. Byhr E. Perforating eye injuries in a western part of Sweden. *Acta Ophthalmol* 1994;72:91–97.
31. Canavan YM, O'Flaherty MJ, Archer DB, Elwood JH. A ten-year survey of ocular injuries in Northern Ireland, 1967–1976. *Br J Ophthalmol* 1980;64:618–625.
32. Garrow A. A statistical inquiry into 100 cases of eye injuries. *Br J Ophthalmol* 1923;7:65–80.
33. Rekhi GS, Kulshreshtha OP. Common causes of blindness: a pilot study in Jaipur, Rajasthan. *Ind J Ophthalmol* 1991;39:108–111.
34. Punnonen E. Epidemiologic and social aspects of perforating eye injuries. *Acta Ophthalmol* 1989; 67:492–498.
35. Hassett PD, Kelleher CC. The epidemiology of occupational penetrating eye injuries in Ireland. *Occup Med* 1994;44:209–211.
36. Niiranen M. Perforating eye injuries: a comparative epidemiologic, prognostic and socioeconomic study of patients treated in 1930–1939 and 1950–59. *Acta Ophthalmol Suppl* 1978;135:1–87.
37. US Department of Labor Statistics: Accidents involving eye injuries. Report 557, April 1980.
38. Jones NP. Eye injuries at work: a prospective, population-based survey within the chemical industry. *Eye* 1992;6:381–385.
39. Saari KM, Parvi V. Occupational eye injuries in Finland. *Acta Ophthalmol Suppl* 1984;161:17–28.
40. Centers for disease control. Leading work-related diseases and injuries—United States. *MMWR* 1984;33:213–215.
41. Dannenberg AL, Parver LM, Brechner RJ, Khoo L. Penetrating eye injuries in the workplace: The National Eye Trauma Registry System. *Arch Ophthalmol* 1992;110:843–848.
42. Patel BCK, Morgan LH. Work-related penetrating eye injuries. *Acta Ophthalmol* 1991;69:377–381.
43. Blomdahl S, Norell S. Perforating eye injury in the Stockholm population: an epidemiological study. *Acta Ophthalmol* 1984;62:378–390.
44. Elman MJ. Racket-sports ocular injuries. The tip of the trauma iceberg. *Arch Ophthalmol* 104: 1453–1454.
45. Larrison WI, Hersh PS, Kunzweiler T, Shingleton BJ. Sports-related ocular trauma. *Ophthalmology* 1990;97:1265–1269.
46. Pashby TJ. Eye injuries in Canadian ice hockey. Phase 2. *Can Med Assoc J* 1977;117:671–678.
47. Pashby TJ. Eye injuries in Canadian hockey. Phase 3: Older players now most at risk. *Can Med Assoc J* 1979;121:643–644.
48. Pashby TJ. Eye injuries in Canadian sports and recreational activities. *Can J Ophthalmol* 1992;27: 226–229.
49. Zagelbaum BM, Hersh PS, Donnenfeld ED, Perry HD, Hochman MA. Ocular trauma in major league baseball players. *N Engl J Med* 1994;330:1021–1023.
50. Pashby TJ. Eye injuries in Canadian sports and recreation activities. *Can J Ophthalmol* 1992;27: 226–229.
51. Schuster M. Baseball-related injuries among children. Boston, Statewide Comprehensive Injury Prevention Program, Bureau of Parent, Child and Adolescent Health. Massachusetts Department of Public Health, 1991.

52. Vinger PF. The eye and sports medicine. In: Tasman WJ, ed. *Duane's Clinical Ophthalmology,* Philadelphia: Lippincott–Raven Publishers, 1994.
53. Martin K, Wilson D, McKeag D. Ocular trauma in college varsity sports. *Med Sci Sports Exerc* 1987;19(suppl):53.
54. Chow AY, Goldberg MF, Frenkel M. Evulsion of the optic nerve in association with basketball injuries. *Ann Ophthalmol* 1984;16:35.
55. Apple DF. Basketball injuries: an overview. *Physician Sportsmed* 1988;16:64.
56. Rose CP, Morse JO. Racquetball injuries. *Physician Sportsmed* 1979;7:73.
57. Reif AE, Vinger PF, Easterbrook M. New developments in protection against eye injuries. *Squash News* 1981;4:10.
58. Genovese MT, Lenzo NP, Lim RK, et al. Eye injuries among pennant squash players and their attitudes towards protective eyewear. *Med J Aust* 1990:153:655.
59. Jones NP. One year of severe eye injuries in sport. *Eye* 1988;2:484.
60. Giovinazzo VJ, Yannuzzi LA, Sorenson JA, et al. The ocular complications of boxing. *Ophthalmology* 1987;94:587.
61. American Academy of Ophthalmology policy statement on boxing.
62. Christoffel KK, Tanz R, Sagerman S, Hahn Y. Childhood injuries caused by non-powder firearms. *Am J Dis Child* 1984;138:557.
63. Sternberg P, deJuan E, Green WR, Hirst LW, Sommer A. Ocular BB injuries. *Ophthalmology* 1984; 91:1269.
64. Preston JD. Review of standard consumer safety specifications for non-powder guns. Engineering Sciences CPSC, Washington, DC, 1980.
65. Delori F, Pomerantzeff O, Cox MS. Perforation of the globe under high-speed impact; its relation to contusion injuries. *Invest Ophthalmol* 1969;8:290–301.
66. Kreshton MJ. Eye injuries due to BB guns. *Am J Ophthalmol* 1964;58:858–861.
67. Young DW, Little JM. Pellet-gun eye injuries. *Can J Ophthalmol* 1985;20:9–10.
68. Bowen DI, Magauran DM. Ocular injuries caused by airgun pellets: an analysis of 105 cases. *Br Med J* 1973;1:333–337.
69. Sharif KW, McGhee CNJ, Tomlinson RC. Ocular trauma caused by airgun pellets: a ten year survey. *Eye* 1990;4:855–860.
70. Schein OD, Enger C, Tielsch JM. The context and consequences of ocular injuries from airguns. *Am J Ophthalmol* 1994;117:501–506.
71. Dannenberg AL, Parver LM, Fowler CJ. Penetrating eye injuries related to assault: the National Eye Trauma System Registry. *Arch Ophthalmol* 1992;110:849–852.
72. Groessl S, Nanda SK, Mieler WF. Assault-related penetrating ocular injury. *Am J Ophthalmol* 1993;116:26–33.
73. Mader TH, Aragones JV, Chandler AC, et al. Ocular and ocular adnexal injuries treated by United States military ophthalmologists during operations Desert Storm and Desert Shield. *Ophthalmology* 1993;100:1462–1467.
74. Heier JS, Enzenauer RW, Wintermeyer SF, Delaney M, LaPiana FP. Ocular injuries and diseases at a combat support hospital in support of operations Desert Shield and Desert Storm. *Arch Ophthalmol* 1993;111:795–798.
75. Nanda SK, Mieler WF, Murphy ML. Penetrating ocular injuries secondary to motor vehicle accidents. *Ophthalmology* 1993;100:201–207.
76. Soni KG. Eye injuries in road traffic accidents. *Injury* 1973;5:41–6.
77. Mackay GM, Gloyns PF, Hayes HRM, et al. Some aspects of facial injuries in present day cars. In: The Government of the Federal Republic of Germany. Eighth International Technical Conference on Experimental Safety Vehicles. US Department of Transportation, 1981;438–451.
78. Hall NF, Denning AM, Elkington AR, Cooper PJ. The eye and the seatbelt in Wessex. *Br J Ophthalmol* 1985;69:317—319.
79. Larkin GL. Airbag-mediated corneal injury. *Am J Emerg Med* 1991;9:444–446.
80. Mishler KE. Hyphema caused by airbag [Letter]. *Arch Ophthalmol* 1991;109:1635.
81. Monestam E, Bjornstig U. Eye injuries in Northern Sweden. *Acta Ophthalmol* 1991;69:1–5.
82. Schein O, Vinger PF. Epidemiology and prevention of ocular injuries. In Albert DM, Jacobiac F, eds. *Principles and Practice of Ophthalmology.* Philadelphia: WB Saunders, 1994.
83. American National Standards Institute, Inc. 1430 Broadway, New York, NY 10018.
84. American Society for Testing and Materials, Inc. 1916 Race St., Philadelphia, PA 19103.

Management of Ocular Injuries and Emergencies,
edited by Mathew W. MacCumber.
Lippincott–Raven Publishers, Philadelphia ©1998.

3

Ocular Evaluation

Nathan G. Congdon and Mathew W. MacCumber

Glaucoma Service, Wills Eye Hospital, Philadelphia, Pennsylvania 19107–5599;
Department of Ophthalmology, Wilmer Eye Institute, The Johns Hopkins University School
of Medicine, Baltimore, Maryland 21287; and Retina Service, Department of
Ophthalmology, Rush Medical College, Chicago, Illinois 60612

History   29
Examination   30
Visual Acuity   30
External Examination   31
Pupillary Examination   31
Brightness Testing, Color Vision, and Red Desaturation   33
Visual Fields   33
Extraocular Motility   34
Procedure: Forced Duction Testing   34
Examination of the Anterior Segment   35
  Cornea   35 · Conjunctiva   35 · Anterior Chamber   35 · Gonioscopy and
  the Iris   35 · Crystallin Lens   36
Intraocular Pressure   36
Posterior Segment Examination   36
  General Principles   36 · Vitreous   36 · Retina and Choroid   37 · Optic
  Nerve Head   37
Ancillary Testing 37

For special considerations in the evaluation of children with ocular trauma, see Chapter 4. For the evaluation of patients with neuroophthalmic emergencies, see also Chapter 24.

HISTORY

As with any medical encounter, the first step in working up patients with an acute ocular problem is to obtain a thorough history. The most significant aspects of the patient's previous ocular history are the preinjury vision in the affected eye and any history of ocular surgery. Previous ocular surgery can predispose the eye toward infection or serious injuries involving dehiscence of surgical wounds. Any ocular history, including medications, previous injuries, or current conditions affecting the visual potential of the fellow eye is naturally of significance in the case of severe loss of vision.

In evaluating a patient with ocular trauma, certain details of the injury itself will be of great importance. In particular, one should inquire about details that could raise the level of suspicion for intraocular or intraorbital foreign bodies. This might include an injury involving broken glass, explosion, or small projectiles such as BBs. The nature of the ocular injury with respect to blunt or penetrating trauma, is also of important prognostic significance, as blunt injuries can be severe and more likely to lead to blinding sequela. The presumed force of an object striking the eye may be estimated by obtaining details of the event and, in particular, the distance from which a BB or other projectile was fired and the presence or absence of intervening ricochet. The identity of any chemical agent involved in an injury should be determined if possible. If a sample of the substance is available, it should be tested for pH. Contact with a local poison control center can be invaluable in the case of unusual or unfamiliar substances. Additional pieces of medical history that may be of significance in a case of acute trauma include the date of the last tetanus inoculation and the timing of the last oral intake so that surgical intervention and anesthesia may be scheduled appropriately.

EXAMINATION

In general, a complete ophthalmic examination of both eyes should be performed. For splash injuries, irrigation is performed before further evaluation (see Chapter 12). In patients with a nontraumatic red eye, dilated fundus examination can be deferred, particularly if infectious conjunctivitis is suspected.

VISUAL ACUITY

The cornerstone of the examination of the patient with an ophthalmic emergency is the measurement of visual acuity. Physician confirmation is of particular importance in the event of severe vision loss, particularly where no light perception vision is reported. Cases in which litigation is likely to result, such as an on-the-job injury, also mandate physician confirmation of acuity. Visual acuity on presentation is one of the most significant prognostic indicators of eventual visual outcome in cases of severe ocular trauma.

Various methods for determining visual acuity exist, each appropriate to different circumstances. A near card may have to suffice for the severely injured or otherwise immobilized or unstable patient, with appropriate correction being provided for presbyopia or aphakia. Whenever possible, however, measurement of acuity using a Snellen, early treatment diabetic retinopathy study (ETDRS), or other standard target at a measured distance in a quiet area is preferred. The acuity of illiterate patients may be assessed by means of an illiterate E or Landholt C

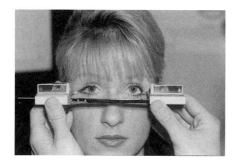

FIG. 3–1. Proper positioning for Hertel measurements.

chart. Preliterate children may be tested with Allen cards, HOTV, letters or the "E game." (For more information on the assessment of acuity in children, see Chapter 4.)

Acuity should be assessed with the patient's spectacles in place wherever possible. In cases of severe visual loss, the normal eye must be patched so the patient does not inadvertently (or intentionally) use the normal eye when the affected eye is tested. Refraction to determine the best-corrected vision in the affected eye, or in the fellow eye in the event of severe visual loss, should be performed at the earliest convenient opportunity.

EXTERNAL EXAMINATION

Many types of ocular injuries and emergencies can be diagnosed by external observation of the face and periorbital area. Specifically, the patient should be examined for the presence or absence of enophthalmos or exophthalmos (with the aid of Hertel measurements if orbital involvement is suspected), ecchymosis, periorbital crepitance, ptosis, and infraorbital hypesthesia (Fig. 3–1). A palpable or tender lacrimal gland may be of significance in a case of suspected acute infection or inflammation. Similarly, the presence of palpable preauricular or submandibular nodes may be of diagnostic importance in acute viral conjunctivitis.

PUPILLARY EXAMINATION

The pupils should be tested carefully as part of the initial ocular assessment. The presence or absence of a relative afferent pupillary defect (RAPD) can be of great prognostic significance in severe ocular injury, particularly to the optic nerve. The size of the pupils may be of importance in assessing the possibility of cranial nerve involvement. The configuration of the pupil also gives clues as to the presence of injury to the iris, vitreous prolapse, or possible intraocular foreign body.

Testing for an RAPD is performed with a swinging flashlight or indirect ophthalmoscope at the highest light setting (Fig. 3–2). If one of the pupils is dilated

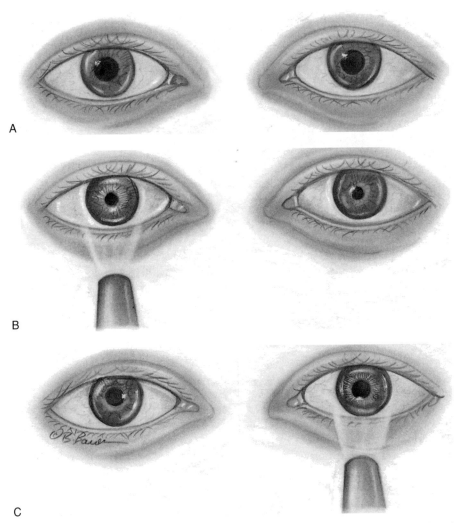

FIG. 3–2. Swinging flashlight test for an RAPD. In this case, there is a left RAPD. **A:** Position of pupils with background lighting only. **B:** A bright light is shined into the right eye; both pupils constrict normally. **C:** The bright light is now shined into the left eye; both pupils dilate and do not return to there previously constricted position until the light is again shined into the right eye.

and nonreactive or poorly reactive because of iris or third-nerve injury, it is still possible to test for an RAPD using the "reverse" method. Rather than examining the direct response to light of each pupil in turn, only the reactive pupil is observed while swinging the flashlight back and forth before each eye. If an RAPD is present in the eye with the poorly reactive pupil, the pupil of the contralateral eye will redilate when the light is swung from that eye to the fellow eye.

The examiner must remember three important points about the pupillary examination:

1. Anisocoria is never caused by a defect in the afferent (sensory) portion of the pupillomotor pathway.
2. A patient with bilateral abnormalities of the optic nerves may not have evidence of an RAPD, even with marked asymmetry of visual function.
3. Dense cataract, vitreous hemorrhage, and other marked opacities of the optical media are believed to rarely if ever cause an RAPD.
4. In the monocular patient this test cannot be performed.

BRIGHTNESS TESTING, COLOR VISION, AND RED DESATURATION

When both pupils are nonreactive, irregular, or obscured, relative brightness testing provides an alternate, albeit more crude, test of relative afferent function. A bright light (e.g., from the indirect ophthalmoscope) is shined in the normal eye along the visual axis. The patient is instructed that this has a value of 100% or $1.00. The light is then shined in the affected eye along the visual axis and the patient is asked if the light has the same value or less. If less, the patient is asked to quantify the relative amount, e.g., 50% or $0.50.

Color vision testing provides another sensitive test of optic nerve function. Hardy-Rand-Rittler, Ishihara, or another set of pseudoisochromatic plates can be used. Patients should be asked about congenital color blindness. When color plates are unavailable, any bright red object can be used (e.g., the top of the dilating drop bottle) to test for red desaturation. The patient is asked to look at the red object with each eye while the opposite eye is covered. When optic nerve disease is present, patients report the red color appearing grayish or washed out when compared with color seen by the normal eye.

VISUAL FIELDS

In the setting of an emergent ocular problem, gross visual field abnormalities often can be detected rapidly and effectively by confrontation. The patient should cover one eye with a patch or occluder and direct his attention to the center of the examiner's face. Examiner and patient should be at the same height, and care should be taken that the patient's head is held level. Fingers from one or both hands are presented to the patient centrally and in each of the four quadrants. Visual neglect without frank scotoma may be detected if fingers from both hands are presented simultaneously in different quadrants. A red test object also may be presented in cases of suspected optic nerve abnormality. The examiner must monitor the patient for central fixation at all times. Testing is then repeated for the opposite eye.

Early Humphrey or Goldmann visual field testing may be useful in distinguishing acute vision loss from retinal, retinal vascular, optic nerve, chiasmal, and central nervous system etiologies. In addition, formal visual field tests are the most sensitive way to follow traumatic optic neuropathies.

EXTRAOCULAR MOTILITY

Assessment of ocular motility can be of significance in the event of known or suspected orbital injury or injury involving the cranial nerves. Forced duction testing may help to distinguish between a paretic versus a restrictive etiology but are deferred when an open globe is suspected.

Procedure: Forced Duction Testing

Forced duction testing is depicted in Fig. 3–3.

1. Administer topical anesthetic (e.g., proparacaine).
2. Place a cotton-tipped applicator soaked in 4% lidocaine or 10% cocaine on the conjunctiva over the extraocular muscle to be tested for restriction. Leave in place for at least 1 minute.
3. Grasp the muscle insertion with toothed forceps (e.g., Graefe's fixation forceps) and rotate the eye toward the direction opposite the muscle being tested (e.g., superior for the inferior rectus; temporal for the medial rectus). Any resistance to passive rotation indicates a restrictive process.

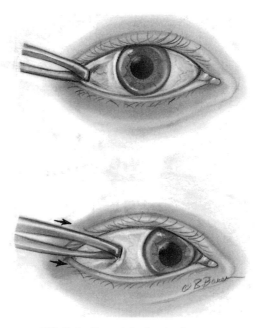

FIG. 3–3. Forced duction testing.

EXAMINATION OF THE ANTERIOR SEGMENT

In patients who are sufficiently stable and mobile, accurate examination of the anterior segment is best performed with the aid of a slit-lamp biomicroscope.

Cornea

Examination of the anterior segment begins with the evaluation of the cornea. Fluorescein is used both to examine for epithelial defects and at a 2% concentration to test for leakage of aqueous from the eye (Seidel test). The cornea should be examined carefully at the slit lamp for the presence or absence of foreign bodies, which may be removed with the aid of a needle or corneal bur. A high index of suspicion for open globe trauma should be maintained during the examination of all but the most superficial corneal wounds. Corneal abrasions, ulcerations, or other irregularities should be documented and measured for height, width, and depth.

Conjunctiva

The conjunctiva is examined for hemorrhagic chemosis, which can be an important indicator of open globe trauma to the eye. The fornices and inverted lid also should be carefully probed for the presence of foreign bodies, provided that there is no suspicion for an open globe. Conjunctival lacerations can be carefully examined under topical anesthesia to rule out underlying scleral lacerations or foreign bodies. Papillary or follicular reactions should be noted.

Anterior Chamber

The depth of the anterior chamber can be a clue to the presence of a scleral rupture, posteriorly dislocated lens, or iridodialysis, all of which can lead to a deepening of the chamber. Choroidal hemorrhage, anteriorly dislocated lens, prolapsed vitreous, or corneoscleral wound leak may be heralded by a shallow chamber. The anterior chamber is also examined for cells, flare, hyphema, hypopyon, and foreign body.

Gonioscopy and the Iris

Gonioscopy generally should be avoided in the event of a possible open globe or acute traumatic hyphema. However, it may be of critical importance when there is a suspected foreign body or occult site of penetration in the anterior chamber angle. It is generally best to use four mirror lenses that require only gentle pressure and no contact solution beyond anesthetic. The iris is examined for evidence of irregularity suggestive of iridodialysis or sphincter tears.

Crystallin Lens

The lens is examined for abnormalities of position such as subluxation, disloca-tion, or extrusion and for the presence or absence of traumatic cataract, capsular rupture, and leakage of cortical material.

INTRAOCULAR PRESSURE

While an abnormally low intraocular pressure may be an important clue to the presence of an occult rupture site, it is equally important to remember that elevated intraocular pressure does not rule out the possibility of a ruptured globe. Low in-traocular pressure also may be seen with ciliary body shutdown in cases of trau-matic iritis on cyclodialysis, and when a retinal detachment is present.

Acute elevation of intraocular pressure may occur in the setting of angle-closure glaucoma (either primary or secondary to tumor, inflammation, or other cause), traumatic (angle-recession) glaucoma, pigmentary glaucoma, uveitis, hyphema, and various combinations of positional and inflammatory factors related to the crystalline lens, among other causes. Usually careful examination of the affected and fellow eyes at the slit lamp, together with an accurate history, allow the correct etiology to be determined.

POSTERIOR SEGMENT EXAMINATION

General Principles

It is important that the posterior segment be examined carefully at the earliest possible time because subsequent examination may be degraded by corneal de-compensation, vitreous hemorrhage, intraocular infection or hyphema, progressive traumatic cataract, or other conditions affecting the clarity of the ocular media. Scleral depression is invaluable in ruling out a retinal tear or other peripheral reti-nal pathology; however, scleral depression should be performed only when an open globe injury has been ruled out. Scleral depression also should be avoided in the setting of acute hyphema or recent ocular surgery. When mydriatics are used to facilitate examination in the severely injured patient, their use should be docu-mented in the chart, particularly in the case of head injuries.

Vitreous

The vitreous is examined for the presence or absence of foreign bodies, red and white blood cells, and pigment (tobacco dust). Posterior vitreous detachment, indi-cated by the presence of a Weiss ring, should be noted. Vitreous streaming towards the anterior segment or pars plana may indicate an occult rupture site.

Retina and Choroid

Important findings in the retina include holes, tears, dialysis, intraretinal or sub-retinal hemorrhage, and retinal detachment. Traumatic changes in the retina often include commotio retinae, which is due to damage to photoreceptor outer segments. Important findings in the choroid include choroidal detachment. All posterior segment findings should be documented with a detailed fundus drawing.

Optic Nerve Head

The optic nerve head should be examined for any swelling or hemorrhage. The size of the optic cup may be significant if abnormally large, small, or irregular in shape.

ANCILLARY TESTING

Imaging studies are of particular importance if the view of the posterior segment is obscured or the orbit is involved. Refer to Chapter 5 (Radiographic and Echographic Imaging Studies) for further information.

Management of Ocular Injuries and Emergencies,
edited by Mathew W. MacCumber.
Lippincott–Raven Publishers, Philadelphia ©1998.

4

Special Issues in Pediatric Ocular Trauma

Arman K. Fard and Michael X. Repka

*Department of Ophthalmology, Wilmer Eye Institute, The Johns Hopkins University
School of Medicine, Baltimore, Maryland 21287*

Basic Considerations 39
History 40
Examination 41
  Visual Acuity 43 · External Examination 46 · Pupillary Examination 46
  Intraocular Pressure 47 · Ocular Motility 47 · Visual Field Testing 47
  Examination of the Anterior Segment 47 · Dilated Fundus Examination 48
  Ancilliary Testing 48
Birth Trauma 48
  Neonatal Eyelid Closure 48 · Corneal Damage (Breaks in Descemet's Membrane) 49 · Retinal Hemorrhages 50
Child Abuse 50
  Battered Child Syndrome 50 · Shaken Baby Syndrome 51
Amblyopia 52
  Management 53

BASIC CONSIDERATIONS

Ocular trauma is a leading cause of blindness in American children. The incidence of trauma in the United States shows a bimodal distribution with one peak in adolescents and young adults and another in those more than 75 years of age (1). Studies have shown that children comprise a disproportionate number of those affected by ocular trauma, with 29% of ocular trauma occurring in children less than 10 years of age (2). Thirty-five percent of hospital admissions for ocular injuries are children younger than 15 years of age (3). Hyphema constitutes about half of all admissions for ocular trauma (4). The management of other important topics in trauma, including intraocular foreign bodies, hyphema, and open globe injuries, are discussed elsewhere in this book.

Other serious diseases may be noticed first after even subtle trauma. An injury may bring to light preexisting strabismus, leukocoria, or proptosis (5). A full discussion of these disorders is beyond the scope of this text, but a differential diag-

TABLE 4–1. *Possible preexisting disorders initially noticed after trauma*

Leukocoria	Proptosis
Retinoblastoma	Orbital teratoma
Retinopathy of prematurity	Rhabdomyosarcoma
Cataract	Strabismus
Toxocariasis	Congenital eso-, exo-, or hyperdeviation
Vitreous hemorrhage	Paralytic (III, IV, VI nerve palsy)
Retinal detachment	Strabismus syndrome (Duane, etc.)

nosis is listed in Table 4–1. One should consider nontrauma etiologies in the evaluation of the injured patient.

This chapter addresses specific conditions unique to the pediatric population and the examination of the child under stress. The routine ocular examination of a healthy child is often a challenge. When this is compounded by the stress of systemic or ocular trauma, a clinician's skill and patience are often tested. It is imperative for the physician to be patient, touch last, and, above all else, do no harm. Many children feel the same level of anxiety about eye drops as they do for needle sticks. Administration of drops should be reserved for last.

HISTORY

A careful history may elucidate a diagnosis and aid in the selection of management. Keep in mind that a child may fabricate a history if involved in a forbidden activity when injured. It also may be difficult to obtain accurate information in cases that may have resulted from poor supervision or child abuse. Some of the key information that needs to be gathered is listed as follows:

TABLE 4–2. *Prophylactic management of tetanus: should tetanus toxoid or immunoglobulin be given?*

Type of wound		No. of adsorbed tetanus toxoid (doses)	
		Uncertain or less than three	Three or more
Nontetanus prone	Td[a]	Yes	No[b]
Age <6 h			
Depth <1 cm			
No signs of infection	TIG	No	No
No contaminants			
Tetanus prone	Td[a]	Yes	No[c]
Age >6 h			
Depth >1 cm			
+signs of infection	TIG	Yes	No
+contamination			
(dirt, feces, saliva)			

Td, tetanus and diptheria toxoid; TIG, tetanus immunoglobulin.
[a]For children <7 years of age, DTP is preferred to tetanus toxoid alone.
[b]Yes, if >10 years since last dose.
[c]Yes, if >5 years since last dose.

1. The mechanism of injury
2. The time of injury
3. Caregiver during the injury
4. The child's visual status before the injury
5. Any history of eye surgery, prior injury, patching, or glasses
6. The child's general medical status before the injury
7. Any medicines or allergies
8. The child's tetanus immunization status (6) (Table 4–2)
9. Involvement of projectiles such as BBs or sharp objects (pen, knife, etc)
10. Loss of consciousness with the injury
11. Loss of vision, double vision, floaters, or flashes of light

EXAMINATION

It is important to establish a routine to assure a complete assessment. In an emergency setting, the physician may feel the pressure to evaluate the patient quickly; however, approaching the child in a hurried fashion may cause the child to become angry and uncooperative. Taking time and appearing to play with and entertain the child may ultimately save time and aggravation.

1. Find out what the child likes to be called and use that name.
2. Make a game of the examination: make funny noises, whistle, use toys.
3. With older children, ask about school, sports, or hobbies and explain the examination to them.
4. Talk softly and keep your distance.
5. Perform the noncontact parts of the examination first.
6. At all times ensure that no pressure is placed on the globe.

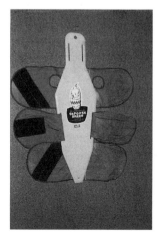

FIG. 4–1. Papoose board.

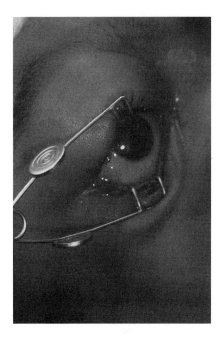

FIG. 4–2. Eyelid speculum.

If an infant or toddler is extremely uncooperative, restraining in a papoose (Fig. 4–1) may become necessary. A wire eyelid speculum (Fig. 4–2) may be needed to retract the eyelids. Use only when certain that the globe is not ruptured or lacerated. Instillation of a drop of proparacaine 0.5% in each eye before placement of the wire lid retractors reduces discomfort. If a wire lid retractor is not available, a sterilized bent paper clip may work adequately. The physician should explain the importance of a thorough eye examination to the parents or guardians as well as each of the steps in the process.

Toddlers also may be restrained in the position shown in Fig. 4–3. If available, it will be more efficient if an assistant holds the patient while the physician performs the examination. This may be done in the following fashion:

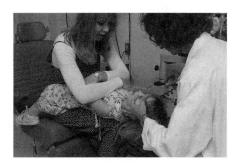

FIG. 4–3. Method used to restrain a toddler. The assistant and parent sit at the same level facing each other. The child lies supine with legs straddling the parent's waist. The child's head is on the assistant's lap, while the parent holds the hands. The assistant holds the child's head.

1. The assistant and parent sit at the same level facing each other.
2. The child lies supine with legs straddling the parent's waist.
3. The child's head is placed on the assistant's lap.
4. The parent holds the child's hands.
5. The assistant holds the child's head still while the physician examines.

A papoose board is not practical for a child over 5 years of age. Physical restraints may not be adequate to allow examination of a struggling child. Also, examination of the anterior segment may be difficult if the eyes elevate (Bell's phenomenon).

In cases where physical restraints are not practical or do not allow an adequate examination, appropriate conscious sedation should be used. The American Academy of Pediatrics (7) has outlined the goals of conscious sedation in pediatric patients as follows:

1. To control behavior
2. To guard the patient's safety
3. To minimize pain and discomfort
4. To minimize negative psychologic response by the use of amnestics and analgesics
5. To return the patient to a safe discharge status

Sedation of the pediatric patient may be complicated by vomiting, anaphylaxis, seizure, hypoventilation, apnea, airway obstruction, or cardiorespiratory arrest. The physician should be familiar with the appropriate management of such complications and be able to act quickly. Sedation should only be performed in a facility where the child's vital signs are monitored and resuscitation and ventilatory equipment are at hand. It is advisable that a qualified person other than the ophthalmologist be present to monitor the patient while sedated.

Before initiation of sedation, a complete history and physical examination should be performed. Vital signs, including temperature, blood pressure, heart rate, and respiratory rate, should be assessed carefully. Informed consent must be obtained from the parents explaining the risks and benefits of sedation. Most institutions have strict policies on the use of conscious and deep sedation for examination. Some of the common drugs (8,9) used for conscious sedation are listed in Table 4–3.

It is important to make sure the child does not have any other injuries, such as intracranial injuries, which preclude the use of sedation. Conditions that may be associated with increased general anesthesia risk include asthma, Down's syndrome, Marfan's syndrome, sickle-cell disease, or congenital heart disease.

Before discharge, the child's cardiovascular function and airway patency should be stable. Protective reflexes must be intact and the patient easily arousable.

Visual Acuity

1. Measure the visual acuity of each eye separately. This is achieved by occluding an eye with opaque tape or patch.

TABLE 4-3. *Commonly used drugs for conscious sedation*

Drug/action	Dosage/administration	Comments
Chloral hydrate hypnotic	PO/PR: 25–100 mg/kg Maximum dose: 2.0 g	Hypnotic Nonsedative, nonamnestic, nonanalgesic Primarily causes immobility Do not combine with narcotics
Midazolam hydrochloride (Versed) short acting benzodiazepine	IV/PO: 0.05 mg/kg slowly over 2 min May be repeated ×4 (maximum dose 0.2 mg/kg)	CNS depressant Produces sedation, anxiolysis, amnesia No analgesic properties
Fentanyl citrate (Sublimaze) narcotic/opioid	IV: 1 µg/kg slowly over 2 min Maximum total dose 3.0 µg/kg	Potent analgesic Minimal sedation, no amnesia May be antagonized by naloxone
Morphine sulfate narcotic/opioid	IV: 0.05–0.1 mg/kg slowly over 2 min	Potent analgesic No amnesia May be antagonized by naloxone
Meperidine hydrochloride (Demerol) narcotic/opioid	IV: 0.5–1.0 mg/kg slowly over 2 min	Ten times less potent than morphine Minimal sedation, no amnesia May be antagonized by naloxone
Pentobarbital (Nembutal) barbiturate	IM/PO: 2–6 mg/kg Maximum dose: 150 mg	Hypnotic Nonsedative, nonamnestic, nonanalgesic Primarily causes immobility Do not combine with narcotics
Ketamine hydrochloride dissociative	IV: 1–3 mg/kg slowly over 2 min IM: 3–5 mg/kg	Dissociative anesthesia Hallucinations/excitement can occur postanesthesia. Combination with barbiturates/opioids prolongs recovery.

PO, orally; PR, rectally; IV, intravenously; CNS, central nervous system.
Use smaller doses in debilitated or chronically ill children.
Wait 5 min between successive doses to assess the effect of previous administration.

2. With a cooperative child, Allen pictures (Fig. 4–4), tumbling E, HOTV, or the Snellen letters are used. Make sure the child knows the alphabet if smaller letters are used. Younger children have their acuity assessed by fixation behavior.
3. Normal fixation acuity:
   By 6 weeks of age: able to fixate with some smooth pursuit
   By 10 to 12 weeks of age: fixate with accurate smooth pursuit (fix and follow)

   Normal optotype acuity:

   3 years: 20/40
   4 to 5 years: 20/30
   6 years and up: 20/20
4. If vision is too poor to be measured with standard charts, a gross assessment of visual acuity such as counting fingers at a specific distance, hand motion, light perception, or no light perception should be obtained.

In determining the visual acuity of infants and children up to 3 years of age, the following points should be borne in mind:

1. They may not be able to perform objective testing.
2. Their ability to fixate and follow should be assessed.
3. A colorful toy, or even the examiner's or parent's face may serve as a fixation target. Never use a light as a target.
4. Move the target slowly side to side.
5. Observe the infant's eye fixating the target and then following the target.
6. Use your thumb or patch to occlude one eye, testing each eye separately.
7. Make sure when assessing the child's ability to follow that he or she is following the visual stimulus not an auditory stimulus of a squeaky toy or the examiners whistling.
8. Normal milestones for fixation acuity are listed above.

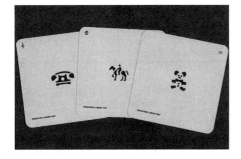

FIG. 4–4. Allen pictures used for acuity testing in children 3 to 6 years of age. To reduce confusion, present the pictures up close initially, so the child may identify the pictures in his or her own words. (The bird may be called a dinosaur, or the telephone a spaceship)

External Examination

If a child is anxious, perform the tactile examination last.

1. Observe the child's alertness and gross appearance.
2. Inspect the eyelids for symmetry.
3. Assess the depth and tissue involvement of any lacerations with particular attention to the lacrimal system.
4. Palpate the bony orbital rim for any "step-off's" or irregularities in the bones, suggesting a fracture.
5. Look for a protruding (exophthalmos) or sunken (enophthalmos) appearance of the eye: enophthalmos suggests ruptured globe or orbital fracture with tissue herniation into maxillary or ethmoid sinuses. Exophthalmos suggests orbital hemorrhage.
6. Assess the face for any sensory deficits (hypoesthesia): infraorbital suggests floor fracture, and supraorbital suggests roof fracture.
7. Feel for any crepitus in the lids and adnexa (subcutaneous emphysema) which would be suggestive of a floor or medial wall fracture.
8. If child abuse is suspected, the examiner should be alert for suggestive signs (Table 4–4).

Pupillary Examination

1. Assess the size, shape, and symmetry of each pupil.
2. Direct pupillary light reaction should be observed with the patient gazing at a distant object.
3. Care must be taken not to mistake the near pupillary reflex for reaction to light.
4. The presence of a relative afferent pupillary defect (Marcus Gunn pupil) is elicited by the swinging flashlight test (see Chapter 3).

If an open globe is suspected, examination by the physician should be stopped at this point to prevent further injury to the eye. A large hard shield (not a pressure patch) should be taped over the eye to the orbital rim and remainder of the examination performed under general anesthesia or monitored sedation. Perform indicated radiographic studies (usually orbital CT scanning).

TABLE 4–4. *Systemic signs of child abuse*

Fractures or bruises in different stages of healing
Bruises in the shape of hand prints or belt buckle
Cigarette burns
Bite marks
Tears of the floor of the mouth
Dehydration

Intraocular Pressure

1. Goldmann applanation tonometer, Perkins tonometer, Tono-Pen or careful finger tip palpation (in comparison with a normal eye) may be used.
2. Crying, struggling, or eyelid closure causes an artifactual increase in intraocular pressure.
3. An accurate intraocular pressure measurement is especially important if a cloudy cornea or hyphema is present. (Ketamine anesthesia may be required.)

Ocular Motility

1. Assess motility in all cardinal gazes.
2. Use an attractive test object:
   Use a toy.
   Flick your finger in front of the light source.
   Place a red lens, colored filter, or translucent lollipop in front of the light source.
   Use your face as a fixation target.
3. Limitation of ocular rotation may be due to entrapment, paresis, or avulsion (rare) of an extraocular muscle. These can be differentiated by forced duction testing.
4. Forced duction testing (see Fig. 4–3), in children, is usually performed with sedation or anesthesia and not in the examination setting.
   A negative test (the eye moves without restriction in a given direction) indicates ocular motor paresis or muscle avulsion.
   A positive test (the inability to forcibly move the eye) suggests entrapment, orbital edema, or hemorrhage.

Visual Field Testing

1. Older children may cooperate with confrontational visual field testing by counting fingers in each quadrant (see Chapter 3).
2. Younger children are examined by moving a target into the visual field. A large target is used to maintain central fixation, while another usually smaller object is brought in from the periphery. The child will switch fixation to the peripheral object once in view. This is a gross test and is best for detecting dense hemianopic field deficits.

Examination of the Anterior Segment

1. The child may need to kneel on the chair, stand on the chair's step, or sit on a parent's lap for a conventional slit-lamp examination.
2. Alternatively, a portable slit lamp may be used if available.
3. Use the dimmest light possible (narrow beam, all filters on).
4. Look at the eye with the injury first—you may only get one look.

5. If a slit lamp is not available, an indirect ophthalmoscopy lens (20 D) with a light source may provide adequate magnification for a screening of the anterior segment structures.
6. If a corneal abrasion is suspected, fluorescein dye should be applied and the cornea examined using a blue handlight (if slit-lamp examination is not possible). A Woods lamp, available in most emergency rooms, also can be used. Fluorescein will appear bright green in areas of corneal epithelial loss.

Dilated Fundus Examination

1. If the child has concomitant head injuries, make sure the pupillary signs are not being used for assessment of neurologic status before dilation.
2. Instillation of proparacaine 0.5% before dilation drops reduces discomfort, reduces reflex tearing, increases drug penetration, and makes the child more cooperative.
3. Mydriasis can be achieved with phenylepherine 2.5% and tropicamide 1%.
4. In children with darker irides, cyclopentolate 1% may be needed.
5. Keep the light intensity of the ophthalmoscope low.
6. With an uncooperative child, focus on one area of the fundus and allow the child's eye movements to bring different views of the retina to your field of view.
7. Minimum examination should include vitreous, optic nerve, macula, and vascular arcades.

Ancilliary Testing

1. Radiographic studies (particularly CT scanning) are often indicated if posterior segment, orbit, or head injury is suspected (see Chapter 5 for further information).
2. Sedation is usually required for young children (see above).

BIRTH TRAUMA

Delivery may be associated with ocular and periocular injuries (10). These include lid edema, subconjunctival hemorrhage, corneal edema, corneal abrasion, hyphema, vitreous and retinal hemorrhage. The use of forceps during delivery increases the likelihood of injury.

Neonatal Eyelid Closure

Diagnosis

1. Periorbital ecchymosis and edema are present after birth.
2. May result from periorbital swelling from obstetrical trauma.

3. Need to rule out other causes of lid closure or swelling, such as congenital ptosis or conjunctivitis.

Management

1. In most cases the injury is self-limited, requiring no treatment.
2. Persistent eyelid closure may produce monocular axial myopia, leading to anisometropic amblyopia (11).
3. The patient should be followed periodically to assess visual development and the presence of astigmatism.
4. Correction of refractive error may be necessary to prevent anisometropic amblyopia.

Corneal Damage (Breaks in Descemet's Membrane)

Forceps delivery may cause corneal damage. Occasionally there may be a corneal abrasion, but the pathology most associated with forceps injury are breaks in Descemet's membrane, leading to a cloudy cornea (12).

Diagnosis

1. Initially appears as unilateral corneal clouding due to corneal stromal edema.
2. Intraocular pressure is normal.
3. Vertical breaks in Descemet's membrane are evident after clearing of the corneal haze.
4. Other causes of corneal clouding in infancy should be considered and excluded (Table 4–5).

Management

1. Corneal edema usually clears within weeks without intervention.
2. Vertically oriented ruptures in Descemet's membrane may lead to high corneal astigmatism, corresponding to the orientation of the defect.

TABLE 4–5. *Causes of cloudy cornea in infancy*

Forceps injury
Congenital rubella
Congenital syphilis
Infantile glaucoma
Congenital hereditary endothelial dystrophy
Corneal ulcer
Sclerocornea
Peter's anomaly
Dermoid
Mucopolysaccharidosis, especially I-H, I-S, IV

3. Increased axial length and high myopia is associated with some of these injuries (12).
4. The combination of anisometropia and astigmatism in such patients may lead to deprivation amblyopia.
5. Patching and corrective spectacles or contact lenses may be needed to prevent amblyopia.

Retinal Hemorrhages

Diagnosis

1. Are seen in about 20% of newborn infants within 24 hours of birth (13).
2. Are resolved quickly—are seen in fewer than 3% of infants by day 5 of life.
3. Are more likely seen after forceps or vacuum extraction deliveries.
4. Are more common in first babies.
5. Are seen in fewer than 1% of cesarean deliveries.
6. Are not associated with intracranial hemorrhage (14).

Management

1. These should be observed to assure resolution. This usually occurs within a month.
2. Diagnostic or therapeutic intervention is usually not necessary.
3. Need to rule out child abuse as cause if found after patient is at home.

CHILD ABUSE

The National Committee for Prevention of Child Abuse estimates that almost 3 million cases of child abuse are reported every year in the United States. Ocular injuries occur in approximately 40% of abused children (15). Therefore, the ophthalmologist must be able to recognize the ophthalmologic signs of child abuse. Prompt recognition may prevent severe morbidity and even death. Child abuse should be included in the differential diagnosis of every child with traumatic injuries.

Battered Child Syndrome

Diagnosis

1. Child abuse should be suspected when:
   - there are discrepancies in the caregiver's history of events
   - no explanation is given by the caregiver
   - the child has a previous history of failure to thrive
   - the child has a history of multiple visits, particularly to different hospitals
   - there is a delay in presentation to the hospital

- there is a disproportionate amount of soft tissue injury for the reported trauma
- the nature of the injury is incompatible with the reported history
- the child has a history of minor trauma, minor fall, or spontaneous choking

2. Social factors associated with child abuse include:
   - caregiver immaturity
   - history of parental substance abuse
   - parental history of violent behavior or mental illness
   - financial or marital problems
3. Systemic signs of child abuse are detailed in Table 4–4.
4. Ocular injuries from physical abuse are listed in Table 4–6.

Shaken Baby Syndrome

Diagnosis

1. Intraocular and intracranial hemorrhages are present in the absence of significant external signs of trauma (16).
2. Is most often seen in children less than 3 years of age.
3. Associated symptoms include vomiting, lethargy, irritability.
4. Retinal hemorrhages are mostly intraretinal; however, subretinal, preretinal, and vitreous hemorrhages are possible (Fig. 4–5).
5. Other causes of retinal hemorrhage need to be considered:

   Leukemia
   Cardiopulmonary resuscitation
   Accidental trauma
   Malignant hypertension
   Idiopathic thrombocytopenia
   Increased intracranial pressure

6. In a child under 3 years of age, in the absence of verifiable life-threatening trauma, the presence of retinal hemorrhages with head injury is nearly pathognomonic for child abuse. Buys et al. (17) in a study of 79 children admitted to

---

TABLE 4–6. *Ophthalmic manifestations of child abuse*

External/ocular motility: nystagmus, motility abnormalitis, proptosis, orbital floor
    fracture
Periorbital: ecchymosis, lid laceration, periorbital edema
Conjunctiva: conjunctivitis from a sexually transmitted organism,
    subconjunctival hemorrhage
Cornea: abrasion, ulceration, laceration, edema, scarring
Anterior chamber: hyphema
Iris: cyclodialysis, traumatic mydriasis, iridodenesis
Lens: cataract, subluxation, dislocation
Vitreous: hemorrhage, detachment
Retina: hemorrhage, detachment, retinoschisis, dialysis, chorioretinal scar,
    perimacular folds, circumferential retinal fold

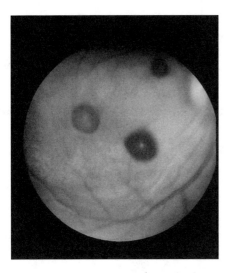

FIG. 4–5. Preretinal hemorrhages in shaken baby syndrome. (Courtesy of Dr. T. Deutsch.) *For a color representation of this figure, please see the color insert facing p. 256.*

an intensive care unit with head trauma reported retinal hemorrhages in only those with nonaccidental head trauma.

Management of Suspected Child Abuse

1. Social worker needs to be notified immediately for the evaluation of child abuse.
2. Pediatric service or child abuse team should be consulted.
3. If child abuse is suspected, patient should be admitted for evaluation, including skeletal survey, x-rays, genital examination.
4. Do not confront parents.
5. Treat ocular problems such as corneal abrasion, lid laceration, hyphema, etc.
6. Retinal hemorrhages may persist from days to weeks depending on the severity of the injury.
7. Severe visual morbidity with shaken baby syndrome may be secondary to macular folds, retinal detachment, optic nerve atrophy, or cortical blindness (18).
8. Dense vitreous hemorrhage not clearing within the first month usually require removal with specialized vitrectomy to prevent deprivation amblyopia.

AMBLYOPIA

In any child younger than 8 years of age, the development of amblyopia in the injured eye is common. Therefore, the effort to optimize the visual outcome must first be to restore the anatomic integrity of the eye and second to prevent amblyopia. The primary effort must include expeditious repair of the retinal detachment, removal of the cataractous lens, and/or repair of the corneal laceration. After the best structural outcome has been obtained, attention should be directed to amblyopia prevention.

The types of amblyopia encountered after trauma include strabismic, refractive, and stimulus deprivation.

Management

Strabismic Amblyopia

Example: entrapped or avulsed muscle, or paralysis of cranial nerve III, IV, or VI.

1. If deviation is small, may try prisms.
2. Consider surgery to restore proper alignment of the eyes after 6 to 9 months.
3. Penalization of the better seeing eye:
   - Occlusion therapy—patching the "good" eye 1 week per year of chronologic age; up to 4 weeks before next examination.
   - Atropine penalization—atropine sulfate 1% (0.5% for children less than 3 years of age) three to six times a week for 8 weeks before next examination.

Refractive Amblyopia

Example: corneal astigmatic changes, dislocated lens, or aphakia.

1. Corrective spectacles or contact lenses.
2. Penalization or occlusion of the better seeing eye (see above).

Deprivation Amblyopia

Example: traumatic cataract, corneal laceration, hyphema, or vitreous hemorrhage.

1. Perform the necessary operation to allow a clear retinal image, such as cataract extraction, penetrating keratoplasty or vitrectomy.
2. Apply contact lens correction as soon as possible.
3. Begin penalization or occlusion of the better seeing eye.
4. Consider early intraocular lens placement for traumatic cataract (19).

REFERENCES

1. Klopfer J, Tielsch JM, Vitale S, See L, Canner JK. Ocular trauma in the United States. *Arch Ophthalmol* 1992;110:838.
2. Maltzman BA, Pruzon H, Mund ML. A survey of ocular trauma. *Surv Ophthalmol* 1976;21:285.
3. Niiranen M, Ilkka R. Eye injuries in children. *Br J Ophthalmol* 1981;65:436.
4. Rudd JC, Jaeger EA, Freitag SK, Jeffers JB. Traumatically ruptured globes in children. *J Pediatr Ophthalmol Strabismus* 1994;31:307.
5. Wright KW, ed. *Pediatric Ophthalmology and Strabismus*. St. Louis: CV Mosby; 1995:495–497.
6. Moore FE, ed. American College of Surgeons' Committee on Trauma. *Early Care of the Injured Patient*. Philadelphia: Decker; 1990.

7. Committee on Drugs. Guidelines for monitoring and management of pediatric patients during and after sedation for diagnostic and therapeutic procedures. *Pediatrics* 1992;89:1110.

8. Committee on Drugs and Committee on Environmental Health. Use of chloral hydrate for sedation in children. *Pediatrics* 1993;92:471.

9. McEvoy GK, ed. *Drug Information 95*. Bethesda, MD: American Hospital Formulary Service; 1995.

10. Holden R, Morsman DG, Davidek GMB, O'Conner GM. External ocular trauma in instrumental and normal deliveries. *Br J Obstet Gynecol* 1992;99:132.

11. Hoyt CG, Stone RD, Fromer C, Billson FA. Monocular axial myopia associated with neonatal eyelid closure in human infants. *Am J Ophthalmol* 1981;91:197.

12. Angell LK, Robb RM, Berson FG. Visual prognosis in patients with ruptures in Descemet's membrane due to forceps injuries. *Arch Ophthalmol* 1981;99:2137.

13. Sezen F. Retinal haemorrhages in newborn infants. *Br J Ophthalmol* 1970;55:248.

14. Smith WL, Alexander RC, Judisch GF, Sato Y, Kao S. Magnetic resonance imaging evaluation of neonates with retinal hemorrhages. *Pediatrics* 1992;89:332.

15. Tongue AC. The ophthalmologist's role in diagnosing child abuse. *Ophthalmology* 1991;98:1009.

16. Caffey J. On the theory and practice of shaking infants: its potential residual effects of permanent brain damage and mental retardation. *Am J Dis Child* 1972;124:161.

17. Buys YM, Levin AV, Enzenauer RW, et al. *Ophthalmology* 1992;99:1718.

18. Han DP, Wilkinson WS. Late ophthalmic manifestations of the shaken baby syndrome. *J Pediatr Ophthalmol Strabismus* 1990;27:299.

19. Koenig SB, Ruttman MS, Lewandowski MF, Schultz RO. Pseudophakia for traumatic cataracts in children. *Ophthalmology* 1993;100:1218.

Management of Ocular Injuries and Emergencies,
edited by Mathew W. MacCumber.
Lippincott–Raven Publishers, Philadelphia ©1998.

5

Radiographic and Echographic Imaging Studies

Daniel P. Joseph, Cathy DiBernardo, and Neil R. Miller

Department of Ophthalmology, Washington University at Barnes, St. Louis, Missouri 63110 and Department of Ophthalmology, Wilmer Eye Institute, The Johns Hopkins University School of Medicine, Baltimore, Maryland 21287

Basic Considerations 55
   Ordering Imaging Studies 56
Studies 56
   Computed Tomographic Scanning 56 · Magnetic Resonance Imaging (MRI) 57 · Magnetic Resonance Angiography 59 · Echography 59 Cerebral Angiography 60 · Plain Radiographs 60 · Dacryocystography 61
Specific Diagnoses and Relevant Radiologic Findings 62
   Aneurysm 62 · Choroidal Detachment 62 · Endophthalmitis 63 · Foreign Bodies 65 · Infectious and Noninfectious Inflammatory Disorders: Wegener's Granulomatosis, Tuberculosis, Sarcoidosis, Pseudotumor, and Mucormycosis 66 · Orbital Fractures 68 · Orbital Cellulitis 68 · Orbital Hemorrhage or Hematoma 69 · Optic Neuritis 69 · Retinal Detachment 69 Open Globe 70 · Subperiosteal Abscess 71 · Subperiosteal Hematoma 71 Thyroid Orbitopathy 74 · Traumatic Optic Neuropathy and Canal Fracture 74 Traumatic Carotid-Cavernous Fistula 74 · Vitreous Hemorrhage 74

BASIC CONSIDERATIONS

The main imaging techniques used in ophthalmology today are computed tomographic (CT) scanning, magnetic resonance imaging (MRI), and ultrasonography. Although the information provided by the two-dimensional images of MRI and CT scans can be appreciated by nonradiologists, the images obtained from these studies should always be interpreted in consultation with a radiologist. Echography provides one- or two-dimensional images displayed in real time on an oscilloscope screen. Interpretation requires consideration of eye position, probe position, and knowledge of the echogenic characteristics of ocular and related structures (1–3). Conventional radiography has almost been completely replaced by CT scan; however, conventional x-rays are still appropriate in certain clinical settings (4). The interpretation of conventional x-rays requires knowledge of each particular projection used (5).

Ordering Imaging Studies

Imaging studies should be ordered only after a complete history has been taken and a thorough examination has been performed. The differential diagnosis will then determine which study to order, whether intravenous injection of contrast material needs to be given, and whether special sections are necessary. Consultation with other services such as otolaryngology, neurosurgery, or plastic surgery may be needed before ordering a study to be certain that the correct study is obtained and performed in an appropriate manner.

This chapter is organized in two main sections. The first section considers the following modalities individually: CT, MRI, ultrasound, dacryocystography, arteriography, and plain radiography. The second section reviews characteristic radiologic and echographic findings for several specific ocular emergencies.

STUDIES

Computed Tomographic Scanning

In the setting of acute ocular trauma, CT scanning is the imaging study of choice. It is available in most emergency facilities and provides simultaneous assessment of facial, sinus, orbital, ocular, and cranial bony and soft tissue structures with minimal disturbance to the patient. Aside from availability, CT scanning has several advantages over MRI in this setting. First, CT scanning can be performed in patients with known or presumed iron-containing foreign bodies and in patients with pacemakers or on external life support. Second, CT scanning is less likely to produce claustrophobia. Finally, CT scanning produces less motion artifact, is quicker, and is less expensive than MRI. An advantage that CT scanning has over ultrasonography is that it requires no contact with the eyelids or globe.

There are many clinical indications for orbital CT scanning in patients with acute blunt or sharp trauma. The most common settings in which a CT scan should be obtained emergently are hemorrhagic chemosis, suspected foreign body, suspected rupture, and suspected orbital fracture with or without motility disturbance. Because fresh blood can be recognized on a noncontrast-enhanced CT, CT is also the preferred means of initial evaluation of suspected intracranial or orbital hemorrhage (6).

An optimum ocular/orbital CT study can be obtained with 1.5- to 2.0-mm thick axial sections and 2.0- to 4.0-mm thick coronal sections of the orbit. The radiologist can generally choose the appropriate study parameters once he or she is made aware of the clinical setting and the information required of the scan. Axial sections provide the most information regarding the structural integrity of the eye. This is largely because a single section in the appropriate plane can image the cornea, sclera, anterior chamber, lens, vitreous cavity, and optic nerve. However, coronal sections are essential when evaluating the extraocular muscles and the walls of the orbit and for localizing foreign bodies. If there is doubt regarding their usefulness, include them on the study requisition form. Occasionally, the information required of a CT scan will be accessible with only coronal views. For example, direct coronal images are generally better than axial scans in assessing the inferior and superior rectus muscles, orbital roof and floor, intracranial optic nerves, optic chiasm, and various sellar and parasellar structures (7).

In order to obtain coronal CT scans, the radiologist must place the patient in the prone position with the head resting on the chin, or in a supine position with the head extended back on its vertex. Such positioning may be impossible in uncooperative or combative patients, young children, unconscious patients, elderly patients, or for other reasons related to the injury itself. In these cases, coronal reconstructions may be necessary. This technique provides reasonable anatomic information if very thin (1.5 to 2.0 mm) axial scans are taken; however, it is our opinion that the best reconstructed images are still suboptimal compared with direct coronal scans and should not be used unless direct coronal images cannot be obtained.

A technique called spiral CT scanning is performed with the patient moving through the CT scanner while the x-ray source and detector rotate rapidly and continuously. The data acquired with this type of scanner are achieved with shorter scan times and less radiation exposure, and they may provide higher quality coronal reconstructions (8). Using a special monitor and computer software package, CT scans obtained with this technique also can be viewed three-dimensionally.

Contrast enhancement of CT images using intravenously injected iodine-containing compounds is generally not needed when evaluating a patient in the setting of ocular trauma. However, contrast is essential when evaluating a patient with a suspected cerebral aneurysm, orbital varix, arteriovenous malformation (e.g., carotid-cavernous fistula), optic neuritis, or other lesions suspected of being highly vascular or inflammatory.

Magnetic Resonance Imaging (MRI)

The role of MRI in acute ocular trauma is still being defined. The main factors that currently limit practical application of this technique are availability and scan time (motion artifact). In addition, specific contraindications for the use of MRI in patients with ocular trauma include iron-containing intraocular or orbital foreign bodies, severe claustrophobia, cochlear implants, intracranial magnetic vascular clips, and cardiac pacemakers.

Conditions where MRI is the preferred modality include vascular lesions, intracranial conditions, intraocular tumors, cavernous sinus thrombosis, and lesions of the optic nerve, including inflammatory and demyelinating conditions (9–13). MRI has the distinct advantage over CT scanning of being able to provide sagittal, coronal, axial, and oblique sections without repositioning the patient. MRI is also superior to CT in its image quality of most soft tissues. Although MRI is at a disadvantage compared with CT when assessing bone for fracture, when the soft tissue of interest is surrounded by bone, such as in the posterior fossa or the pituitary region, MRI actually provides better images than does CT.

MR image quality is dependent on intrinsic properties and extrinsic parameters. The intrinsic properties are determined by nuclear and chemical composition of the tissue of interest. For example, bone, vitreous, fat, blood, brain, and muscle all have specific nuclear and chemical properties that largely determine the magnetic resonance of each tissue. The extrinsic parameters can be set by the machine operator to provide three types of pulse sequences: T1, T2, and proton density-weighted images. These sequences are defined by specific parameters of pulse repetition and signal acquisition times. Various artifacts can lead to image degradation (motion artifact is probably the most frequently encountered). In general, the details of normal anatomy are best appreciated on T1-weighted images. These sequences provide the most contrast between fat, vitreous, and extraocular muscles. Fat is bright, vitreous is dark, and muscle is an intermediate intensity on T1-weighted images. Pathology is generally best outlined by T2 or proton density-weighted images. T2-weighted images have a lower signal-to-noise ratio and require a longer acquisition time than do T1-weighted images. The latter feature makes T2 images more prone to motion artifact. In T2-weighted images, fat is dark, vitreous is bright, and extraocular muscles display an intermediate density. Proton density-weighted pulse sequences provide the highest signal-to-noise ratio but require the longest acquisition time. This feature makes proton density-weighted images most prone to image degradation secondary to motion artifact. The contrast between different tissues obtained with proton density imaging tends to be lower than with the T1- or T2-weighted images because the proton density of different tissues only varies by about 20% (14). A good MRI study usually consists of T1- and T2-weighted images.

Image resolution is determined in part by the number of pixels of information per volume imaged and by the amount of noise that coexists with a given level of signal (i.e., signal-to-noise ratio). For examination of small ocular or anterior orbital lesions, it may be desirable to improve on the spatial resolution and reduce the signal to noise ratio of the MRI. This can be accomplished in practice by using a surface coil. The closer proximity of the coil to the area of interest improves the signal-to-noise ratio and increases the number of pixels per unit volume imaged (15,16). The use of head or ocular surface coils has made it possible to obtain thinner sections and improve image resolution. However, the advantages of surface coils may not always be realized because surface coils also increase the susceptibility to motion artifact originating from globe or head motion with subsequent degradation of images.

Image enhancement during MRI is possible with intravenous administration of paramagnetic contrast material such as gadolinium-DPTA. This is often combined with fat suppression techniques to allow enhancing lesions in the orbit to be distinguished from orbital fat with its characteristically intense signal. This technique is especially useful when evaluating lesions of the intraorbital optic nerve (10).

Magnetic Resonance Angiography

Conventional arteriography is the study of choice for detecting of intracranial vascular lesions such as aneurysms and arteriovenous malformations; however, it is an invasive procedure with a definite morbidity and mortality that depends in part on the age and health of the patient. Magnetic resonance angiography (MRA), on the other hand, is a noninvasive and safe method of evaluating such lesions and can be performed at the same time as standard MRI (17). Normally, vessels with flowing blood image as voids in the MRI scan. MRA uses a set of pulse sequences that allow flowing blood to be differentiated from stationary soft tissues. Unfortunately, MRA is prone to a variety of artifacts that complicate interpretation and limit resolution of images created by nonvascular structures and by pulsatile flow of cerebrospinal fluid. In addition, for reasons related to geometry or decreased flow velocity, flowing blood may not always create a signal on MRA. This form of imaging will no doubt continue to evolve, and as it does, the use of MRA in the evaluation of aneurysms and other vascular lesions will continue to be refined. In the meantime, conventional arteriography remains the study of choice in the evaluation of known or presumed intracranial or intraorbital vascular lesions.

Echography

Echography provides excellent images of the eye and in the hands of an experienced echographer can provide reliable and detailed information about the ocular and orbital structures. When ophthalmoscopic evaluation is limited or not possible, echography is useful in determining the density of vitreous opacities and hemorrhage, and the extent of retinal or choroidal detachments (1,2,18). Additionally, ultrasound is reliable in localizing choroidal and scleral rupture sites as well as radio-opaque and radiolucent intraocular and orbital foreign bodies (19,20). Orbital structures, including the lacrimal gland, extraocular muscles, optic nerve, orbital soft tissue, and bony structures, can be visualized using this modality (3,21).

Ophthalmic ultrasound has several practical advantages compared with CT and MRI. Because of the relatively high frequency of the sound waves (10 MHz), the resolution is 0.1 to 0.01 mm. In addition, ultrasound uses real-time imaging, which aids in the detection of motion and blood flow. Finally, the equipment needed to perform echography is easily transportable to a patient's bedside or to an operating room when necessary, making it one of the most efficient and rapid means of diagnostic imaging in many different settings. Unfortunately, ultrasonography requires direct contact with the eyelids, globe, or both, and it therefore may not be appropriate for initial evaluation in situations that could lead to extrusion of intraocular contents. Thus, a ruptured globe may be a relative contraindication to ultrasound examination, depending on the severity of the injury and the experience of the ultrasonographer.

The most common and useful mode of operation in ophthalmic echography is B-scan (brightness modulation), which provides two-dimensional images of the eye and orbit. This type of scanning details the topography (shape, location, and extension) of intraocular and orbital structures. Cross-sections and radial sections of the eye and orbit can be obtained by changing the orientation of the ultrasound probe, thus providing the maximum amount of information about intraocular and orbital pathology.

Standardized A-scan (amplitude modulation) displays a series of spikes along a baseline. The height of the spikes obtained using this mode correlates with the density of the structure displayed, whereas the distance between spikes corresponds to the distance between structures. This modality makes it possible to differentiate one pathologic process from another. For example, a series of spikes that are of low amplitude relative to the tallest initial spike of the A-scan indicates that the structure being examined has low reflectivity (e.g., myositis), whereas a series of spikes that are nearly the same height as the initial spike on the A-scan indicate that the structure has high reflectivity (e.g., muscle swelling associated with thyroid orbitopathy).

A form of echography called color flow Doppler imaging permits evaluation of blood flow of the eye and orbit (22). Using this technique, B-scan images are color coded, depending on the direction and velocity of blood flow. Clinical applications of this technique include evaluation of ocular arterial and venous occlusion, and various lesions that can develop after trauma, such as traumatic carotid-cavernous sinus fistulas.

Cerebral Angiography

Cerebral angiography (arteriography) is usually necessary to complete the workup of vascular lesions of the orbit, intracranial aneurysms, carotid-cavernous fistulas, and other vascular malformations. For example, in the case of an aneurysm, arteriography usually is required before surgery to demonstrate the neck of the aneurysm, its precise location, and any additional aneurysms. Because angiography tends to underestimate the true size of a partially thrombosed aneurysm, however, it may be appropriate to perform CT or MRI scanning before surgery in certain cases (23). Such decisions should be left to the neuroradiologist and the neurosurgeon.

Plain Radiographs

The role of conventional plain radiographs in the evaluation of patients with eye trauma has been diminished considerably by the development of CT scanning and MRI. However, if CT or MRI is not immediately available, plain x-rays may be helpful in screening for radio-opaque foreign bodies, orbital fractures, and sinus disease. For example, if a patient presents with a history of being injured by a metal projectile (BB or pellet), a plain film is an excellent way to screen for the presence of an intraorbital foreign body (4). In such cases, posterior-anterior and lateral films may be the only diagnostic studies that are required. Also of particular value during the evaluation of an eye for a subtle intraocular foreign body is the use of dental x-ray film against the medial canthus to obtain a bone-free image across the globe.

Evaluation of the orbit for fractures using conventional radiographic techniques usually requires five main projections: the Caldwell projection, the Waters projection, the submental vertex (or basal) projection, and the right and left oblique projections.

The Caldwell projection is obtained by tilting the beam toward the feet so that it makes about a 25-degree angle with the canthal–meatal line (a line drawn between the lateral canthus and the meatus that is extended anteriorly and posteriorly). The Caldwell projection provides a good view of the superior and lateral orbital rims, the medial wall of the orbit, and the ethmoid and frontal sinuses.

The Waters projection is obtained by positioning the central beam at right angles to the film and extending the neck until the canthal–meatal line makes about a 37-degree angle with the central beam. This projection provides the best view of the orbital floor and roof. It is the most useful view for evaluating blowout fractures.

The submental vertex or basal projection is obtained by hyperextending the neck so that the canthal–meatal line is parallel to the film surface. The central beam is then oriented at a right angle to the film. This projection provides a good view of the sphenoid and ethmoid sinuses, the nasopharynx, the nasal cavities, and the zygomatic arch.

The right and left oblique views are obtained by positioning the patient so that the canthal–meatal line is at a right angle to the film. The central beam is then angled about 32 degrees toward the feet and about 37 degrees to the right or left of the mid-sagittal plane. These projections provide images of the optic foramina. For patients over 6 years of age, a diameter greater than 6.5 mm and an asymmetry greater than 1 mm are considered abnormal.

Dacryocystography

Dacryocystography is usually performed by obtaining plain x-rays of the orbital region after cannulation and injection of contrast material into the lacrimal drainage apparatus. Computerized digital subtraction techniques can then be used to eliminate bone shadows (24). Abnormal findings associated with trauma include canalicular obstruction (upper, lower, and common limbs), nasolacrimal obstruction, and abnormal sac silhouette. This technique is rarely used in the setting of trauma. A variation of conventional dacryocystography can be performed using CT scanning after topical administration of iodinated-contrast material (25).

SPECIFIC DIAGNOSES AND RELEVANT RADIOLOGIC FINDINGS

This section provides examples of several specific conditions that may be encountered in the emergency room setting and the characteristic findings of the appropriate diagnostic imaging techniques. The topics discussed here are not meant to be all inclusive or comprehensive. The reader is referred to the pertinent chapters of this book for more detailed information on a given subject.

Aneurysm

Conventional arteriography is the most sensitive method for diagnosing an aneurysm. However, CT scanning and MRI provide a more accurate assessment of the size of an aneurysm when a thrombus is present within the lumen (23).

Arteriography: Findings include saccular out-pouching or fusiform dilation of a vessel wall.

CT: Findings include a homogeneous enhancing mass, laminated clots, and calcification of aneurysm wall.

MRI: Hypointensity (signal void) represents blood flow. Areas of thrombus, calcification, and surrounding tissue appear as a heterogeneous region with areas of hyper-, hypo-, and isointensity.

Choroidal Detachment

Ultrasound is the preferred modality of imaging choroidal detachments for initial evaluation and follow-up examination. However, choroidal detachments also may be detected by CT scan during a workup in cases of blunt or penetrating injury to the eye. If hemorrhage and blood clot formation occur in the suprachoroidal space, serial ultrasound examinations are useful to monitor the clot for dissolution before a drainage procedure.

Ultrasound: On B-scan choroidal detachments appear as dome-shaped, often bullous lesions that do not extend to the optic disk. They may be localized or involve the entire fundus (Fig. 5–1). On A-scan the choroidal detachment produces a maximally high, thick, double-peaked spike separate from the fundus spikes. The height of the chain of spikes between the surface of the choroid and the sclera is the most reliable indication of the density of the hemorrhage and clot formation in the suprachoroidal space. A series of tall spikes represents a newly formed clot (Fig. 5–1). A series of low spikes is observed after lysis of the clot.

CT: Findings include crescentic, clover leaf, or ring-shaped hyperintensity in the vitreous cavity attached to the vortex veins, ciliary body, and short posterior ciliary arteries and nerves (Fig. 5–2). Underlying fluid may be serous or hemorrhagic, with images appearing isodense or hyperintense relative to vitreous, respectively (26).

MRI: The pattern of findings are similar to those described for CT. Acute hemorrhage appears hypointense on both T1- and T2-weighted images. As the age of the

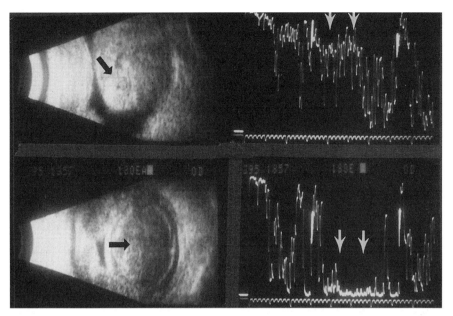

FIG. 5–1. Ultrasound of acute and chronic hemorrhagic choroidal detachments. Top (*left and right*): Acute hemorrhagic choroidal detachments. Note echodense nature of the clotted blood on B-scan (*black arrow*) and very high reflectivity on standardized A-scan (*white arrows*). Bottom: Same eye as above, 7 days later. Lysis of the clot leads to a decrease in the echo density of the choroidal detachment on both contact B-scan (*black arrow*) and standardized A-scan (*white arrows*).

hematoma increases, the signal becomes hyperintense, first on T1-weighted images (subacute), then later on both T1- and T2-weighted images (26).

Endophthalmitis

Patients present with a wide spectrum of ocular signs. The most useful role of echography is documentation of findings at the onset of symptoms and continued follow-up to assess improvement or worsening of the infection. If the fundus cannot be visualized, ultrasound is of critical importance to rule out choroidal detachments before performing a vitreous tap or injection of intravitreal antibiotics. CT scan is useful in situations where there is a history of trauma, suspected foreign body, or the cause of endophthalmitis is unknown.

Ultrasound: Findings include mild to dense vitreous opacities that appear as mobile echodense condensates (Fig. 5–3); membrane formation that, when located posteriorly, can be difficult to distinguish from a retinal detachment; retinal detachment; and choroidal detachment.

CT: Scleral/uveal thickening associated with a variable degree of increased density in the vitreous (Fig. 5–4). Periocular tissues also have variable increased density.

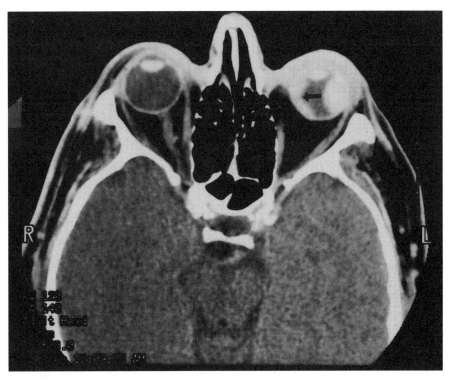

FIG. 5–2. Axial CT scan of acute hemorrhagic choroidal detachments in a patient with a corneal laceration. Note the hyperdense uveal contours that presumably attach to a vortex vein (*arrow*).

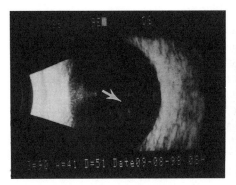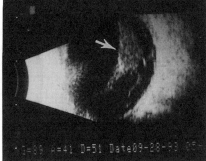

FIG. 5–3. B-scan ultrasound images of a patient presenting with endophthalmitis. Left: Initial presentation with vitreous opacities (*arrow*). Right: One week later with increased vitreous opacities and membrane formation (*arrow*).

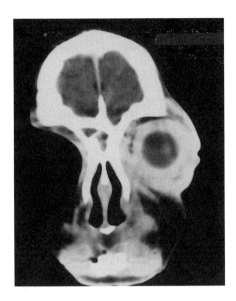

FIG. 5–4. Coronal CT scan of a patient presenting with endophthalmitis showing soft-tissue swelling around the globe and orbit. Vitreous condensates are evident as diffuse opacities in the vitreous of this eye with advanced endophthalmitis.

Foreign Bodies

CT scan is the most sensitive technique for identifying and localizing most metallic intraocular and orbital foreign bodies. Detection by CT depends on the size, composition, and number of foreign bodies (27–30). The lower limit of resolution of steel and copper are reported to be as small as 0.06 mm^3; aluminum is somewhat more difficult to detect and requires larger volumes (1.5 mm^3). The ability to detect glass is similar to that for aluminum. Because of its extremely low density, which is similar to fat and air, wood can be quite difficult to detect in the absence of a high index of suspicion from the history. MRI may be useful in identifying nonmagnetic foreign bodies (31–33). Ultrasound is a valuable adjunct to the detection and localization of both metallic and nonmetallic foreign bodies (19). The resolution depends on the echogenicity of the material; the lower limit of resolution is approximately 0.2 mm in diameter.

CT: Metal foreign bodies are hyperintense and may be associated with scatter artifact (Fig. 5–5). Wood is radiolucent and can be difficult to distinguish from air (Fig. 5–6). Other materials such as cement, glass, and plastic may appear hypo-, hyper-, or isodense relative to surrounding ocular structures.

Ultrasound: Foreign bodies in the globe or orbit generally produce an extremely bright signal on B-scan (Fig. 5–7) with an associated shadow or comet tail artifact depending on the composition of the foreign body (e.g., cement produces a shadow, round BB produces a comet tail). On standardized A-scan, foreign bodies produce a single extremely high spike.

When an object has perforated the globe both anteriorly and posteriorly, echographically a hemorrhagic track can be identified extending from the point of entry

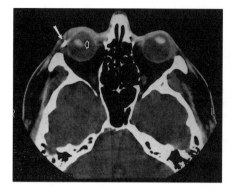

FIG. 5–5. Axial CT scan of a patient struck in the eye with a piece of metal. The hyperdense metallic foreign body adjacent to the globe (*arrow*) did not penetrate the eye, as indicated by the uniform corneoscleral contour. The lens is dislocated into the vitreous cavity (*open arrow*).

to the exit site. The fundus near the exit wound is usually markedly thickened, with elevation of the adjacent retina. There also may be blood and a hemorrhagic track through the orbital tissue.

Plain films: These studies are useful to screen for intraorbital or intraocular radiopaque densities (metal foreign bodies). Dental x-ray film positioned against the medial canthus to obtain a bone-free image across the globe is particularly sensitive for detecting a subtle intraocular foreign body.

Infectious and Noninfectious Inflammatory Disorders: Wegener's Granulomatosis, Tuberculosis, Sarcoidosis, Pseudotumor, and Mucormycosis

CT: Sarcoid and pseudotumor are characterized by thickening of the uveal scleral coat, perioptic soft-tissue densities, enlargement of the lacrimal gland, and dif-

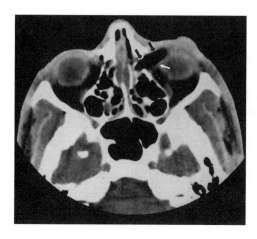

FIG. 5–6. Axial CT scan of a patient who fell on a stick. A radiolucent foreign body composed of wood presses against the globe inferonasally and penetrates the medial wall of the orbit (*arrows*).

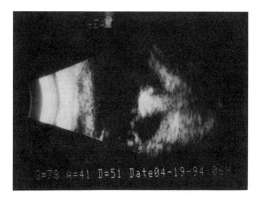

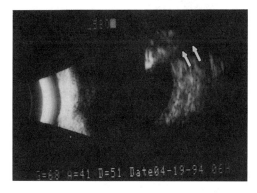

FIG. 5–7. B-scan ultrasound of a patient with a large metallic foreign body in the eye. Transverse (top) and longitudinal (bottom) sections demonstrate anterior location of the large echodense object in the vitreous cavity with echolucent shadow (*arrows*).

fuse enlargement of one or more extraocular muscles (13,34–36). Tuberculosis is characterized by nonspecific infiltrations with low-attenuation areas, bone destruction with sclerosis, sequestrum formation, and tuberculous formation (13). Wegener's granulomatosis is characterized by proptosis, a retro-orbital soft-tissue mass, destruction of the nasal septum, turbinates, and bone (37). A hypointense mass may be observed on T2-weighted MRI. Mucormycosis (or aspergillosis) is characterized by diffuse poorly defined mucosal thickening, sclerosis and/or bone destruction of the sinuses, speckled radiodensities within opacified sinuses, isodense orbital infiltrations of variable size, lateral displacement of the medial rectus, increased density of the orbital apex, and axial globe displacement (35,38).

Ultrasound: Normal orbital tissue is composed of connective tissue and large cells producing high reflectivity echographically. Inflammatory lesions are generally low reflective by ultrasound and therefore easily defined. Inflammatory pseudotumor can be localized or diffuse and can involve single or multiple orbital structures. In the case of myositis, the affected muscle or muscles are generally markedly enlarged from the inserting tendons to the muscle bellies and have extremely low reflectivity (1,34).

Orbital Fractures

CT scan is the study of choice; floor and medial wall fractures are the most common sites.

CT (axial and coronals): Disruption of the bony orbit; orbital contents may herniate into the adjacent sinuses (e.g., maxillary or ethmoid; Fig. 5–8); air fluid levels or complete opacification of adjacent sinuses may suggest an occult floor fracture in the axial section.

Follow the course of muscle in nondisplaced fractures to rule out entrapment where a portion of the muscle is visible on the sinus side of the orbital wall. Clinical correlation is imperative. Coronal studies are imperative (Fig. 5–8).

Ultrasound: Findings include orbital emphysema (nearly complete attenuation of sound waves beyond the air pocket), discontinuity of orbital walls (bone is very bright), and soft tissue prolapse (21).

Orbital Cellulitis

CT (include sinus cuts): Findings include increased density and thickening of the eyelids, proptosis, intraconal mottled infiltrations of orbital fat, increased vascular markings, and associated sinus disease, especially ethmoiditis. The presence

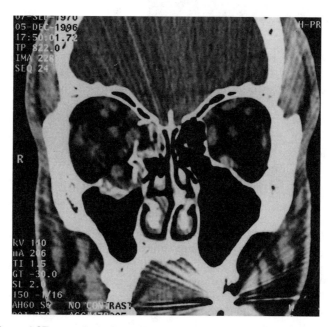

FIG. 5–8. Coronal CT scan of a patient with right orbital floor and medial wall fractures. There is prolapse of the medial and inferior rectus muscles into the fractures.

of a subperiosteal infiltrate is indicated by displacement of the periorbita into the orbital cavity with enlargement and inward displacement of the medial or superior rectus muscles (35,39).

Ultrasound: Usually diffuse swelling of the orbital structures is noted; reflectivity of most structures is usually unaltered. However, areas of low reflectivity may indicate abscess (34).

Orbital Hemorrhage or Hematoma

CT (axial and coronals): Findings include proptosis, stretching of the optic nerve, and diffuse densities within orbital fat early in evolution. After the formation of a clot, a discreet hyperintense mass in the orbit may be observed (36). As the age of the hemorrhage increases beyond 2 to 3 days, the mass becomes isodense compared with surrounding soft tissue.

Ultrasound: Hematomas are characterized by low reflective lesions within the orbital soft tissue (Fig. 5–9). It may be impossible to distinguish from abscess initially. Hemorrhage may be distinguished from abscess on follow-up examinations because the hemorrhage may show a shift to higher reflectivity and decrease in size.

MRI: Extremely fresh hemorrhage is not well seen on MRI. Old blood may image brightly on both T1- and T2-weighted images (36,40).

Optic Neuritis

MRI: Hyperintense tissue changes in white matter of brain or along optic nerve; occasional diffuse enlargement of intraorbital nerve; lesions enhance after intravenous injection of paramagnetic contrast material (10).

CT: Diffuse enlargement and slight nerve enhancement after intravenous injection of contrast material may be observed.

Retinal Detachment

Ultrasound: The detached retina appears as a dense, thick, often folded, slightly mobile continuous membrane that inserts into the optic disk. The retina can be detached in a localized area or totally detached, producing a funnel-shaped membrane (Fig. 5–10). On standardized A-scan retinal detachments almost always produce a maximally high spike separate from the fundus spikes.

CT or MRI: The retina is beyond the limits of resolution of these modalities; however, a retinal detachment may be detected if it separates two compartments of fluid with different densities. A retinal detachment may be observed as a V-shaped structure with the apex at the disk and its extremities toward the ciliary body; subretinal fluid may have the same signal intensity as vitreous fluid (serous detachment) or may be more dense as in the case of hemorrhagic or exudative detachments (26). The appearance of a retinal detachment may be difficult to distinguish from a choroidal detachment (see above).

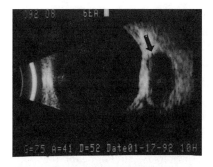

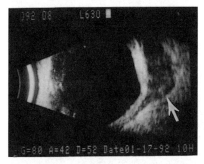

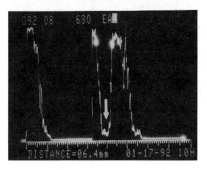

FIG. 5–9. B-scan ultrasound of a patient with orbital hemorrhage. Top: In cross section the hemorrhage appears as a discrete area of low reflectivity posterior to the globe (*arrow*). Center: Longitudinal section shows extent of hemorrhage from the anterior orbit (*arrow*). Bottom: Standardized A-scan showing typical low reflectivity of fresh orbital hemorrhage (*arrow*).

Open Globe

CT: Findings include axial length asymmetry greater than 1 mm, globe deformity (Fig. 5–11), intraocular air, intraocular foreign body, lens absence, and flat anterior chamber. Subtle globe deformities must be judged in the context of comparable views of the fellow eye.

Ultrasound: Findings include abnormal scleral contour or scleral folds (Fig. 5–12). The rupture or penetration site may be imaged directly as a discontinuity of the sclera, with a hemorrhagic tract in the vitreous leading up to the rupture site (Fig. 5–13).

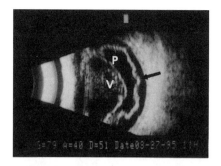

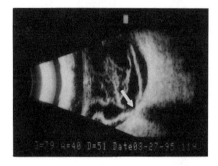

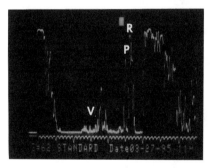

FIG. 5–10. B-scan ultrasound of a patient with a retinal detachment. Top: Transverse section showing dispersed vitreous hemorrhage (V), posterior vitreous detachment (P), and a dense thick folded retinal detachment (*arrow*). Center: Longitudinal section showing the attachment of the retina to the optic disk (*arrow*). Bottom: A-scan showing low chain of spikes representing the vitreous hemorrhage (V); the posterior vitreous detachment is represented by the medium to high spike (P); the retinal detachment is represented by a maximally high spike (R).

Subperiosteal Abscess

CT: Findings include a low-density mass along the orbital wall with or without involvement of underlying bone; gas may be present in the abscess. There also may be lateral displacement and thickening of adjacent muscle, most commonly the medial rectus (35,39). The rim of the abscess may enhance.

Subperiosteal Hematoma

CT: Findings include a hyperdense homogeneous mass with a broad base abutting bone. The lesion is generally sharply defined and nonenhancing. Fat is dis-

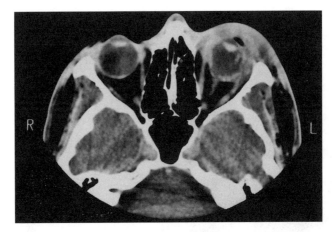

FIG. 5–11. Axial CT scan of a patient struck in the left eye with a bungi chord. The rupture site was not apparent on clinical examination. The CT scan shows disruption of the normal corneoscleral contour: soft-tissue swelling, orbital hemorrhage, and vitreous opacities (hemorrhage).

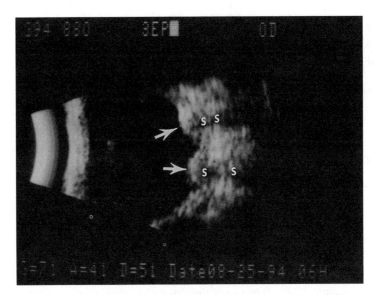

FIG. 5–12. B-scan ultrasound of a patient with a ruptured globe showing multiple folds of the posterior sclera (*arrows*). These folds can produce a shadow (S) and could be confused with an intraocular foreign body.

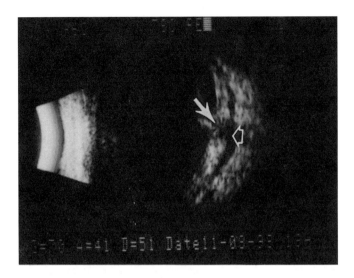

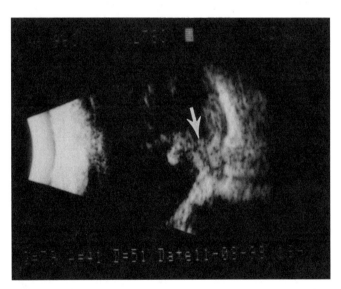

FIG. 5–13. B-scan ultrasound of a patient with a posterior rupture site. Top: A transverse section at decreased gain shows a large scleral rupture (*white arrow*) and blood in the orbit surrounding the globe (*open arrow*). Bottom: Longitudinal section at higher gain showing hemorrhagic track extending through the vitreous to the impact and rupture site (*white arrow*).

placed peripherally toward the center of the eye. Axial sections display lateral medial wall lesions. Coronal sections display roof and floor lesions.

MRI and ultrasound also may be useful in diagnosing a subperiosteal hematoma with similar spatial characteristics as noted for CT above. The imaging characteristics of a hematoma have been discussed above.

Thyroid Orbitopathy

Unlike myositis, where usually only one or two muscles of one orbit are involved, thyroid disease typically involves numerous muscles in both orbits.

CT and MRI: Spindle-shaped enlargement of muscle belly sparing tendons (typically inferior or medial recti but can affect any or all muscles), bunching of muscles in the apex, exophthalmos, compression of nerve, fatty expansion of orbital contents, and deviation of lamina papyracea (13).

Ultrasound: Echographically multiple muscles in both orbits are enlarged and highly reflective; the inserting tendons usually appear normal, unlike myositis (see above).

Traumatic Optic Neuropathy and Canal Fracture

CT: Findings may include nerve avulsion, bone chips contusing nerve, air in middle cranial fossa, swelling of the intraorbital portion of the nerve. Ipsilateral tripod fractures and multiple facial fractures are frequently associated with canal fractures (41).

Ultrasound: Disk elevation is usually present, and fluid or hemorrhage can be demonstrated within the nerve sheath. In optic nerve avulsion a collection of dense membranous opacities emanating from the region of the disk may be observed.

If the intracanalicular portion of the nerve itself is in question, MRI may be the best imaging study. CT images of intracanalicular nerve are susceptible to degradation of the image due to volume averaging from adjacent bone. MRI gives clear images of the intracanalicular portion of the optic nerve because the adjacent bone is not imaged.

Traumatic Carotid-Cavernous Fistula

Angiography: Findings include abnormal blood flow from the intracavernous portion of the internal carotid artery directly into the cavernous sinus, with drainage centrally into the superior and/or inferior ophthalmic veins, or posteriorly into the inferior petrosal sinus (42).

CT: Findings include an enlarged cavernous sinus, proptosis, or dilated superior ophthalmic vein (36).

MRI: Findings include an enlarged cavernous sinus and a dilated superior ophthalmic vein which appears as an image flow-void channel. Axial proptosis may be present.

Ultrasound: The superior ophthalmic vein can be massively dilated, and nonspecific congestive changes (a widened echographic pattern as compared with the unaffected orbit), enlarged muscles, and expansion of retrobulbar fat volume may be noted.

Vitreous Hemorrhage

Ultrasound: Acute dispersed hemorrhage may be minimally echogenic. In subacute and chronic hemorrhages the vitreous cavity may be filled with echoes (Fig.

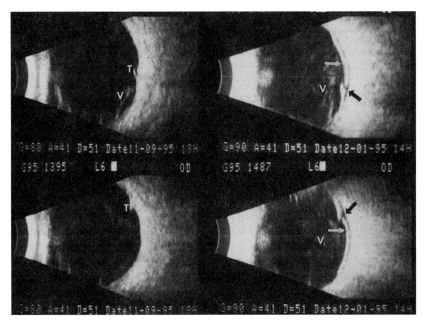

FIG. 5–14. Ultrasound of vitreous hemorrhage secondary to retinal tear. Top left: At initial presentation, echography showed mild vitreous hemorrhage (V) and cross-section of a focal horseshoe tear (T) located in the superotemporal quadrant of the eye. Bottom left: Longitudinal section of the retinal tear (T). The patient was followed for 3 weeks, and the hemorrhage worsened. Top right: Cross-section showing an increase in density of vitreous hemorrhage (V). The tear is even more apparent (*black arrow*). A shallow retinal detachment has developed (*white arrow*). Bottom right: Longitudinal section showing the same findings.

5–14). Associated findings may include retinal tear, retinal or choroidal detachments, foreign bodies, lens dislocation, scleral rupture, orbital hemorrhage, or fracture (see above).

CT: Findings depend on the age of the hemorrhage. Acutely, diffuse blood may appear as diffuse hyperdensities in the vitreous. Newly formed clots appear as discreet hyperdensities. As the blood clot age increases beyond 2 to 3 days, the CT image becomes isodense.

MRI: Acute hemorrhages are hypointense on both T1- and T2-weighted images. As the age of the blood increases, first the T1-weighted image becomes hyperintense followed in several days by a transition of the T2-weighted image from hypo- to hyperintense.

REFERENCES

1. Coleman DJ, Woods S, Rondeau MJ, Silverman RH. Ophthalmic ultrasonography. *Radiol Clin North Am* 1992;30:1105.
2. Kwong JS, Munk PL, Lin DTC, Vellet AD, Levin M, Buckley AR. Real-time sonography in ocular trauma. *Am J Radiol* 1992;158:179.

3. Ossoinig KC. Standardized echography. Basic principles, clinical applications, and results. *Int Ophthalmol Clin* 1979;19:127.
4. Otto PM, Otto RA, Virapougse C, et al. Screening test for detection of metallic foreign objects in the orbit before magnetic resonance imaging. *Invest Radiol* 1992;27:308.
5. Hanafee WN. Plain views of the orbit. *Radiol Clin North Am* 1972;10:167.
6. Rubenfeld M, Taylor S, Wirtschafter JD. Assessment of acute trauma. *Ophthalmol Clin North Am* 1984;7:277.
7. Koorneef L, Zonneveld FW. Role of direct multiplanar high resolution CT in the assessment and management of orbital trauma. *Radiol Clin North Am* 1987;25:753.
8. Heiken JP, Brink JA, Vannier MW. Spiral (helical) CT. *Radiology* 1993;189:647.
9. Bilaniuk LT, Atlas SW, Zimmerman RA. Magnetic resonance imaging of the orbit. *Radiol Clin North Am* 1987;25:509.
10. Miller DH, Newton MR, van der Poel JC, et al. Magnetic resonance imaging of the optic nerve in optic neuritis. *Neurology* 1988;38:175.
11. Rubenfeld M, Wirtschafter JD. The role of medical imaging in the practice of neuro-opthalmology. *Radiol Clin North Am* 1987;25:863.
12. Savino PJ, Grossman RI, Schatz NJ, Sergott RC, Bosley TM. Highfield magnetic resonance imaging in the diagnosis of cavernous sinus thrombosis. *Arch Neurol* 1986;43:1081.
13. Weber AL, Mikulis DK. Inflammatory disorders of the paraorbital sinuses and their complications. *Radiol Clin North Am* 1987;25:615.
14. Wehrli FW, Kanal E. Orbital imaging: factors determining magnetic resonance appearance. *Radiol Clin North Am* 1987;25:419.
15. Schenck JF, Hart HR Jr, Foster TH, Edelstein WA, et al. Improved MR imaging of the orbit at 1.5 T with surface coils. *Am J Neur Radiol* 1985;6:193.
16. Zimmerman RA, Bilaniuk LT, Yanoff M, et al. Orbital magnetic resonance imaging. *Am J Ophthalmol* 1985;100:312.
17. Pernicone JR, Thorp KE, Ouimette J, Siebert JE, Potchen EJ. Magnetic resonance angiography in intracranial vascular disease. *Semin Ultrasound CT MRI* 1992;13:256.
18. Jack RL, Coleman DJ. Diagnosis of retinal detachment with B-scan ultrasound. *Can J Ophthalmol* 1973;8:10.
19. Coleman DJ, Trokel SL. A protocol for B-scan and radiographic foreign body localization. *Am J Ophthalmol* 1971;71:84.
20. Rubsamen PE, Cousins SW, Winward KE, Byrne SF. Diagnostic ultrasound and pars plana vitrectomy in penetrating ocular trauma. *Ophthalmology* 1994;101:809.
21. Forrest CR, Lata AC, Marcuzzi DW, Bailey MH. The role of orbital ultrasound in the diagnosis of orbital fractures. *Plast Reconstr Surg* 1993;92:28.
22. Williamson TH, Harris A. Color Doppler ultrasound imaging of the eye and orbit. *Surv Ophthalmol* 1996;40:255.
23. Taveras JM, Wood EH. *Diagnostic Neuroradiology.* Vol. 2. 2nd ed. Baltimore: Williams & Wilkins; 1976.
24. Galloway JE, Kavic TA, Raflo GT. Digital subtraction macrodacryocystography. *Ophthalmology* 1984;91:956.
25. Zinreich SJ, Miller NR, Freeman LN, Glorioso LW, Rosenbaum AE. Computed tomographic dacryocystography using topical contrast media for lacrimal system visualization. *Orbit* 1990;9: 79.
26. Mafee MF, Peyman GA. Retinal and choroidal detachments: role of magnetic resonance imaging and computed tomography. *Radiol Clin North Am* 1987;25:487.
27. Kadir S, Aronow S, Davis KR. The use of computerized tomography in the detection of intra-orbital foreign bodies. *Comput Tomogr* 1977;1:151.
28. Lindahl S. Computed tomography of intraorbital foreign bodies. *Acta Radiol* 1987;28:235.
29. Tate E, Cupples H. Detection of orbital foreign bodies with computed tomography: current limits. *Am J Radiol* 1981;137:493.
30. Topilow HW, Ackerman AL, Zimmerman RD. Limitations of computerized tomography in the localization of intraocular foreign bodies. *Ophthalmology* 1984;91:1086.
31. Green BF, Kraft SP, Carter KD, Buncic JR, Nerad JA, Armstrong D. Intraorbital wood: detection by magnetic resonance imaging. *Ophthalmology* 1990;97:608.
32. Lagouros PA, Langer BG, Peyman GA, Mafee MF, Spigos DG, Grisolano J. Magnetic resonance imaging and intraocular foreign bodies. *Arch Ophthalmol* 1987;105:551.

33. LoBue TD, Deutsch TA, Lobick J, Turner DA. Detection and localization of nonmetallic intraocular foreign bodies by magnetic resonance imaging. *Arch Ophthalmol* 1988;106:206.
34. Harr DL, Quencer RM, Abrams GW. Computed tomography and ultrasound in the evaluation of orbital infection and pseudotumor. *Radiology* 1982;142:395.
35. Osguthorpe JD, Hochman M. Inflammatory sinus diseases affecting the orbit. *Otolaryngol Clin North Am* 1993;26:127.
36. Armington WG, Bilaniuk LT. The radiologic evaluation of the orbit conal and intraconal lesions. *Semin Ultrasound CT MR* 1988;9:455.
37. Haynes BF, Fishman ML, Fauci AS, Wolff SM. The ocular manifestations of Wegener's granulomatosis: fifteen years experience and review of the literature. *Am J Med* 1977;63:131.
38. Centeno RS, Bentson JR, Mancuso AA. CT scanning in rhinocerebral mucormycosis and aspergillosis. *Radiology* 1981;140:383.
39. Zimmerman RA, Bilaniuk LT. CT of orbital infection and its cerebral complications. *Am J Radiol* 1980;134:45.
40. Gomori JM, Grossman RI, Goldberg HI, Zimmerman RA, Bilaniuk LT. Intracranial hematomas: imaging by high-field MR. *Radiology* 1985;157:87.
41. Guyon JJ, Brant-Zawadski M, Seff SR. CT demonstration of optic canal fractures. *Am J Neuroradiol* 1984;5:575.
42. Miller NR. *Walsh and Hoyt's Clinical Neuro-Ophthalmology.* Vol. 4. 4th ed. Baltimore: Williams & Wilkins;1991.

Management of Ocular Injuries and Emergencies,
edited by Mathew W. MacCumber.
Lippincott–Raven Publishers, Philadelphia ©1998.

6

Timing Guidelines for Emergent Surgery

Sharon Fekrat and Eugene de Juan, Jr.

*Department of Ophthalmology, Wilmer Eye Institute, The Johns Hopkins University
School of Medicine, Baltimore, Maryland 21287*

Basic Considerations 79
Overview 80
  Immediate Surgical Intervention 80 · Urgent Surgical Intervention (within
  next 24 hours) 80 · Semielective Surgical Intervention (within 72 hours) 81
  Elective Surgical Intervention (nonemergent) 81
Corneal Laceration 81
Corneoscleral Laceration 81
Endophthalmitis (of any cause) 82
Giant Cell Arteritis (Temporal Arteritis) 83
Infectious Keratitis with Corneal Perforation 83
Intraocular Foreign Body 83
Lid Laceration(s) 84
Nonarteritic Anterior Ischemic Optic Neuropathy 85
Orbital Bone Fracture with and without Muscle Entrapment 85
Orbital Bone Fracture with Optic Nerve Compression 85
Orbital Cellulitis Secondary to Sinusitis 85
Orbital Foreign Body 86
Perforating Injury 86
Posterior Penetrating Injury 87
Retinal Detachment 87
Traumatic Retrobulbar Hemorrhage 87
Sickle Cell Hyphema and Elevated Intraocular Pressure 88

BASIC CONSIDERATIONS

How soon should a surgical procedure be performed for an ocular emergency requiring surgical intervention when the patient presents to the ophthalmologist in
the evening or late at night? This is an important issue confronting the ophthalmologic community in the face of health-care reform and increasing financial limitations. We offer some guidelines.

TABLE 6–1. *Ophthalmologic emergencies requiring an operative procedure*

Corneal laceration
Corneoscleral laceration
Endophthalmitis (of any cause)
Giant cell arteritis (temporal arteritis)
Infectious keratitis with corneal perforation
Intraocular foreign body
Lid laceration(s)
Nonarteritic anterior ischemic optic neuropathy
Orbital bone fracture with and without muscle entrapment
Orbital bone fracture with optic nerve compression
Orbital cellulitis secondary to sinusitis
Orbital foreign body
Perforating injury
Posterior penetrating injury
Retinal detachment
Traumatic retrobulbar hemorrhage
Sickle cell hyphema and elevated intraocular pressure

Despite the information in this section, the treating physician must remember that each clinical scenario encountered should be approached on an individual case-by-case basis and that none of the guidelines in this chapter should be followed strictly. There are exceptions in every clinical scenario, and the final decision concerning surgical intervention should remain with the attending physician.

In some challenging surgical cases, it may be beneficial to the patient to perform the surgical repair at a time when the surgeon, anesthesiologist, and nursing staff are alert and when experienced operating room personnel and all necessary equipment are at one's disposal.

Please refer to the appropriate chapters in this text for details regarding the suggested medical and surgical management of each of these emergency situations (Table 6–1).

OVERVIEW

Immediate Surgical Intervention

- Endophthalmitis of any cause
- Intraocular foreign body (IOFB) (recent, first 24 hours) or with high risk of endophthalmitis
- Orbital cellulitis secondary to sinus disease
- Orbital bone fracture with optic nerve compression
- Traumatic retrobulbar hemorrhage, if canthotomy and cantholysis ineffective
- Orbital bone fracture with muscle entrapment

Urgent Surgical Intervention (within next 24 hours)

- Open globe injury without IOFB
- Lid laceration(s)

- IOFB (remote, second 24 hours) or with low risk of endophthalmitis
- Sickle cell hyphema with elevated intraocular pressure meeting specific criteria
- Macula-on retinal detachment extending into the temporal vascular arcades, particulary when a superior detachment

Semielective Surgical Intervention (within 72 hours)

- Macula on retinal detachment peripheral to temporal vascular arcades
- Macula off retinal detachment with duration of less than 5 to 7 days
- Selected orbital foreign bodies

Elective Surgical Intervention (nonemergent)

- Macula off retinal detachment with duration longer than 5 to 7 days
- Orbital bone fracture without muscle entrapment
- Nonarteritic anterior ischemic optic neuropathy
- Giant cell arteritis (temporal arteritis)

CORNEAL LACERATION

Surgical repair may be postponed until the following day (up to an 18-hour delay after presentation) in those traumatized eyes with a simple corneal laceration, while initiating intravenous antibiotics in the interim, unless there is an IOFB present (recent, less than 24 hours), evidence of endophthalmitis, or a high risk of developing endophthalmitis. If the latter situations exist, intravenous antibiotics should be started and surgical intervention should be immediate.

CORNEOSCLERAL LACERATION

1. Surgical intervention may be postponed until the following day (up to an 18-hour delay after presentation) in traumatized eyes with a simple corneoscleral laceration while initiating intravenous antibiotics in the interim, unless there is an IOFB (recent, less than 24 hours), evidence of endophthalmitis, or a high risk of developing endophthalmitis. If the latter situations exist, intravenous antibiotics should be begun and surgical intervention should be immediate.
2. Barr retrospectively studied 106 patients with corneoscleral lacerations and found no statistically significant difference between the length of time from the injury to surgical repair and the final visual acuity (1). The final visual acuity was not affected by delaying the surgery for ≥36 hours after the injury in the study. There was no statistically significant correlation between the time from injury to repair and the length of the laceration, amount of hyphema, fundus visibility, presence of uveal prolapse, or the likelihood of enucleation within 10 days of the injury. Variation in anterior chamber depth was not examined. No cases of sympathetic ophthalmia were observed in an average follow-up of 18 months. Of the four eyes (3%) that developed endophthalmitis, two were re-

paired within 24 hours of injury, and the remaining two were repaired 48 to 52 hours after the injury. This was not a randomized prospective study, however.

3. Few data are available regarding the risk of developing endophthalmitis if the primary repair is delayed. This is difficult to study in a controlled fashion because it may seem intuitive that delayed intervention in an open globe may be associated with an increased risk of endophthalmitis. Thompson and co-workers (2) demonstrated a small trend toward a higher incidence of infection with delayed surgical repair compared with earlier repair (6.5% versus 2.3%, p < 0.1) in a retrospective review of 259 patients. The timing of "early" surgical repair was not specified in this study. There was no difference in the development of infection when patients with an open globe from penetrating trauma received intravenous antibiotics early (within 12 hours after injury) when compared with those that received delayed administration (more than 12 hours after injury) (5.6% versus 3.6%). Whether the patients receiving intravenous antibiotics underwent primary repair early or late, however, was also not evaluated in this study. The investigators did not mention whether prophylactic intravitreal antibiotics were administered. The injection of prophylactic intraocular antibiotics at the time of primary repair of a penetrating injury to prevent endophthalmitis is controversial.

ENDOPHTHALMITIS (of Any Cause)

1. Previous experimental and clinical studies have recognized the importance of timing of therapeutic intervention in endophthalmitis (3–12). The Endophthalmitis-Vitrectomy Study (EVS) evaluated eyes with endophthalmitis after cataract extraction with intraocular lens implantation or after secondary intraocular lens implantation, a visual acuity of less than 20/50, and a hypopyon or clouding of media to obscure second-order retinal vessels (13). In this study, 420 eyes were randomized to either immediate pars plana vitrectomy (PPV), immediate PPV and intravenous antibiotics, immediate needle aspiration or single-port vitrectomy removing no more than 0.3 cm³ (vitreous tap) and intravenous antibiotics, or vitreous tap alone. All patients received topical, oral, and subconjunctival steroids and intravitreal, subconjunctival, and topical antibiotics.

Intravenous antibiotics were found to be of no benefit in any subgroup in this study population. PPV was not superior to a vitreous tap if the visual acuity was better than light perception. If the visual acuity was light perception, then PPV demonstrated a significant benefit over a vitreous tap.

Perhaps these results also may apply to those eyes with endogenous or traumatic endophthalmitis, although only postsurgical endophthalmitis cases were evaluated in the EVS.

2. Based primarily on EVS results, a vitreous tap with the injection of intravitreal antibiotics (vancomycin and ceftazidime) should be performed immediately in all closed globes with vision better than light perception. All closed globes with

vision of light perception should undergo immediate PPV and intravitreal antibiotic injection.

3. If the globe is open and there is evidence of endophthalmitis, the presenting visual acuity may actually have been better than light perception if it were not for the presence of a ruptured globe. Thus, the EVS data regarding visual acuity upon presentation cannot be used for therapeutic decision making in these cases. All of these patients should be taken immediately to the operating room for primary closure of the globe, aqueous and vitreous cultures, injection of intravitreal antibiotics (i.e., vancomycin and ceftazidime), and consideration of PPV. Intravenous antibiotics are also suggested.

GIANT CELL ARTERITIS (TEMPORAL ARTERITIS)

1. In a patient in whom giant cell arteritis is the most likely diagnosis, a temporal artery biopsy may be postponed until the following day(s), even when acute visual loss is the presenting symptom.
2. In the interim, intravenous corticosteroids (or oral prednisone depending on the clinical scenario) must be started acutely (see Chapter 24). The biopsy may be performed at any time within the following 8 days without significant alteration of the histopathologic findings (14,15). Even if corticosteroids have been administered for more than 8 days, the clinical usefulness of a temporal artery biopsy is not to be overlooked.

INFECTIOUS KERATITIS WITH CORNEAL PERFORATION

1. This clinical scenario should be approached as an open globe with endophthalmitis.
2. Because the globe is open and there is an obvious source of endophthalmitis, intravenous antibiotics should be started and surgery performed to repair the globe, to obtain appropriate cultures, and to administer intraocular antibiotics as soon as possible. Intraocular antibiotic injection may need to be repeated during follow-up.

INTRAOCULAR FOREIGN BODY

1. There is no study available to date that demonstrates that removal of an IOFB with injection of intravitreal antibiotics should be performed within a certain period after the traumatic event.
2. Because 8% to 13% of eyes with any retained IOFB develop endophthalmitis with 66% of these losing light perception (16) and because up to 26% of eyes with a retained IOFB contaminated with organic matter from a rural setting develop endophthalmitis (17), we support the early use of prophylactic antibiotics (subconjunctival, topical, intravenous, and intravitreal) (18) in eyes with IOFB, preferably within 12 hours after trauma (16). The potential for intraocular an-

tibiotic toxicity (19) after intravitreal antibiotic administration must always be weighed against the suspicion of infection.

3. We feel that an IOFB that has been in the eye for less than 24 hours or poses a high risk of causing endophthalmitis should be removed as soon as possible. The operating surgeon, however, may opt to remove an IOFB present for greater than 24 hours in an eye, without high risk or any evidence of endophthalmitis, the following day. A computed tomography (CT) scan and/or ultrasound may be obtained in the interim and intravenous antibiotics begun. The precise role of the use of only intravenous antibiotics and not intravitreal antibiotics in suppressing a possible intraocular infection is not clear. Intraocular penetration of these antibiotics may be limited (20–23).

4. Although not statistically significant, Camacho and colleagues showed that eyes subjected to vitrectomy to remove an IOFB within 72 hours after the trauma did better (66% with improvement in visual acuity compared with that on presentation) than did those treated later (55% improved) (24).

5. No matter how well tolerated an IOFB is, the risk of endophthalmitis remains high. Well-tolerated (inert) foreign bodies include carbon, coal, glass, lead, plaster, platinum, porcelain, rubber, stone; however, a toxic coating may be present. It may not always be possible to discern the type of IOFB preoperatively.

LID LACERATION(S)

1. Surgical repair of an eyelid laceration may usually be postponed until the following day or two. In the interim, the wound should be thoroughly irrigated with sterile balanced saline solution and the lacerated tissues covered by a gauze soaked in an antibiotic solution. Delayed repair is especially beneficial for those lacerations at significant risk for contamination such as those from human bites.

2. Irrigation of the wound(s) in uncooperative children, especially those due to punctures and animal or human bites, may pose a problem, thus necessitating general anesthesia and earlier surgical intervention. Parenteral antibiotics may be a temporary option in children who require general anesthesia for wound irrigation. Each case should be handled individually.

3. In adults and cooperative children, the majority of lacerations may be repaired in a minor surgery room upon presentation or the following day.

4. Lacerations that may require operating room repair include:
   • those associated with ocular trauma requiring surgery. The timing is dictated by coexisting ocular injuries.
   • those involving the lacrimal drainage apparatus. In an 11-year study on canalicular lacerations by Kennedy and co-workers, there were no statistically significant associations found between the time interval from injury to surgical repair and the presence of postoperative epiphora (25).
   • those involving the levator aponeurosis of the upper eyelid or superior rectus muscle.

- those in which the medial canthal tendon has been avulsed.
- those associated with an orbital foreign body. The timing of repair may be dictated by the timing of the removal of the IOFB.
- those associated with extensive tissue loss especially greater than one-third of the eyelid, severe distortion of anatomy, or with ischemic portions present.
5. If orbital fat is exposed, consider the use of parenteral antibiotics while awaiting repair.

NONARTERITIC ANTERIOR ISCHEMIC OPTIC NEUROPATHY

Any type of surgical intervention, specifically optic nerve sheath decompression, is still controversial and is of no proven benefit. A prospective, randomized trial to assess the benefit of surgical intervention within 7 days after the onset of symptoms suggested that decompression surgery was no more beneficial than careful follow-up (26).

ORBITAL BONE FRACTURE WITH AND WITHOUT MUSCLE ENTRAPMENT

1. If an extraocular muscle is entrapped in a trap door fracture as demonstrated radiographically and confirmed by forced ductions, repair of the fracture with release of the muscle should be considered as soon as possible to prevent irreversible ischemia and subsequent diplopia.
2. Positive forced ductions alone without radiographic confirmation suggests that the motility restriction may be likely due to incarceration of a small muscle fiber, hematoma, edema, or surrounding connective tissue. In these cases, surgical repair would be recommended at 10 to 14 days after trauma.
3. If forced ductions are negative, the patient may be observed. If the patient has persistent diplopia in primary gaze or when attempting to read, if cosmetically unacceptable enophthalmos exists, or if a large fracture is present, surgical repair is currently recommended 10 to 14 days after trauma.

ORBITAL BONE FRACTURE WITH OPTIC NERVE COMPRESSION

If fracture of an orbital bone results in compression of the optic nerve, immediate orbital exploration with alleviation of direct pressure on the nerve by the bony fragment is necessary. Intravenous corticosteroids should be administered upon diagnosis but should not delay surgical decompression (see Chapter 24).

ORBITAL CELLULITIS SECONDARY TO SINUSITIS

1. Otolaryngology consultation should be obtained immediately after confirmation of the diagnosis. Emergent surgical drainage of the sinus(es) and any asso-

ciated subperiosteal abscess is recommended in most cases, especially if the optic nerve or central retinal artery is threatened. Cavernous sinus thrombosis is a devastating and life-threatening complication that may be avoided by early drainage of the offending sinus and/or abscess.

2. The otolaryngology consultants may prefer an ophthalmologist to be present in the operating room when the orbit is entered and the orbital fat examined via biopsy.

ORBITAL FOREIGN BODY

1. Surgical exploration and removal of an orbital foreign body usually can be postponed until the following day or even later unless indications for earlier removal exist. Intravenous antibiotics should be administered in the interim. Depending on the location of the foreign body and its composition, it may not require removal at any time.

2. Poorly tolerated orbital foreign bodies include copper and organic materials such as wood and vegetable matter. Fairly well-tolerated orbital foreign bodies include copper alloys that are less than 85% copper such as brass and bronze. Well-tolerated orbital foreign bodies include stone, glass, plastic, iron, steel, lead, and aluminum.

3. Indications for surgical exploration and extraction of an orbital foreign body include:
   - coexistent orbital infection requiring earlier intervention, although parenteral antibiotics may allow intervention to be postponed until the following morning but may alter culture results.
   - optic nerve compression requiring immediate intervention. A trial of intravenous corticosteroids may allow intervention to be postponed until the morning, although no studies document this.
   - presence of a poorly-tolerated foreign body when well localized.
   - large or sharp-edged foreign body, irrespective of composition, that can be easily extracted.
   - fistula formation.
   - passage of the foreign body through the globe (perforating injury) to the orbit in some cases.

PERFORATING INJURY

1. Perforation of the globe (through and through ocular injuries) requires primary repair of the anterior penetrating site after the timing recommendations for corneoscleral lacerations described above are appropriate.

2. The use of prophylactic intravitreal and/or intravenous antibiotics is controversial.

3. After primary repair of the anterior site as far posteriorly as possible, the secondary reparative procedure including a vitrectomy may be deferred for 7 to 10 days to allow the posterior penetration site to heal. No randomized, controlled

trial has been performed to delineate the most appropriate timing for the secondary repair (27–30).

POSTERIOR PENETRATING INJURY

1. If the globe is open and there is an IOFB (recent, less than 24 hours) or evidence of or high risk of endophthalmitis, intravenous antibiotics should be started and surgical intervention should be performed immediately.
2. If no IOFB or evidence of endophthalmitis is present and the risk of endophthalmitis is low, primary repair may be postponed until the following day. Intravenous antibiotics should be administered in the interim.
3. A pars plana vitrectomy at the time of initial repair of the penetrating wound is indicated if there is an IOFB requiring vitreous techniques for removal. However, there is controversy as to whether a vitrectomy should be performed at the time of primary repair in these eyes when no IOFB is present, when there is an established infective endophthalmitis, or when other posterior segment pathology such as retinal detachment coexists (27–31).

RETINAL DETACHMENT

1. One randomized study suggests that a macula-on retinal detachment may be repaired the following day (32). Hartz and co-workers retrospectively compared the final visual outcome for patients who had emergency surgery with those who had scheduled surgery after taking into account patient factors related to prognosis (32). There were no differences between emergency and scheduled patients in ocular or systemic complications, rate of reattachment, rate of decreased visual acuity after surgery, visual outcome adjusted for prognosis, or length of hospital stay. None of the 18 patients with an attached macula experienced macular involvement while awaiting scheduled surgery. If the detachment is within the macula but not involving the fovea, one may push for earlier repair if feasible. Patients should be counseled on restrictions on activity (particularly to avoid reading) and maintenance of appropriate head position to decrease risk of retinal detachment progression. Consideration should be given to hospital admission with bilateral patching until surgery can be performed.
2. A macula-off retinal detachment should usually be repaired within a few days to a few weeks, depending on its age. If the macula has been detached for a short duration of 5 to 7 days, then earlier repair is warranted. All cases should be individualized. For example, if the patient is monocular, earlier repair is indicated irrespective of the configuration of the detachment.

TRAUMATIC RETROBULBAR HEMORRHAGE

1. A lateral canthotomy and cantholysis may be performed in the minor surgery room upon presentation (see Chapter 9) if the intraocular pressure cannot be ad-

equately controlled with medical management or if signs of optic nerve compression are present.

2. If a canthotomy and cantholysis do not lead to a reduction in intraocular pressure or if signs of optic nerve compression persist, emergent orbital decompression surgery or paracentesis may be necessary.

SICKLE CELL HYPHEMA AND ELEVATED INTRAOCULAR PRESSURE

To avoid optic atrophy, any patient with any variety of sickle cell disease or trait should undergo an anterior chamber washout within 24 hours if the intraocular pressure by applanation tonometry has been greater than 25 mm Hg for 24 hours or more and could not be adequately lowered by maximum medical treatment or a single anterior chamber paracentesis (33,34). Repeated anterior chamber paracentesis as a method of controlling repeated increases in intraocular pressure in these patients is not recommended.

REFERENCES

1. Barr CC. Prognostic factors in corneoscleral lacerations. *Arch Ophthalmol* 1983;101:919.
2. Thompson WS, Rubsamen PE, Flynn HW Jr, Schiffman J, Cousins SW. Endophthalmitis after penetrating trauma. Risk factors and visual acuity outcomes. *Ophthalmology* 1995;102:1696.
3. Peyman GA, Carroll CP, Raichand M. Prevention and management of traumatic endophthalmitis. *Ophthalmology* 1980;87:320.
4. Peyman GA, Raichand M, Bennett TO. Management of endophthalmitis with pars plana vitrectomy. *Br J Ophthalmol* 1980;64:472.
5. Diamond JG. Intraocular management of endophthalmitis: a systemic approach. *Arch Ophthalmol* 1981;99:96.
6. Puliafito CA, Baker AS, Haaf J, Foster CS. Infectious endophthalmitis; review of 36 cases. *Ophthalmology* 1982;89;1055–1066.
7. Verbraeken H, van Laethem J. Treatment of endophthalmitis with and without pars plana vitrectomy. *Ophthalmologica* 1985;191:1.
8. Weber DJ, Hoffman KL, Thoft RA, Baker AS. Endophthalmitis following intraocular lens implantation; report of 30 cases and review of the literature. *Rev Infect Dis* 1986;8:12.
9. Nobe JR, Gomez DS, Liggett P, et al. Post-traumatic and postoperative endophthalmitis; a comparison of visual outcomes. *Br J Ophthalmol* 1987;71:614.
10. Vastine DW, Peyman GA, Guth SB. Visual prognosis in bacterial endophthalmitis treated with intravitreal antibiotics. *Ophthalmic Surg* 1979;10:76.
11. Davey PG, Barza M, Stuart M. Dose response of experimental pseudomonas endophthalmitis to ciprofloxacin, gentamicin, and imipenem: evidence for resistance to late treatment of infections. *J Infect Dis* 1987;155:518.
12. Brinton GS, Topping TM, Hyndiuk RA, Aaberg TM, Reeser RH, Abrams GW. Posttraumatic endophthalmitis. *Arch Ophthalmol* 1984;102:547.
13. Endophthalmitis Vitrectomy Study Group. Results of endophthalmitis vitrectomy study: a randomized trail of immediate vitrectomy and of intravenous antibiotics for the treatment of postoperative bacterial endophthalmitis. *Arch Ophthalmol* 1995:113:1479.
14. Fauchald P, Rygvold O, Oystese B. Temporal arteritis and polymyalgia rheumatica. Clinical and biopsy findings. *Ann Intern Med* 1972;77:845.
15. Fulton AB, Lee RV, Jampol LM, Keltner JL, Albert DM. Active giant cell arteritis with cerebral involvement. Findings following four years of corticosteroid therapy. *Arch Ophthalmol* 1976;94:2068.

16. Mieler WF, Ellis MK, WIlliams DF, Han DP. Retained intraocular foreign bodies and endophthalmitis. *Ophthalmology* 1990;97:1532.
17. Boldt HC, Pulido JS, Blodi CF et al. Rural endophthalmitis. *Ophthalmology* 1989;96:1722.
18. Seal DV, Kirkness CM. Criteria for intravitreal antibiotics during surgical removal of intraocular foreign bodies. *Eye* 1992;6:465.
19. Campochiaro PA, Conway BP. Aminoglycoside toxicity—a survey of retinal specialists. Implications for ocular use. *Arch Ophthalmol* 1991;109:946.
20. Abel R Jr, Boyle GL, Furman M, Leopold IH. Intraocular penetration of cefazolin sodium in rabbits. *Am J Ophthalmol* 1974;78:779.
21. Peyman GA, May DR, Homer PI, Kasbeer RT. Penetration of gentamicin into the aphakic eye. *Ann Ophthalmol* 1977;9:871.
22. Barza M Kane A, Baum J. Oxacillin for bacterial endophthalmitis: subconjunctival, intravenous, both, or neither? *Invest Ophthalmol Vis Sci* 1980;19:1348.
23. Barza M. Antibacterial agents in the treatment of ocular infections. *Infect Dis Clin North Am* 1989;3:533.
24. Camacho H, Mejia LF. Extraction of intraocular foreign bodies by pars plana vitrectomy; a retrospective study. *Ophthalmologica* 1991;202:173.
25. Kennedy RH, May J, Dailey J, Flanagan JC. Canalicular laceration: an 11 year epidemiologic and clinical study. *Ophthalmic Plast Reconstr Surg* 1990;6:46.
26. Kelman S, Rismundo V. Ischemic optic neuropathy decompression trial (IONDT). University of Maryland, Department of Ophthalmology.
27. Spalding SC, Sternberg P Jr. Controversies in the management of posterior segment ocular trauma. *Retina* 1990;10(suppl):76.
28. de Juan E Jr, Sternberg P Jr, Michels RG. Timing of vitrectomy after penetrating ocular injuries. *Ophthalmology* 1984;91:1072.
29. Punnonen E, Laatikainen L. Long-term follow-up and the role of vitrectomy in the treatment of perforating eye injuries without intraocular foreign bodies. *Acta Ophthalmol* 1989;67:625.
30. Punnonen E, Laatikainen L. Prognosis of perforating eye injuries with intraocular foreign bodies. *Acta Ophthalmologica* 1989;66:483.
31. DeBustros S, Michels RG, Glaser BM. Evolving concepts in the management of posterior segment penetrating ocular injuries. *Retina* 1990;10(suppl):72.
32. Hartz AJ, Burton TC, Gottlieb MS, et al. Outcome and cost analysis of scheduled versus emergency scleral buckling surgery. *Ophthalmology* 1992;99:1358.
33. Deutsch TA, Weinreb RN, Goldberg MF. Indications for surgical management of hyphema in patients with sickle cell trait. *Arch Ophthalmol* 1984;102:556.
34. Goldberg MF. Sickled erythrocytes, hyphema, and secondary glaucoma. I. The diagnosis and treatment of sickled erythrocytes in human hyphemas. *Ophthalmic Surg* 1979;10:17.

Management of Ocular Injuries and Emergencies,
edited by Mathew W. MacCumber.
Lippincott–Raven Publishers, Philadelphia © 1998.

7

Preoperative Preparation and Anesthesia

William E. Vickers and Marc A. Feldman

*Department of Anesthesiology, Wilmer Eye Institute, The Johns Hopkins University
School of Medicine, Baltimore, Maryland 21205*

Patient Assessment   91
Patient Preparation   94
Anesthesia Plan   94

Management of the ocular emergency patient for surgery requires (a) a thorough assessment, (b) medical and psychological preparation of the patient, and (c) development of an anesthesia plan, including induction, maintenance, emergence, analgesia, and postoperative management.

PATIENT ASSESSMENT

The purpose of the preoperative assessment is to improve the patient's medical status, to anticipate potential problems, and to assess and reduce risk (1). Elements of the preoperative assessment include the nature of the injury, the degree of urgency of the procedure, a systems assessment, last oral intake status, and laboratory testing.

Patients with traumatic ocular injury can have coexisting head, facial, or other trauma. The initial assessment must follow the ABCs of *A*irway, *B*reathing, and *C*irculation. Patients with facial trauma should be immediately assessed for injuries to the airway. Early consultation with anesthesiology and otolaryngology can prevent poor outcomes. Signs of respiratory distress include stridor, nasal flaring, and thoracic retractions. Intraabdominal hemorrhage can be subtle, and the presence of impending circulatory shock must be considered. Head trauma can be associated with cervical spine injuries. These injuries may make the neck unstable and predispose the patient to cervical spinal cord injury with extremes of positioning. Cervical spine radiologic studies should be performed, and the neck should be stabilized with a cervical collar if such an injury is suspected. A neurologic examination is conducted to assess for acute intracranial trauma that could be associated with the development of elevated intracranial pressure. Vital signs should be stabilized before further assessment is undertaken.

The nature of the injury will also determine the urgency of the surgical procedure. Some ocular injuries are true emergencies and must be treated immediately. Other procedures are urgent and should be performed within one to several hours. Others can be scheduled more electively. The degree of urgency, then, can determine the nature and time for preoperative assessment.

The essential elements of the patient history and physical examination are listed in Tables 7–1 and 7–2. The patient's general state of health and exercise tolerance dictates his or her ability to tolerate anesthesia and surgery. Some high-risk patients may require medical or cardiology consultation before surgery. Patients with unstable angina may require a dobutamine echocardiogram or cardiac catheterization before surgery, if time permits. Some of these patients may require invasive hemodynamic monitoring intraoperatively, as well as postoperative intensive care. Information regarding previous surgery and anesthesia is particularly helpful. Especially noted are unusual reactions to drugs, ease or difficulty of endotracheal intubation, and any cardiac or pulmonary sequelae after surgery.

The assessment of the hepatic and renal systems is principally only of importance in determining clearance and metabolism of anesthetic drugs and anticipating any electrolyte imbalances caused by reduced glomerular filtration rate. The endocrine disorders of diabetes, hyperthyroidism, and pheochromocytoma may be triggered under anesthesia, and patients with hyperglycemia from diabetes may have intravascular volume deficits and be at increased risk of poor central nervous system outcome in the event of hypotension during anesthesia. The gastrointestinal assessment focuses on the possibility of gastroesophageal reflux or bowel obstruction, leading to an increased risk of aspiration. These conditions can be treated pe-

TABLE 7–1. *Essential elements of the medical history interview*

Chief complaint: The reason for the surgery, the mechanism of the injury
General state of health, exercise tolerance (flights of stairs or distance walked), weight gain or loss
Previous surgeries and anesthetics
Current medications
Allergies and drug reactions
Drug use and abuse (alcohol, tobacco, opiates, cocaine)
Menstrual and obstetric history
Central nervous system (seizures, stroke, dementia)
Dental (loose or false teeth)
Cardiovascular (hypertension, angina, heart failure)
Respiratory (COPD, wheezing, cough, sleep apnea)
Hepatic (jaundice, hepatitis)
Gastrointestinal (ulcers, bowel obstruction, hiatal hernia, gastroesophageal reflux, last oral intake)
Musculoskeletal (arthritis)
Endocrine (diabetes, adrenal, or thyroid disorder)
Hematologic (bleeding or clotting problems, anemia)

TABLE 7–2. *Essential elements of the physical examination*

Weight and height, blood pressure, pulse, respiration, and temperature
Mental status and gross neurologic: Alertness, orientation to person, place, and time, moving
  all extremities
Auscultation of the heart and lungs
Examine the extremities for edema, cyanosis, veins for venous access
Mouth and airway: Neck mobility, mouth opening, dentition, uvula visible

rioperatively to decrease the overall risk of aspiration. The hematologic assessment should look for patients with a history of underlying coagulopathies, anemias such as sickle cell disease, and the patient's ideas and feelings concerning possible blood transfusion received during the surgery.

The patient's overall physical status is assessed using the American Society of Anesthesiologists (ASA) Physical Status Classification. Anesthetic morbidity and mortality have been shown to correlate with ASA physical status. The classification is listed in Table 7–3.

The patient is carefully questioned regarding last oral intake. The emphasis is placed on withholding oral intake stems from the risk of pulmonary aspiration, which has a mortality rate of 5% to 10%, with significant morbidity including an average hospital stay of 21 days, most of which is spent in the intensive care unit. The risk of aspiration is generally low: it approaches one in 800 cases in emergent surgery, but small aspiration may occur anywhere between 4% and 26% of all general anesthetics (2–4). Trauma patients in pain or shock have higher gastric volumes secondary to decreased gastric emptying from sympathetic outflow and medication with narcotics. Patients should have no solid food for at least 6 hours to allow for sufficient gastric emptying. In true emergencies, the benefit of earlier surgery usually outweighs the risk of aspiration.

Laboratory testing is based on the results of the patient history and physical examination (Table 7–4). Routine chemistries, blood cell counts, electrocardiogram, and chest radiographs add a substantial cost to overall patient care and are not of clear benefit. In general, a chest x-ray is only indicated if an abnormality is suspected. An electrocardiogram may be indicated if a patient is greater than 40 years of age or if there are known cardiac risk factors. An assessment of hemoglobin or hematocrit may be indicated, especially with traumatic injuries involving significant blood loss. Electrolytes should be measured in patients on diuretic therapy or

TABLE 7–3. *American Society of Anesthesiologists Physical Status Classification*

ASA 1 Normal, healthy patient with no systemic disease
ASA 2 Mild systemic disease (diet-controlled diabetes or hypertension, anemia, bronchitis)
ASA 3 Severe systemic disease that limits activity (angina, COPD, complicated diabetes)
ASA 4 Life-threatening systemic disease (heart failure, unstable angina, renal failure)
ASA 5 Moribund patient not expected to survive 24 hours

TABLE 7–4. *Recommended laboratory testing*

Complete blood count: All emergency patients
Electrocardiogram: Over 40 years of age or with risk factors (hypertension, diabetes, high cholesterol)
Serum electrolytes: Diuretic therapy, dehydration, prolonged vomiting
Pregnancy testing: Urine or blood beta-hCG testing for women of child-bearing age

if there is a suspected disturbance. Pregnancy testing should be performed in women of child-bearing age.

PATIENT PREPARATION

The patient assessment provides the tools for proper patient preparation for surgery. Patient rapport and cooperation are elicited through the preoperative interview. The medical history and prior anesthesia experiences and concerns are reviewed with the patient. The anesthetic alternatives, their associated risks, and benefits are discussed. The timing of the surgery and recovery are described. Discussion of methods of postoperative pain management help relieve patient anxiety. Informed consent is obtained.

Patient interview and discussion are usually enough to allay anxiety. The occasional patient may benefit from oral diazepam or other anxiolytic. Patients with significant pain preoperatively can be helped with codeine or other oral analgesia. Intramuscular morphine can provide excellent analgesia but must be used with caution due to potential respiratory depression. Metoclopramide may be given to speed gastric emptying and as an antiemetic. Cimetidine, ranitidine, or oral nonparticulate antacids may be given to neutralize gastric pH, to decrease the risk of pulmonary acid aspiration.

Exacerbations of chronic medical problems may be treated preoperatively to smooth the perioperative course. Medical consultation may be indicated if time permits. Acute hypertension may be treated with beta-blockers or other antihypertensives. Patients with asthma may benefit from nebulized bronchodilators or a short course of steroid therapy.

ANESTHESIA PLAN

Traditionally, ocular surgical emergencies were managed with general anesthesia. With modern techniques, however, local anesthesia and intravenous sedation may be alternatives. The choice of general versus regional anesthesia is made on the basis of patient, surgical, and anesthetic factors. High patient anxiety, prolonged procedures, and difficulty communicating or obtaining patient cooperation require general anesthetic techniques. Severe cardiopulmonary disease may make regional anesthesia a safer choice. A large corneal or scleral laceration may require general anesthesia because a regional anesthesia technique may lead to increased pressure on the globe from the injection of local anesthetic or the activity of eyelid or extraocular muscles. Small, sealed injuries to the globe may be managed with topical or peribulbar local anesthetics. A facial nerve block may be important to prevent eyelid squeezing during the procedure.

Children nearly always require general anesthesia. Topical anesthetics can be very helpful before placement of intravenous catheters. In younger patients with difficult intravenous access, an inhalational induction by mask can be the best choice.

The patient with an open globe injury presents a dilemma for the anesthesiologist who wants to protect the patient from aspirating stomach contents and to protect the eye from losing vitreous. A rapid sequence intravenous induction is needed to protect the airway, but concerns arise from the use of succinylcholine with its associated rise in intraocular pressure (5–8). Factors to consider in the choice of muscle relaxant are listed as follows:

- Size of the perforation: A very small puncture to the globe would have higher resistance to vitreous loss with succinylcholine.
- Pulmonary status: If the patient has decreased functional residual capacity, hypoxia will occur soon, and a nondepolarizing muscle relaxant might not have time to be effective.
- NPO status: What is the reasonable assessment of aspiration risk? When was the last solid food taken?
- Duration of the procedure: If the surgery is short, the patient may require postoperative mechanical ventilation if a large dose of a nondepolarizing muscle relaxant is used.
- Precurarization: Use of small doses of nondepolarizing muscle relaxants, such as curare or pancuronium, as a pretreatment before succinylcholine may attenuate, but not eliminate, the increase in intraocular pressure (9).

As more evidence accumulates, the concern over the effects of succinylcholine on intraocular pressure appears more theoretical (10,11). If a rapid sequence induction is needed, succinylcholine with precurarization is a reasonable choice.

The goals of general anesthesia include a smooth intubation with stable intraocular pressure, avoidance of severe oculocardiac reflexes, maintenance of a motionless field, and an equally smooth emergence and extubation. This can be accomplished with inhalational anesthesia, balanced narcotic anesthesia, or intravenous agents, with or without muscle relaxants.

If intravitreal gas is to be used as part of a retinal repair, nitrous oxide must be avoided. Nitrous oxide diffuses into enclosed gas spaces and can increase intraocular pressure dramatically by increasing the size of the gas bubble (12–14).

Antiemetics can be useful. Droperidol or ondansetron given intraoperatively can help prevent postoperative nausea and vomiting. Opioid narcotics such as fentanyl and morphine are excellent analgesics but can exacerbate postoperative nausea. Ketorolac is a parenteral nonsteroidal anti-inflammatory drug with significant analgesic properties. It may be contraindicated in patients at risk for gastrointestinal bleeding or unstable kidney function. Supplementing the general anesthesia with a regional local anesthetic block provides excellent postoperative pain relief and helps to block oculocardiac reflexes.

Many emergent ocular procedures can be done as outpatients. Modern anesthetic techniques with short-acting agents allow for rapid recovery and ambulation. Other patients require inpatient admission for medical or ophthalmic observation. Rare patients with multiple traumatic injuries, cardiac instability, or respiratory failure may require intensive care. Postoperative management should always be considered as part of the perioperative plan.

REFERENCES

1. Barash PG, Cullen BF, Stoelting RK, eds. *Handbook of Clinical Anesthesia.* Philadelphia: JB Lippincott; 1991.
2. Mendelson CL. The aspiration of stomach contents into the lungs during obstretric anesthesia. *Am J Obstet Gynecol* 1946;2:191.
3. Warner MA, Warner ME, Weber JG. Clinical significance of pulmonary aspiration during the perioperative period. *Anesthesiology* 1993;78:56.
4. LeFrock JL, Clark TS, Davies B, et al. Aspiration pneumonia: a ten-year review. *Am Surg* 1979;45:305.
5. Lincoff HA, Breinin GM, DeVoe AG. Effect of succinylcholine on extraocular muscles. *Am J Ophthalmol* 1957;43:440.
6. Cook JH. The effect of suxamethonium on intraocular pressure. *Anaesthesia* 1981;36:359.
7. Pandey K, Badola RP, Kumar S. Time course of intraocular hypertension produced by suxamethonium. *Br J Anaesth* 1972;44:191.
8. Wynands JE, Crowell DE. Intraocular tension in association with succinylcholine and endotracheal intubation. *Can Anaesth Soc J* 1960;7:39.
9. Meyers EF, Krupin T, Johnson M, et al. Failure of nondepolarizing neuromuscular blockers to inhibit succinylcholine induced increased intraocular pressure. *Anesthesiology* 1978;48:149.
10. Libonati MM, Leahy JJ, Ellison N. The use of succinylcholine in open eye surgery. *Anesthesiology* 1985;62:637.
11. Murphy DF, Davis NJ. Succinylcholine use in emergency eye operations. *Can J Anaesth* 1987;34:101.
12. Abrams GW, Edelhauser HF, Aabert TM, et al. Dynamics of intravitreal sulfur hexafluoride gas. *Invest Ophthalmol* 1974;13:863.
13. Fuller D, Lewis ML. Nitrous oxide anaesthesia and intravitreal gas. *Am J Ophthalmol* 1975;80:778.
14. Wolf GL, Capuano C, Hartung J. Nitrous oxide increases IOP after intravitreal sulfur hexafluoride injection. *Anesthesiology* 1983;59:547.

Management of Ocular Injuries and Emergencies,
edited by Mathew W. MacCumber.
Lippincott–Raven Publishers, Philadelphia ©1998.

8

Injuries of the Lid and Lacrimal System

Shannath L. Merbs and Nicholas T. Iliff

*Wilmer Eye Institute, The Johns Hopkins University School of Medicine,
Baltimore, Maryland 21287*

Basic Considerations 97
Diagnosis 98
Management 98
General Considerations 98 · Simple Lacerations Involving Skin Alone or
Skin and Orbicularis 100 · Lacerations Involving the Eyelid Margin 101
Lacerations Involving the Medial Canthus and Lacrimal System 102 · Lacerations Involving the Lateral Canthus 103 · Trauma to the Levator Muscle or
Aponeurosis and Deeper Structures 106

BASIC CONSIDERATIONS

Injury to the eyelids and lacrimal apparatus after penetrating and blunt trauma and bites is common. Penetrating trauma with a sharp object tends to produce a clean wound without tissue loss. Blunt trauma can produce abrasions, irregular lacerations, and partial avulsions. Bites, in addition to being contaminated, usually produce tearing of tissues without tissue loss. Each case is unique, requiring a tailored approach.

Knowledge of the anatomy and function is crucial to the successful management of these cases. Eyelid function depends on smooth contour and margins, absence of restriction from scarring and fibrosis, and the ability to make extremely rapid movements. Precise and delicate realignment of structures requires knowledge of the exact surgical anatomy and reconstructive procedures applicable to eyelids.

Normally functioning eyelids and lacrimal system are important for maintaining the health of the globe. Additionally, the aesthetic importance of the eyelids cannot be overstressed. For these reasons, even seemingly minor lacerations to the vital structures can present a great challenge.

DIAGNOSIS

1. Obtaining a detailed history—focusing on the cause, location, and time of injury and whether safety glasses were worn—is essential in determining the degree of contamination and the presence of foreign bodies. A patient's tetanus immunization history determines the need for a tetanus toxoid booster or tetanus immune globulin. Time of the last oral intake must be determined if surgical intervention is needed. Animal bites should be reported to the local or state public health department. Accurate documentation also is essential, particularly if future legal action is anticipated.

2. A complete ocular examination should be performed to rule out associated intraocular trauma, although the full examination of a child may need to be deferred until the patient is under anesthesia. Even a minor penetration of the eyelid should arouse suspicion of a penetrating injury to the globe. Management of the lid laceration is undertaken after management of any globe injury (1).

3. The clinician should determine and document the extent of the orbital and eyelid injuries (1). Initial evaluation of the extent of lacerations requires gentle cleaning and separation with a cotton swab. The edges of the lid lacerations often adhere to each other in relatively normal orientation, disguising a more serious injury. Photographs should be obtained, if possible, to document the nature and extent of the injuries.

4. The nature and extent of the eyelid injury influences the choice of surgical procedure. The presence and degree of tissue loss should be estimated. Involvement of the lid margin should be determined. A laterally displaced punctum suggests a laceration involving the lacrimal drainage system (2). Involvement of the medial canthal tendon and a naso-orbital fracture can result in rounding of the medial canthus or telecanthus (3). Visible orbital fat confirms penetration of the orbital septum (4). The presence of some levator function, despite limitation secondary to lid edema, suggests an intact levator.

5. Computed tomographic imaging can aide in evaluation if the mechanism of injury and the depth of resultant periorbital injuries suggest a possible orbital fracture or the presence of an orbital foreign body (see Chapter 5). Magnetic resonance imaging may be useful if a wooden foreign body is suspected (5).

6. After the examination, a lubricating ointment can be applied to the cornea if no corneal laceration is present. A saline dressing and protective shield should be applied to the eyelid laceration to prevent drying of tissues and further injury before the repair. In general, protruding foreign bodies should not be disturbed until the time of repair.

MANAGEMENT

General Considerations

1. Timing of repair of eyelid injuries should ideally be within 24 hours of injury (1). However, eyelid injuries can easily be repaired up to several days later. Life-

threatening and vision-threatening injuries take precedence over periorbital injuries, but protection of the cornea to prevent ulceration must be a priority. In cases of significant tissue loss, primary closure should be undertaken if possible. Skin grafting at the time of primary closure is rarely necessary. Definitive repair, which may include skin grafts and tissue flaps, should be delayed as long as possible to allow scars to mature.

2. Antibiotic prophylaxis is not usually necessary for most uncomplicated lacerations of the eyelid and lacrimal system. Application of an antibiotic-steroid ointment is helpful in lubricating the eye, decreasing inflammation, and minimizing crusting around sutures to facilitate suture removal. For grossly contaminated wounds or bites, antibiotics should be given for prophylaxis against infection. Amoxicillin-clavulanate (Augmentin, SmithKline Beecham), 40/mg/kg/day up to 500 mg three times daily, is effective against anaerobes and penicillinase-producing staphylococci (6). For surgery involving the sinuses, preoperative antibiotic prophylaxis with a single dose of cefazolin (Ancef, SmithKline Beecham), 1 to 2 g intravenously, is usually sufficient (6).

3. Tetanus prophylaxis is considered for all patients (7). Primary immunization consists of a series of three tetanus injections given before 7 years of age. A tetanus booster (0.5 ml of tetanus, diphtheria intramuscularly) is necessary for adult patients every 10 years. For contaminated or puncture wounds, immunized patients should receive a booster if it has been more than 5 years since their last booster. Patients with uncertain immunization status and a clean, nonpuncture wound should receive a tetanus booster and completion of their immunization series. Patients with uncertain immunization status and a tetanus-prone wound should receive a tetanus injection and a 250-IU dose of tetanus immune globulin intramuscularly.

4. Rabies prophylaxis is also important for patients who sustain animal bites (8). If a pet watched for 10 days develops rabies, if a wild animal cannot be found but is suspected to have rabies, or if rabies is found on examination of the animal in question, rabies prophylaxis should be administered. Initially, 20 IU/kg of rabies immune globulin is given half intramuscularly and half infiltrated at the wound. Additionally, 1 ml of human diploid cell rabies vaccine is given intramuscularly on days 0, 3, 7, 14, and 28.

5. Adequate wound cleansing is necessary to remove foreign material embedded in the wound and to minimize bacterial contamination. Normal saline, irrigated with force through a 19-gauge needle on a 30-ml syringe, reduces bacterial counts and experimental wound infection by 90% (9).

6. The choice of suture material is determined by the site where it is to be used. Nonabsorbable 8-0 silk is used for the eyelid skin and lid margin. Nonabsorbable 6-0 nylon is used for the more robust skin of the brows. Skin sutures can be removed in 4 to 7 days, but the lid margin sutures should be left in place from 7 to 10 days. In children or patients in whom suture removal is difficult, 7-0 chromic sutures can be used. Absorbable 6-0 polyglactin 910 sutures (Vicryl) are used to repair the tarsus.

7. The choice of anesthesia can be local, regional, or general. Local anesthesia by infiltration of the surrounding tissue through the wound with 1% or 2% lidocaine with 1:100,000 epinephrine is used for small lacerations. We rarely use regional anesthesia, which requires multiple injections including the infraorbital, supraorbital, infratrochlear, and supratrochlear nerves for sufficient anesthesia of the periorbital area and lacrimal system. General anesthesia is used in children and in cases of extensive injury. In cases requiring lacrimal intubation, 10% cocaine or Afrin (Schering–Plough)-soaked material placed beneath the inferior turbinate may reduce bleeding.

Simple Lacerations Involving Skin Alone or Skin and Orbicularis

1. Lacerations involving skin alone or skin and orbicularis muscle require skin closure alone with fine suture technique. Deep sutures should not be used except possibly in lacerations involving the brow. Wound edges on eyelid skin are approximated with interrupted 8-0 silk sutures for irregular lacerations. Flaps, corners, and identifiable landmarks should be sutured first. Running 8-0 silk sutures can be used for linear lacerations. Skin sutures can be removed in 4 to 7 days.
2. Triangular or curved linear lacerations of eyelid skin result in contraction of the skin flap, whic99h at first glance may seem to represent a loss of soft tissue. However, frequently the tissue can be readily stretched to fill the defect, and true tissue loss is not the case. For small losses of eyelid skin and orbicularis, primary closure is usually possible, particularly in the upper lid, where redundancy of tissue is the usual situation. Where primary closure is likely to cause lid retraction or lagophthalmos, slight undermining of the surrounding tissue can be used to mobilize a skin–muscle flap (Fig. 8–1).
3. Lacerations involving larger losses of eyelid skin may require skin grafts, which can be taken from the opposite upper eyelid or from retroauricular or supraclav-

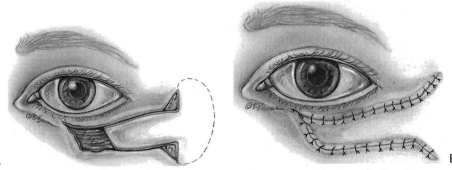

A   B

FIG. 8–1. A: Skin-muscle flap. Undermining of the skin and orbicularis allows advancement of the flap to close the area of the avulsed eyelid skin. Burow's triangles are removed to facilitate flap advancement. **B:** The skin and orbicularis are reapproximated with 8-0 silk suture.

icular areas. However, the best skin available for grafting should not be used in the acute setting and should be saved if at all possible if later reconstructive maneuvers are needed.

Lacerations Involving the Eyelid Margin

1. The lid margin and tarsus require precise realignment to prevent contour irregularities, notching, or trichiasis. All sutures have to be placed in a fashion that will not cause corneal abrasion. Scar contraction tends to work against attempts at restoring normal contour. Tissue may be limited, restricting excision of lacerated or shredded edges. In most cases of margin lacerations, a fine reapproximation of the cut edges is preferable to trimming of edges. It can be difficult to achieve fine, straight cuts through the lid margin and tarsus of a swollen hemorrhagic lid, and tissue may be removed, which results in additional stress on the repair postoperatively. In many cases, it may be preferable to close the wound primarily and revise scarring with re-excision at a later date under more controlled circumstances.

2. Reconstruction begins with tarsal reapproximation (Fig. 8–2). A 6-0 polyglactin suture on a small-diameter needle (e.g., Ethicon S28 or S29) is placed 3 mm from the lid margin and tied with the knot on the anterior surface of the tarsus and the posterior loop of the suture just anterior to the conjunctiva. This prevents any possibility of corneal abrasion. Alignment of the lid margin is examined, and the remainder of the tarsal plate is similarly closed. At most, three to four sutures in the upper tarsus and two sutures in the lower tarsus are typically needed.

3. The lid margin is repaired next. Sutures aligning the lashes and the tarsal plates are placed, as is a third suture in the area of the gray line if needed. Tra-

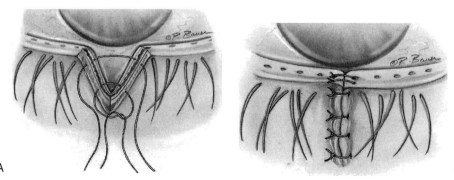

A   B

FIG. 8–2. A: Eyelid margin repair. The tarsal plate is reapproximated with two to three 6-0 Vicryl mattress sutures placed as illustrated. Placing all tarsal sutures before tying any suture can facilitate closure. **B:** The skin is reapproximated with interrupted 8-0 silk sutures. The sutures at the level of the gray line and meibomian orifices are cut short so as not to rub on the cornea.

ditionally, the ends of the sutures are left long so they can be brought onto the anterior surface of the lid and secured with another suture to prevent their rubbing on the cornea. However, we have found that carefully and closely trimming the 8-0 silk suture ends also prevents corneal abrasions and eliminates the possibility of the long ends working loose and abrading the cornea. The suture bites in the lid margin should be large enough to provide some bulging of the tissues, for there will be loosening as swelling decreases and contraction of tissues occurs, which can result in a small notch if the tissues were not initially bunched. Lid contour should be normal after closure of the tarsus and lid margin.

4. Skin and, if involved, levator tendon are then reapproximated. The lid margin sutures should be left in place from 7 to 10 days.

5. For tissue loss of one fourth to one third of the upper or lower eyelid, direct closure of a full-thickness eyelid avulsive injury is possible. Lateral canthotomy and cantholysis allows closure of slightly larger defects (Fig. 8–3). Even larger defects of the middle of the eyelid can be repaired by undermining the skin and orbicularis laterally and creating a subciliary incision to create a myocutaneous flap which can be pulled medially and sutured to remaining medial eyelid (Fig. 8–3). Other more severe tissue losses require reconstructive flaps or grafts, the discussion of which is beyond the scope of this text (10).

6. Avulsion of the lid margin and lashes in the absence of significant loss of tarsal tissues requires little initial surgical care in most cases. The margin often heals in a fashion smooth enough to prevent corneal injury. If there has not been significant loss of tarsus in a vertical direction, lagophthalmos may not be a prob-

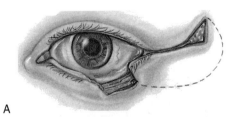

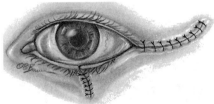

A

C

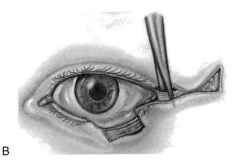

B

FIG. 8–3. A: Canthotomy and cantholysis for repair of a full-thickness eyelid defect. If the eyelid margin edges cannot be reapproximated without excessive tension, a horizontal incision (canthotomy) is made through the lateral canthus to the rim and extended laterally through the skin and orbicularis. A triangle of skin is removed at the end of the incision to prevent formation of a "dog ear." **B:** The lower arm of the lateral canthal tendon is cut with canthotomy scissors (cantholysis). **C:** The lid margin is then advanced and reapproximated as described in Fig. 8–2.

lem. Acute reconstruction is not needed and is best left to a later date when the situation is completely stabilized.

Lacerations Involving the Medial Canthus and Lacrimal System

1. Repair of the laceration should include internal stenting of the canaliculus (Fig. 8–4). Both the upper and lower lacrimal canaliculi should be probed and irrigated if examination shows that the eyelid injury is at or medial to the punctum. High-powered loupes or an operating microscope is useful to locate the proximal end of the canaliculus. If the laceration is close to the medial canthus, or if swelling of the surrounding tissues is present, identification of the proximal end may be difficult. Allowing tissue swelling to subside with time may help with identification. Irrigation of air or a milky corticosteroid solution through the opposite canalicular system may also help locate the proximal cut end.
2. A bicanalicular stent is used, such as the Guibor design (Concept), with stainless-steel probes swaged onto the silicone tubing. The probe is lubricated with an ophthalmic ointment and is first passed vertically through the punctum of the involved canaliculus. While stretching the lid, the probe in rotated 90 degrees to the horizontal plane and advanced out through the laceration. The probe is then placed into the proximal end of the canaliculus and advanced along the horizontal plane into the lacrimal lacerated sac. When it rests against the medial orbital wall, it is rotated to the vertical plane and advanced through the nasolacrimal duct. A grooved director under the inferior turbinate is used to externalize the probe from the nares. The process is repeated for the uninvolved canaliculus. The silicone tubes are brought from the nares and tied together using 6-0 silk suture. The knot is retracted back into the laceration, and a second knot is placed proximal to the first, forming a smaller loop in the silicone tubing. The first knot is removed, and the second knot is pulled through the canalicular system so that the knot rests in the lacrimal sac, keeping the tubes in place (11). The silicone tubes are then trimmed 1 cm proximal to the nares. The canthal ligament and connective tissue adjacent to the canaliculus are sutured with 6.0 polyglactin 910, allowing the reapproximation of the canaliculus.
3. Superficial injuries of the medial canthal area not involving the lacrimal drainage system can be repaired by primary closure using 8.0 silk for skin closure and 6.0 polyglactin 910 if closure of the deep layers is required.
4. Laceration of the medial canthal ligament is repaired by reapproximating the lacerated ends of the ligament with 6-0 polyglactin 910. Avulsion of the medial canthal ligament from the anterior lacrimal crest is repaired by suturing the tendon to the periosteum with a 5-0 or 6-0 nonabsorbable suture (nylon or polyester).

Lacerations Involving the Lateral Canthus

Direct closure of lateral canthal lacerations is possible if at least 70% of the upper and lower lid margins remain. The lateral tarsus is secured to the inner aspect of the lateral orbital rim periosteum with 5-0 or 6-0 mersilene.

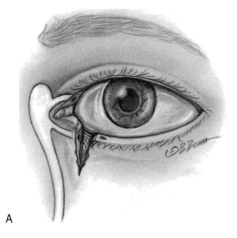

A

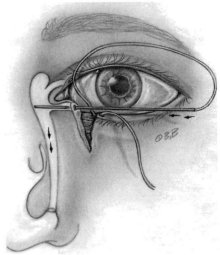

B

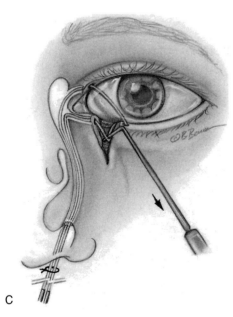

C

FIG. 8–4. A: Silicone intubation for repair of a laceration involving the lacrimal system. The involved (inferior) punctum is displaced laterally. **B:** The involved punctum is intubated by minimally advancing the probe perpendicular to the lid margin, then rotating the probe until it is parallel to the lid margin and advancing the probe out through the laceration. The probe is then placed into the cut end of the canaliculus and advanced horizontally into the lacrimal sac. The probe is rotated vertically while it is resting against the medial wall of the sac. With the probe resting against the brow, it is advanced into the nose. The probe should advance without resistance and care should be taken as not to create a false passage. The probe is externalized from the nose using a grooved director. The process is repeated for the other punctum and canaliculus. **C:** The tubes are tied together using a 6.0 silk suture. A Steven's hook is used to retract the tubes from the laceration.

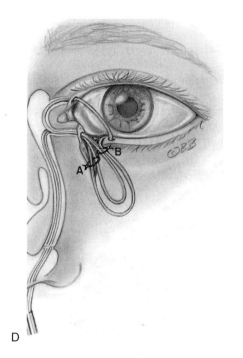

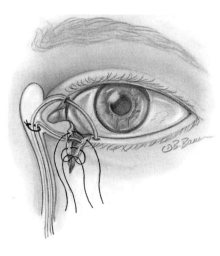

E

D

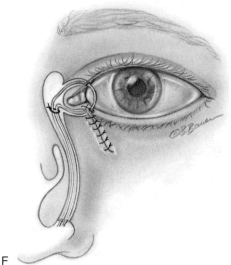

F

FIG. 8–4. *Continued.* **D:** Retraction of the silicone tubes is continued using fingers or a needle holder to bring the suture out through the cut end of the canaliculus. When the first knot (a) is visualized, a second knot (b) is placed making a smaller loop of silicone tubing running between the puncta an lacrimal sac. This second knot (b) prevents the tubes from being externalized into the medial canthal area. The first suture (a) is removed, and the tubes are pulled from the nose until the second knot (b) pops into the lacrimal sac. **E:** The canalicular ends are reapproximated with two 6.0 Vicryl mattress sutures. **F:** The silicone tubes are trimmed 1 cm inside the nares. The skin is closed with 8.0 silk sutures.

Trauma to the Levator Muscle or Aponeurosis and Deeper Structures

1. Lacerations involving the deeper structures of the eyelid require careful evaluation, aided by loupe magnification. The appearance of the orbital septum and levator tendon deep in a wound can be very similar. Prolapsed hemorrhagic fat can obscure normal relationships. From the mid-tarsal area superiorly for about 1 cm, the septum and tendon are closely approximated.

2. The levator muscle should be reapproximated, but the orbital septum should not be closed. An aide in identification and differentiation of these two structures is the gentle traction on the tissue in question. Traction on the septum transmits a pull directly to the periosteum of the orbital rim and should be firm and unyielding. Traction on the levator tendon is transmitted deeper in the orbit and should be somewhat springy in character. The levator tendon can be closed with interrupted 6-0 polyglactin 910 sutures.

3. Full-thickness lacerations of the eyelid, not involving the tissues, present additional difficulties in the identification of structures. Large lacerations of the conjunctiva are closed first with a fine absorbable suture such as 7-0 chromic. The levator tendon is then reapproximated, and lastly, the skin is closed. No other structure (orbicularis, orbital septum, or Mueller's muscle) need be repaired. Intentional or inadvertent closure of the orbital septum can cause mid-lamellar lid shortening and lagophthalmos.

REFERENCES

1. Mindlin AM. Prioritizing the repair of adnexal trauma. *Adv Ophthalmic Plast Reconstr Surg* 19876:91, 1987.
2. Hawes MJ. Trauma of the lacrimal drainage system. In: Linberg JV, ed. *Lacrimal Surgery.* New York: Churchill Livingstone; 1988:241.
3. Beyer CK, Fabian RL, Smith B. Naso-orbital fractures, complications and treatment. *Ophthalmology* 1982;89:458.
4. Stasior GO, Lemke BN. Anatomy of the orbit and ocular adnexa. In: Shingleton BJ, Hersh PS, Denyon DR, eds. *Eye Trauma.* St. Louis: Mosby-Year Book; 1991:261.
5. Green BF, Kraft, SP, Carter KD, Buncic JR, Nerad JA, Armstrong D. Orbital wood. Detection by magnetic resonance imaging. *Ophthalmology* 1990;95:608.
6. Antimicrobial prophylaxis in surgery. *Med Lett* 1993;35:91.
7. Advisory Committee of Immunization Practices. Diptheria, tetanus, and pertussis: guidelines for vaccine prophylaxis and other preventive measures. *MMWR* 1985;34:405.
8. Immunization Practice Advisory Committee. Rabies prevention—United States. *MMWR* 1983:393:1984.
9. Stevenson TR, Thacker JG, Rodenheaver GT, Cleansing of the traumatic wound by high pressure syringe irrigation. *J Am Coll Emerg Phys* 1976;5:17.
10. Bosniak S, ed. *Ophthalmic Plastic and Reconstructive Surgery.* Philadelphia: WB Saunders; 1996.
11. Harris LL, Merbs SL, Iliff NT. (manuscript in preparation).

Management of Ocular Injuries and Emergencies,
edited by Mathew W. MacCumber.
Lippincott–Raven Publishers, Philadelphia ©1998.

9

Orbital Trauma

John B. Kerrison, Mami Aiello Iwamoto, Shannath L. Merbs, and Nicholas T. Iliff

Wilmer Eye Institute, The Johns Hopkins University School of Medicine, Baltimore, Maryland 21287

Basic Considerations   107
Traumatic Orbital Hemorrhage   108
  Diagnosis   108 · Management   108 · Procedure   109
Orbital Fractures   110
Orbital Floor Fracture   110
  Diagnosis   110 · Management   110
Medial Orbital Wall Fracture   111
Orbital Roof Fractures   111
  Procedure   111
Complex Orbital Fractures   113
Traumatic Myopathy   114
  Diagnosis   114 · Management   114
Orbital Foreign Body   115
  Diagnosis   115 · Management   115

BASIC CONSIDERATIONS

Patients with trauma to the orbits have often sustained significant multisystem trauma and require a multidisciplined team that can prioritize and perform treatment plans. Associated life-threatening injuries must be recognized and addressed. Ophthalmic examination is often difficult and limited in this setting; however, maxillofacial trauma is often associated with ocular injury. Thus, injury to the globe must not be overlooked in the setting of orbital trauma.

Orbital trauma may be both blunt and penetrating. The nature and circumstances of the injury should be determined, with specific attention directed to the mechanism of insult, point of impact, and composition of the injuring device; the possibility of retained foreign bodies should be assumed until proven otherwise. Specific inquiry as to the presence of decreased vision, diplopia, and epiphora should

107

be made in addition to whether such symptoms were immediate or of delayed onset with progressive worsening.

Clinical examination should include assessment of visual acuity, pupillary responses, confrontation visual fields, and color vision. On external examination, entrance wounds, proptosis, ptosis, poor levator function, subcutaneous emphysema, or orbital rim step off should be recognized. Infraorbital hypesthesia indicates damage to the infraorbital branch of the trigeminal nerve and may suggest orbital floor fracture. Motility examination assesses alignment and ductions. Forced ductions may be indicated. The globe should be examined carefully. Hyphema is a relative contraindication to orbital surgery because of the potential increased risk of rebleeding. In the setting of orbital congestion, the intraocular pressure may be elevated, compromising retinal perfusion.

Computed tomography (CT) is the imaging study of choice in assessing orbital fracture, hematoma, or retained foreign bodies (see Chapter 5). For the management of preseptal and orbital cellulitis, see Chapter 10.

TRAUMATIC ORBITAL HEMORRHAGE

Orbital hemorrhage may occur after blunt or penetrating injury. It may be generalized or localized subperiosteally, extraconally, within the belly of an extraocular muscle, or intraconally. Orbital congestion may cause elevated intraocular pressure. Importantly, a large enough hemorrhage may impair retinal and optic nerve perfusion. Vision threatening orbital hemorrhages should be recognized and treated expeditiously.

Diagnosis

1. Complaints include pain, diplopia, and decreased vision.
2. Proptosis, hemorrhagic chemosis, and dystopia are present.
3. Intraocular pressure may or may not be elevated.
4. Limited motility may be generalized or present in one field of gaze with localized hematoma.
5. Visual acuity, color vision, and pupillary responses (relative afferent pupillary defect) may be abnormal due to optic nerve or retinal ischemia.
6. The central retinal artery may be pulsating or occluded. Choroidal folds may be present.
7. CT scan of the orbits with axial and coronal views is the study of choice. In the setting of compromised vision, treatment should be instituted before imaging.

Management

1. Orbital hemorrhages may resolve without intervention; however, vision-threatening hemorrhages causing retinal or optic nerve ischemia should be addressed immediately.

2. Be sure that the cornea is well lubricated if lagophthalmos due to proptosis is present.
3. In the setting of elevated intraocular pressure (more than 30 mm Hg with normal optic nerve; more than 20 mm Hg with glaucomatous optic neuropathy) without evidence of visual compromise, the patient may be managed conservatively using topical beta-blockers, iopidine, acetazolamide, or osmotic agents.
4. If retinal perfusion is compromised, lower intraocular pressure and consider orbital decompression by canthotomy or cantholysis (see below). Manage central retinal artery occlusion (CRAO) as in other settings (see Chapter 23).
5. Indications for surgical intervention include inability to control intraocular pressure medically, optic neuropathy, and central retinal artery occlusion. Surgical options include lateral canthotomy and cantholysis, which can be performed in the emergency room. If these are insufficient, an immediate referral to an orbital plastic surgeon is required for consideration of lateral orbitotomy, which should be performed under general anesthesia.

Procedure: Lateral Canthotomy and Cantholysis

1. After informed consent, inject a mixture of 2% xylocaine with 1:100,000 epinephrine into the lateral canthal area.
2. In order to achieve hemostasis, position a straight clamp for 10 seconds, extending it horizontally from the lateral canthal angle beyond the lateral fornix to the orbital rim.
3. Using the Steven scissors, perform a lateral canthotomy in this area (Fig. 9–1*A*).
4. If lateral canthotomy alone does not provide enough decompression, perform lateral cantholysis. Position the Stevens scissors perpendicular to the canthotomy incision and incise the superior and inferior extensions of the lateral canthal ligament (Fig. 9–1*B*).

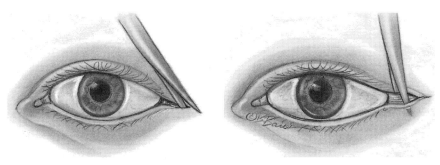

A   B

FIG. 9–1. A: Canthotomy. **B:** Cantholysis.

ORBITAL FRACTURES

The orbit consists of the roof, formed by the frontal bone and lesser wing of the sphenoid bone; the floor, formed by the maxillary, zygomatic, and palatine bones; the lateral wall, formed by the zygomatic bone and the greater wing of the sphenoid; and the medial wall, formed by the ethmoid, maxillary, lacrimal, and sphenoid bones. The medial wall is the thinnest, followed by the orbital floor. The orbital floor is the most commonly fractured area of the orbit. The infraorbital nerve travels in the floor of the orbit and may be affected by floor fractures, leading to infraorbital hypesthesia. Fractures may involve the floor, roof, or medial wall or may be more complex, requiring a multidisciplinary approach.

ORBITAL FLOOR FRACTURES

Orbital blowout fractures are those of the orbital floor not involving the orbital rim (see Fig. 5-8). They occur after blunt trauma to the orbit and may cause enophthalmos and diplopia. Controversy exists as to whether fractures should be repaired within 2 weeks, with the aim of achieving less scarring and better repositioning of the globe, or after 4 to 6 weeks, to allow time to assess the degree of enophthalmos and diplopia, possibly obviating the need for surgery (1–3). Surgery is performed to reduce the chances of enophthalmos, globe malposition, or impaired motility. Thus, surgery is strongly recommended for fractures larger than 200 mm^2 or larger than 100 mm^2 and located 1 cm or more behind the rim (4). Immediate repair should be performed for trapdoor entrapment, which occurs when the inferior rectus muscle herniates into the maxillary sinus and is pinched off by a bone fragment. Diplopia requiring strabismus surgery is infrequent (5,6).

Diagnosis

1. Complaints include pain, binocular double vision, and swelling of the lids upon blowing the nose.
2. Perform complete ophthalmic examination to rule out injury to the globe (rupture, hyphema, traumatic iritis).
3. Test infraorbital sensation.
4. Pay careful attention to impaired upgaze. Consider forced ductions.
5. Palpate gently for crepitus or irregularity of the rim.
6. Although difficult, perform exophthalmometry in order to assess the globe position. It may take a few days for the swelling to subside before enophthalmos is evident.
7. Orbital CT scan with axial and coronal cuts is the study of choice.

Management

1. No nose blowing
2. Nasal decongestant spray two times a day for the first 10 days

3. Ice packs for the first 24 to 48 hours.
4. Some physicians recommend oral steroids (7)
5. Immediate surgical repair is recommended for trapdoor entrapment. Otherwise, surgical repair is recommended for persistent diplopia at 2 weeks, cosmetically significant enophthalmos, and large fractures (see below for repair procedure).

MEDIAL ORBITAL WALL FRACTURE

The lamina papyracea is often fractured along with other orbital structures or in isolation without significant sequelae. Because of the proximity to the ethmoid sinus, orbital emphysema may be present. If air collects in the orbit under a ball valve mechanism after nose blowing, elevated intraorbital and intraocular pressure may compromise optic nerve or retinal blood flow, leading to decreased vision. This can be relieved by aspiration of air through the conjunctiva if there is functional impediment (8). Isolated medial wall fractures do not commonly cause enophthalmos or strabismus. Work-up and management are similar to that for floor fractures (see above). Surgical repair of medial wall fractures is reserved for enophthalmos and medial rectus entrapment.

ORBITAL ROOF FRACTURES

Orbital roof fractures may be associated with pneumocephalus, intracranial injury, and cerebrospinal fluid leak, and they may be complicated by infection, leading to complications involving meningitis or abscess formation. They should be evaluated in conjunction with a neurosurgeon. Traumatic optic neuropathy should be ruled out. Ptosis, pain, and limitation of supraduction, secondary to hematoma, superior rectus entrapment, or depressed bony fragments, may be present. CT scan of the orbits and brain is the imaging study of choice. Indications for surgical repair include bony displacement leading to impaired motility, vision loss, or globe malposition. Simple roof fractures that limit motility and do not involve the inner table of the skull may be explored through a brow incision, upper lid blepharoplasty incision, or existing laceration (9,10). With significant basilar skull fractures involving the inner table with displacement of tissue into the orbit or out of the orbit, a coronal exposure, requiring an incision in the coronal plane from the superior aspect of each ear across the vertex, is indicated to reduce the fracture and release incarcerated tissue (10,11). Neurosurgical procedures can be performed simultaneously.

Procedure: Repair of Orbital Floor (Blowout) Fracture

1. After informed consent is obtained, the patient is taken to the operating room, where general anesthesia is administered. Forced ductions may then be performed and compared with the fellow eye (see Fig. 3-3).

2. A subciliary or transconjunctival forniceal incision can be performed:
   • A subciliary incision is followed by dissections through the pretarsal orbicularis extending inferiorly to the orbital rim anterior to the orbital septum. One may administer a suborbicularis injection of 2% xylocaine with 1:100,000 epinephrine.
   • If an inferior transconjunctival cul de sac incision is preferred, the globe is protected with a malleable retractor as the lower lid is retracted with a Demarres retractor. A scalpel or cautery is then used to incise through the conjunctiva to the periosteum of the orbital rim.
3. Retractors are placed in order to expose the periosteum of the inferior orbital rim. A 6-0 silk lid traction suture is placed in the lid margin of the lower lid and retracted superiorly if a subciliary incision has been used.

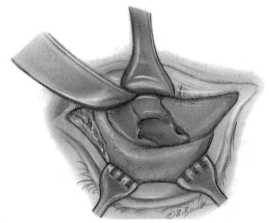

A

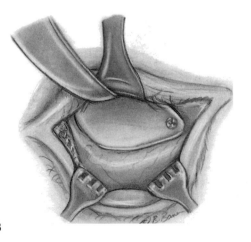

B

FIG. 9–2. Orbital floor (blowout) fracture repair. A transconjuctival approach has been performed. **A:** The periosteum is elevated to expose the fracture. **B:** A nylon implant has been secured to the floor with a titanium screw to cover the defect.

4. The periosteum is incised using a no. 15 Bard-Parker blade and elevated to expose the anterior, medial, and lateral aspects of the fracture (Fig. 9–2A). Identify the infraorbital nerve in order to avoid further damage.
5. Gently lift prolapsed tissue out of the fracture site in a hand-over-hand maneuver. Bone fragments may be removed using small rongeurs in order to facilitate tissue repositioning.
6. Design a nylon 0.5- to 0.8-mm implant that will cover the defect. Keep in mind that the distance from the orbital rim to the optic foramen varies from 45 to 55 mm. Secure the implant to the floor with a single titanium screw or to the rim with wire or 5-0 proline suture material (Fig. 9–2B).
7. Repeat force ductions and release any further incarcerated tissue if restriction is present.
8. Irrigate the operative site with antibiotic solution.
9. Close the skin with running 8-0 silk or 6-0 nylon sutures. If a transconjunctival approach was used, close initially with one 7-0 Vicryl suture. Secure the traction suture to the forehead with sterile strips for 24 to 48 hours to minimize lower lid vertical shortening.
10. Postoperatively, as soon as the patient is awake, check for light perception through the lid as well as visual acuity, color vision, and pupillary reactivity after the traction suture is removed. If evidence of a new postoperative optic neuropathy is present, the possibilities include orbital hemorrhage or impingement on the nerve by the implant. The patient should return immediately to the operating room for exploration.
11. Oral antibiotics are administered for 7 to 10 days.

COMPLEX ORBITAL FRACTURES

These fractures are generally repaired by plastic surgeons, otolaryngologists, or maxillofacial surgeons. The ophthalmologist's role is to determine the presence of ocular trauma or motility restriction. After repair of naso-orbital-ethmoid complex fractures, nasolacrimal obstruction is common and may require repair (12).

LeFort I: This fracture extends horizontally across the maxilla at the base of the nasal septum, not involving the orbit (Fig. 9–3A).

LeFort II: This fracture extends from the nasofrontal suture along the nasal bridge to the medial wall at the level of the cribiform plate, posteriorly into the orbital floor, and through the maxillary sinus. Associated findings include epistaxis, cerebrospinal fluid rhinorrhea, enophthalmos, traumatic optic neuropathy, enophthalmos, and vertical dystopia (Fig. 9–3B).

LeFort III: This fracture is a disarticulation of the facial skeleton from the base of the skull. It extends from the nasofrontal suture to the medial orbital wall at the level of the cribriform plate, along the orbital floor, following the inferior border of the greater wing of the sphenoid, and across the lateral wall, through the zygomatic arch and pterygoid plates (Fig. 9–3C).

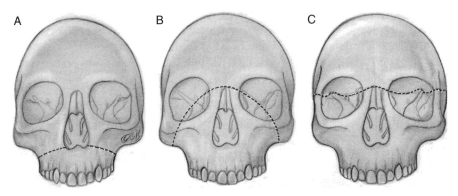

FIG. 9–3. A: LeFort I fracture. **B:** LeFort II fracture. **C:** LeFort III fracture.

Naso-orbital-ethmoid fractures: These involve medial orbital wall, nasal, and ethmoidal bones. Collapse of the sinuses with widening of the nasal bridge, telecanthus, enophthalmos, and medial rectus entrapment may be present.

TRAUMATIC MYOPATHY

Direct injury to extraocular muscle may occur after blunt or penetrating trauma leading to impaired motility. Isolated muscle injury may be secondary to edema, hemorrhage, laceration (13), or avulsion of the muscle from its insertion (14). One of the most commonly lacerated muscles is the inferior rectus.

Diagnosis

1. Consider the possibility of traumatic myopathy with penetrating injuries.
2. Impaired ductions and versions are present with unrestricted motility on forced ductions in the case of lacerations or avulsions. Restriction may develop with time due to contracture of the antagonist of the injured muscle. Deviations are in the range of 30 prism diopters with inferior rectus lacerations.
3. CT of orbits with axial and coronal views is the study of choice.

Management

Repair is performed by reattachment of the lacerated ends of the muscle or tendon. When the muscle is detached at the insertion, the muscle may be retrieved if the attachment to the intermuscular membrane is intact. If the muscle is lost and reattachment is not possible, repair requires muscle transfer or tendon-splitting techniques (12).

ORBITAL FOREIGN BODY

Orbital foreign bodies are divided into three categories: inorganic nonmetallic, metallic, and organic. These injuries often are work-related or occur in young children during play. Intraorbital foreign bodies may be associated with injury to the globe, extraocular muscles, optic nerve, or other soft tissues. In managing these injuries, the primary concerns are the composition of the object, the mechanical effect of the foreign body, injury caused by the foreign body, and the possibility of infection.

Diagnosis

1. A detailed history should be obtained, with particular attention directed to composition of materials involved, time since injury, and whether the foreign body or a portion of it is recovered.
2. Complete ophthalmic examination should be performed, with particular attention directed to possible entry sites: lid puncture wounds and focal subconjuctival hemorrhages in addition to conjunctival, corneal, or scleral lacerations. Protruding foreign bodies generally should not be removed until the time of surgical repair.
3. Orbital CT with axial and coronal views may be used to detect glass and steel fragments as small as 0.5 mm in diameter (15), but CT is not always effective in locating wood, which may be better localized via magnetic resonance imaging (MRI) (16). MRI is contraindicated if a metallic, magnetic foreign body is suspected.

Management

1. Nails should be considered potentially infectious. Bullets can be considered sterile but are of concern because of possible metallic toxicity. Steel and aluminum are well tolerated. Copper causes a sterile, suppurative inflammatory reaction and should be removed. Copper alloys, such as brass or bronze, and copper-coated steel BB pellets are better tolerated. Iron-containing orbital foreign bodies can theoretically cause ocular toxicity but are generally well tolerated. However, their presence is a contraindication to MRI. Although retained lead pellets may lead to increased blood levels of lead or systemic lead toxicity, a small number of lead pellets retained in the orbit are generally well tolerated. BBs and shotgun pellets may or may not contain lead; thus the content of the projectiles should be determined (17).
2. Stone, glass, and plastic are well tolerated.
3. Wood causes an acute suppurative inflammatory response and may cause bacterial or fungal infection. Prompt removal with culture is recommended.
4. Large objects or objects that cause mechanical impairment or compression of the optic nerve should be removed.

5. Tetanus toxoid 0.5 ml intramuscularly should be administered if neccessary (see Table 4–2).

6. Prophylaxis with broad-spectrum antibiotics, even with metallic foreign bodies, should be used (metallic, amoxicillin/clavulanate 250 to 500 mg orally every 8 hours for 10 to 14 days; organic, ceftazidime 2 g intravenously every 12 hours and clindamycin 600 mg intravenously every 8 hours for 4 to 10 days followed by oral antibiotic, e.g., amoxicillin/clavulanate, for completion of a 10- to 14-day course).

7. Indications for surgical management include evidence of infection, severe inflammatory reaction, fistula formation, impingement on structures (i.e., optic nerve compression), and large protruding objects.

REFERENCES

1. Holt JE, Holt GR, Blodgett JM. Ocular injuries sustained during blunt facial trauma. *Ophthalmology* 1983;90:14–18.
2. Manson PN, Iliff NT. Management of blow-out fractures of the orbital floor. II. Early repair of selected injuries. *Surv Ophthalmol* 1991;35:280–292.
3. Putterman AM. Management of blow-out fractures of the orbital floor. III. Conservative approach. *Surv Ophthalmol* 1991;35:292–8.
4. Iwamoto MA, Iliff NT. Management of orbital trauma. In: Tasman W, Jaeger EA, eds. *Duane's Clinical Ophthalmology.* Vol. 6. Philadelphia: JB Lippincott; 1993.
5. Putterman AM, Stevens T, Urist MJ. Non-surgical management of blowout fractures of the orbital floor. *Am J Ophthalmol* 1974;77:232–9.
6. Helveston EM. The relationship of extraocular muscle problems to orbital floor fractures: early and late management. *Trans Am Acad Ophthalmol Otolaryngol* 1977;83:660–2..
7. Millman AI, Della Roca RC, Spector S, et al. Steroids and orbital blow-out fractures. A new systemic concept in medical management and surgical decision making. *Adv Ophthalmic Plast Reconstr Surg* 1987;6:291–300.
8. Segrest DR, Dortzbach RK. Medial orbital wall fractures: complications and management. *Ophthalm Plast Reconstr Surg* 1989;5:75–80.
9. Coleman CC, Troland CE. The surgical treatment of spontaneous cerebrospinal rhinorrhea. *Ann Surg* 1947;125:718–28.
10. Manson PN, Iliff NT. Fractures of the orbital roof. In: Hornblass A, ed. *Oculoplastic, Orbital, and Reconstructive Surgery.* Vol. 2. Baltimore: Williams & Wilkins; 1990.
11. Flanagan JC, McLachlan DL, Shannon GM. Orbital roof fractures. Neurologic and neurosurgical considerations. *Ophthalmology* 1980;87:325–9.
12. Gruss JS, Hurwitz JJ, Nik, et al. The pattern and incidence of nasolacrimal injury in naso-orbital-ethmoidal fractures: the role of delayed assessment and dacryocystorhinostomy. *Br J Plast Surg* 1970;12:339–46.
13. Helveston EM, Grossman RD. Extraocular muscle lacerations. *Am J Ophthalmol* 1976;81:754–60.
14. Mailer CM. Avulsion of the inferior rectus. *Can J Ophthal* 1974;9:262–6.
15. Zinreich SJ, Miller NR, Aguayo JB, et al. Computed tomographic three-dimensional localization and composition evaluation of intraocular and orbital foreign bodies. *Arch Ophthalmol* 1986;104:1477–82.
16. Green BF, Kraft SP, Carter KD, et al. Intraorbital wood: Detection by magnetic resonance imaging. *Ophthalmology* 1990;97:608–11.
17. Keeny AH. Orbital foreign body management. *Trans New Orleans Acad Ophthalmol* 1974;22:14–23.

Management of Ocular Injuries and Emergencies,
edited by Mathew W. MacCumber.
Lippincott–Raven Publishers, Philadelphia ©1998.

10

Infections of the Lacrimal System, Eyelids, and Orbit

Srinivas R. Sadda and Nicholas T. Iliff

*Department of Ophthalmology, Wilmer Eye Institute, The Johns Hopkins University
School of Medicine, Baltimore, Maryland 21287*

Lacrimal System Infections   117
   Basic Considerations   117 · Dacryoadenitis   117 · Canaliculitis   119
   Dacryocystitis   121
Infections of the Lids   124
   Blepharitis   124 · Hordeolum   125 · Preseptal Cellulitis   126
Orbital Cellulitis   130
   Etiology/Microbiology   131 · Diagnosis   131 · Management   132

LACRIMAL SYSTEM INFECTIONS

Basic Considerations

The lacrimal system includes the lacrimal gland and the lacrimal drainage system. This system may be predisposed to infection by two major risk factors: (a) reduced tear production and (b) obstruction of tear outflow (1). All components of the system are susceptible to infection.

Dacryoadenitis

Dacryoadenitis (infection of the lacrimal gland) is a rare entity with both acute suppurative and chronic forms.

Acute Suppurative Dacryoadenitis

Etiology

The most common cause is *Staphylococcus aureus.* Other causes include streptococci, *Chlamydia trachomatis,* and *Neisseria gonorrhoeae* (1). Nonsuppurative forms of acute dacryoadenitis may occur and are typically due to inflammatory pseuodotumor (see Chapter 11).

117

The differential diagnosis includes severe blepharitis, preseptal cellulitis, and orbital cellulitis.

Diagnosis

1. Symptoms: sudden unilateral pain, swelling, and redness at the lateral aspect of the upper eyelid, often with epiphora and discharge. Fever and malaise are not uncommon.
2. Signs: tenderness, erythema, and swelling over the lateral aspect of the upper lid. Enlarged lacrimal gland may be palpable. Purulent discharge may appear beneath the lid. The conjunctiva is often injected, most prominently over the lacrimal gland. The patient may be febrile. Preauricular lymphadenopathy may be present.
3. Perform complete ophthalmic examination, including motility examination, exophthalmometry, and intraocular pressure (rule out preseptal or orbital cellulitis). Palpate the eyelid for fluctuance suggesting abscess formation. Also palpate for preauricular lymph nodes.
4. Check vital signs (especially temperature).
5. Perform Gram stain and culture analyses on any discharge. Also obtain blood cultures and a complete blood count with differential if the patient is febrile.

Management

1. For mild to moderate cases oral antibiotics are usually sufficient. One suggested regimen is Augmentin (SmithKline Beecham) (amoxicillin/clavulanate):
   • Adults: 250 to 500 mg (depending on severity) orally every 8 hours
   • Children: 20 to 40 mg/kg/day orally in three divided doses
2. For severe cases intravenous (i.v.) antibiotics are necessary. One suggested regimen is i.v. oxacillin (2):
   • Adults: 1 to 2 g i.v. every 4 hours
   • Children 100 to 200 mg/kg/day (divided every 6 hours), maximum 12 g/day
   Antibiotics are to be adjusted based on culture/sensitivity data. Antibiotics can be changed from i.v. to oral when clear, consistent improvement is seen. A total of 10 to 14 days of systemic antibiotics should be given.
3. Patients should initially be followed daily to look for signs of orbital cellulitis or abscess formation. Lacrimal gland abscesses require incision and drainage.
4. Systemic steroids are indicated in cases of inflammatory pseudotumor. This diagnosis should be considered in patients who fail to respond to antibiotics (see Chapter 11).

Chronic Dacryoadenitis

Etiology

The cause is usually viral, with mumps being the most frequent instigator (especially in children). Epstein-Barr virus, cytomegalovirus, coxsackievirus, echoviruses, and varicella-zoster virus (VZV) infections also are seen.

A variety of fungi also can cause chronic dacryoadenitis. Granulomatous infection of the lacrimal gland can occur (due to tuberculosis, leprosy, or syphilis) (1). Noninfectious inflammations of the lacrimal gland, such as sarcoidosis, Sjogren's syndrome, tumor infiltration (lymphoma), and primary lacrimal gland tumors also occur, but are not discussed here.

Diagnosis

1. Symptoms: slowly progressive, often painless, swelling at the lateral aspect of the upper lid.
2. Signs: swelling, minimal if any tenderness. With viral infection there is typically no fever or signs of systemic toxicity. With granulomatous infections, findings due to involvement of other areas of the eye and adnexa may be seen (e.g., choroidal granuloma in tuberculosis).
3. Perform a complete ophthalmic examination, including visual acuity, color vision, pupillary responses, visual fields, motility examination, exophthalmometry, biomicroscopy, intraocular pressure, and ophthalmoscopy.
4. Smear (including staining with acid-fast bacillus, KOH, Giemsa) and culture (viral, fungal, mycobacterial) the discharge if present (rare).
5. Consider obtaining results of testing with purified protein derivative with anergy panel, chest x-ray, and rapid plasma reagin (RPR) fluorescent treponemal antibody-absorption (FTA-Abs).
6. Workup for noninfectious causes may be required (this may include computed tomography [CT] of the orbit, internal medicine consultation and systemic investigation (for malignancy), or lacrimal gland biopsy.

Management

1. Symptomatic: warm compresses four times daily, frequent artificial tears; one can also consider topical antibiotics (e.g., Polytrim (Allergan) four times daily) for prophylaxis against bacterial superinfection.
2. Definitive therapy depends on the cause (however, the cause is frequently viral and no additional therapy is available).

Canaliculitis

Primary canaliculitis may or may not be related to obstruction of the nasolacrimal passages. It may follow manipulation of the nasolacrimal passages or may be secondary to implanted material (e.g., silicone or plastic tubing) (1). However, canaliculitis usually occurs without a known antecedent problem. Also, a secondary canaliculitis can develop from contiguous spread of infection from the conjunctiva or lacrimal sac (3).

Etiology

Anaerobic bacteria are the primary cause of canaliculitis, and *Actinomyces israelii* (previously known as streptothrix) and *Propionibacterium proprionicum* (both Gram-positive filamentous bacteria) are by far the most common organisms. Another causative anaerobe is *Fusobacterium nucleotum.* Fungal, viral (e.g., herpes simplex [HSV], herpes zoster [HZV]), chlamydial, and a multitude of other bacterial (e.g., *Nocardia*) infections of the canaliculus also have been reported (3).

Diagnosis

1. Symptoms: epiphora, itching, irritation of eyes.
2. Signs: swelling and pouting of the punctum, unilateral conjunctivitis with conjunctival injection most prominent nasally, mucopurulent material at the medial canthus, follicles, and swollen occasionally tender canaliculus (Fig. 10–1). In advanced cases, canalicular diverticuli can form, and even spontaneous fistulization can occur (3).
3. In one series it has been reported to more frequently involve the lower canaliculus (4), although either upper or lower can be involved.
4. Pressure over the punctum may allow expression of purulent discharge and concretions. Material should be smeared (KOH preparation, Gram stain, Giemsa stain) and cultured (anaerobic, fungal, and aerobic, although aerobic cultures are usually of no value in canaliculitis).
   - The appearance of the concretions also may suggest the causative organisms:
   - Yellowish, cheesy concretions are typical of *Actinomyces israeilii* infections. On Gram stain of the concretions, *Actinomyces israeilii* are seen as thin, branching, Gram-positive filaments.
   - Rubbery concretions may suggest *Candida* infection.
   - Blackish brown debris is characteristic of *Aspergillus niger* (3).
5. A dacryocystogram (not required) may show irregularity of the canalicular epithelium and may show diverticuli or filling defects due to concretions (3).

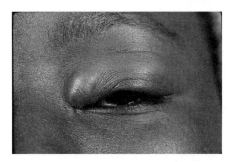

FIG. 10–1. Canaliculitis.

Management

1. The critical aspect of treatment is the removal of as much inspissated material as possible (5). Surgical incision of the canaliculus is indicated: a probe is inserted into the canaliculus and an incision is made into the canaliculus through the adjacent conjunctiva. This is followed by curettage of all concretions. Occasionally, curettage through the punctum is possible.
2. Antibiotic therapy, although controversial, may be helpful. Consider instillation/irrigation of the canaliculus with penicillin G (100,000 U/ml) after surgery and/or curettage of the canaliculus. Topical penicillin drops or erythromycin, both four times daily, are then used for 1 to 2 weeks. Also consider a 7- to 10-day course of oral antibiotics. Antibiotic therapy is adjusted based on culture results: *Actinomyces israellii* is usually sensitive to penicillin, erythromycin, and bacitracin; *Nocardia* is usually susceptible to trimethoprim/sulfamethoxazole.

Dacryocystitis

Infection of the nasolacrimal sac is largely a disease of infants and middle-aged adults. In the latter group, women are affected four times as often as men. In both age groups, nasolacrimal duct obstruction is the major factor leading to infection; in a minority of cases, however, dacryocystitis may develop secondary to spread from contiguous structures (nasal, sinus, or conjunctival infections). Both acute and chronic forms of dacryocystitis can be seen.

Causes of obstruction are numerous:

1. Chronic inflammation/fibrosis
2. Nasal/sinus disease (mechanical obstruction from structural defects [e.g., deviated septum, enlarged inferior turbinate or inflammatory or hypertrophic disease of the nasal mucosa)
3. External compression from neoplasms (e.g., paranasal sinus tumor)
4. Primary tumor of the lacrimal sac
5. Trauma (iatrogenic [nasal/sinus/orbital surgery, probing of the lacrimal duct system] and noniatrogenic [e.g., mid-facial trauma])
6. Systemic diseases (e.g., Wegener's granulomatosis, sarcoid)
7. Congenital variations (e.g., narrow osseous canal)
8. Dacryoliths (3)

Differential diagnosis includes sinusitis, preseptal/facial cellulitis, and orbital cellulitis.

Etiology/Microbiology

Gram-positive cocci are the most frequent causative organisms, with staphylococcal species (aureus and epidermidis) being the most common, followed by *Strep-*

tococcus pneumoniae. Gram-negative infections (usually *Pseudomonas aerugi-nosa* or *Escherichia coli*) also may occur. Anaerobes are rare causes. Fungal infections (most commonly *Candida albicans*) also may be seen (3,6).

Diagnosis

1. Symptoms: pain, swelling, erythema in the medial canthal region. Pain may radiate to the top of the head, jaw, or to the ear (7). In chronic cases, pain may or may not be present, and erythema is usually less apparent.
2. Signs: swelling (initially diffuse, but eventually localizing to a point under medial canthal ligament); erythema of overlying skin, and lower lid and cheek, point tenderness below the medial canthal ligament (Fig. 10–2). Discharge is often not expressible because swelling of the sac closes off the common canaliculus.
3. Complications may ensue if untreated and include mucocele/pyocele, orbital cellulitis, corneal involvement, and perforation through the skin with fistula formation.
4. A complete ophthalmic examination is essential, including evaluation for orbital cellulitis.
5. Smear and culture any discharge.

Management

1. Broad-spectrum systemic antibiotics with staphylococcal coverage should be instituted until the culture and sensitivity data are available. Although a fluoroquinolone (norfloxacin) was effective against the greatest percentage of staphylococcal species (both aureus and epidermidis) in Huber-Spitzy's study (8), a penicillinase-resistant penicillin or second-generation cephalosporin is usually the starting point for therapy. One suggested empirical regimen is Augmentin (SmithKline Beecham), 250 to 500 mg orally three times daily in adults, and 20 to 40 mg/kg/day divided every 8 hours in children. Intravenous antibiotics (e.g., oxacillin) may be required for severe cases and in toxic- appearing patients. Antibiotics are adjusted based on culture results, but a total course of 1 to 2 weeks should be completed.

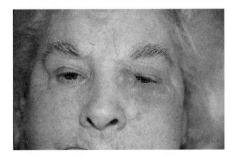

FIG. 10–2. Acute dacryocystitis.

2. Patients with moderate to severe cases also may require incision and drainage to decompress the sac. The sac should then be irrigated with antibiotic solution.
3. Topical antibiotic preparations have a more minor role, but also should be instituted; e.g., bacitracin or erythromycin ointment or Polytrim (Allergan) drops, both four times daily.
4. Warm compresses for 10 to 15 minutes, followed by digital massage over the lacrimal sac four times daily.
5. Patients are followed frequently (up to daily as severity dictates) until clear, consistent improvement is seen (they are then seen less frequently).
6. In chronic dacryocystitis (commonly due to anaerobes such as *Actinomyces*), systemic antibiotics are usually not necessary. However, acute exacerbations can be treated as noted above.
7. Definitive treatment for acute or chronic dacryocystitis is dacryocystorhinostomy (9). This can be performed in the acute phase but is more easily performed after the acute episode has resolved.

Neonatal Dacryocystitis

This condition is almost always secondary to congenital nasolacrimal duct obstruction (CNDO), occurring in approximately 3% of infants with CNDO.

Etiology

Unlike in adults, *Streptococcus pneumoniae* is the most common causative organism. Staphylococcal species are next most common, with micrococci, *Pseudomonas, Acinetobacter,* and diphtheroids being less common (3).

Diagnosis

1. Symptoms: swelling, erythema, and pus in the medial canthal area; epiphora.
2. Signs: the critical finding is an acutely distended lacrimal sac, which helps distinguish this entity from simple CNDO, in which there can be crusting of the lashes and drainage of mucopurulent material with pressure over the sac. Also, erythema and tenderness over the sac is observed. Low-grade fever may be present.
3. Slit-lamp or penlight examination should be performed.

Management

1. Uncomplicated nasolacrimal obstruction can be treated conservatively with digital massage and warm compresses four times daily. Topical antibiotics (e.g., Polytrim, sodium sulfacetamide, erythromycin twice daily) are added if significant discharge is present.

2. Probing of the nasolacrimal duct is the hallmark of treatment in true cases of neonatal dacryocystitis (3,10).

3. Because significant bacteremia/septicemia has been reported with probing (11), systemic and topical antibiotics (as in older patients) should be used. Antibiotic therapy may be initiated before probing. For Augmentin (amoxicillin/clavulanate) in neonates, we suggest 20 to 40 mg/kg/day divided every 8 hours. For i.v. oxacillin we recommend 150 to 200 mg/kg/day divided every 6 hours. For premature infants, consult hospital pharmacy for dosing.

INFECTIONS OF THE LIDS

Blepharitis

Blepharitis may be divided into anterior (predominantly involving the bases of lashes) or posterior (primarily involving the meibomian glands). Blepharitis also may be classified, as recommended by McCulley et al., according to the cause of dysfunction into six categories: staphylococcal, seborrheic, seborrheic with staphylococcal superinfection, seborrheic with meibomian seborrhea, seborrheic with focal secondary meibomanitis, and primary meibomanitis (12). A variety of other organisms aside from staphylococci also may produce blepharitis. Moreover, blepharitis may be caused by allergic reactions (particularly cosmetics).

Differential diagnosis includes keratoconjunctivitis sicca, infectious conjunctivitis, and underlying malignancy (which should be considered in patients with persistent or recurrent unilateral disease).

Etiology/Microbiology

The relationship between infectious organisms and blepharitis is often unclear because many of these organisms are found in equal frequency in both normal individuals and patients with blepharitis. However, the total amount of microbial growth is typically greater in patients with blepharitis (13). Staphylococcal species (especially *S. epidermidis*) are the most common. *Propionibacterium acnes* and corynebacterium species also are seen more commonly in patients with blepharitis than in normal individuals and may be pathogenic.

Other infectious causes of lid infection or blepharitis include viruses (e.g., molluscum contagiosum, HSV, VZV), tuberculosis, leprosy, syphilis (chancre, maculopapular rash, gumma), *Chlamydia, Rickettsia,* fungi (e.g., *Candida,* ringworm, coccidioidomycosis, blastomycosis, sporotrichosis, cryptococcosis, rhinosporidiosis), and parasites (e.g., phthiriasis from *Phthirus pubis,* leishmaniasis, loa loiasis, onchocerciasis, and roundworms [ascariasis]) (14,15).

Diagnosis

1. Symptoms: mild ocular irritation frequently with foreign body sensation, eyelid erythema, crusting, tearing, itching; usually bilateral.

2. Signs: erythema of the lid margins, scale, crusts, collarettes around the cilia, madarosis or trichiasis (if chronic), notching of the lid margin, plugging of meibomian gland orifices. May have an associated papillary conjunctivitis. Punctate epithelial keratopathy (PEK), most prominently at the inferior limbus. Less commonly may be associated with phlyctenules, marginal infiltrates/ulcers (due to staphylococcal hypersensitivity), and Salzmann's nodules (14,15). Features of rosacea may be seen: rhinophyma, mid-facial erythema/"malar rash," telangiectasias, and recurrent papules/pustules on the face.

3. Some signs may suggest specific diagnosis (e.g., umbilicated papule in molluscum, or nits on the lashes in phthiriasis).

Treatment

Goals are to control symptoms and prevent secondary complications:

1. Eyelid hygiene measures are the cornerstone of treatment:
   - Warm compresses: to be applied over closed eyelids for 10 to 15 minutes with the cloth rewarmed (by running through hot water) as it cools. This helps increase the fluidity of the meibum and loosens the debris from the bases of the lashes.
   - To remove the secretions, follow compresses with lid scrubs: baby shampoo diluted with water (one drop baby shampoo in cup of water) on a cotton ball or clean cloth (we prefer this over a cotton-tipped applicator).
   - These measures should be performed two to four times daily.
2. Topical antibiotic (erythromycin or bacitracin) following lid scrubs twice daily.
3. Tetracycline 250 mg orally four times daily or doxycycline 100 mg orally twice daily is added for patients with rosacea or chronic blepharitis not responding to conservative measures. For pregnant or breast-feeding women and children under 12, erythromycin is substituted. Alternatively, topical fusidic acid 1% gel twice daily may be used, and this has been found to be more effective than oxytetracycline in patients with rosacea and blepharitis. Of note, the combination of fusidic acid and oral tetracycline derivatives has been found to be less effective than either alone (16).
4. Artificial tears five to six times daily in patients with PEK.
5. Specific therapy in certain patients: e.g., for phthiriasis, mechanical removal of nits and application of yellow mercuric oxide 1% ophthalmic ointment or physostigmine ointment.
6. Intense acute therapy is usually required for 2 to 6 weeks. Antibiotics should be tapered as soon as possible once patient responds to treatment. Maintenance therapy (e.g., warm compresses and lid scrubs daily or every other day) is usually required.

Hordeolum

A hordeolum (stye) is an acute localized inflammation of the glands of Zeis (external or anterior hordeolum) or meibomian glands (internal or posterior hordeolum). A chalazion is a cyst of the meibomian gland that, if inflamed or infected, can become an internal hordeolum.

Etiology

Hordeola are usually infectious (most commonly staphylococcal species), often presenting in association with blepharitis. However, sterile inflammation of an obstructed gland also may occur.

Diagnosis

1. Symptoms: acute onset of a localized eyelid mass or bump often with erythema, mild pain, and tenderness.
2. Signs: palpable, frequently visible nodule within the lid, often with overlying erythema and even pustular appearance. Localized eyelid tenderness.
3. Sebaceous cell carcinoma is in the differential and must be considered in cases of recurrent chalazion. Preseptal cellulitis also must be ruled out.

Management

1. Warm compresses for 15 minutes three to four times daily.
2. Gentle massage over hordeolum three times daily.
3. Erythromycin ointment twice daily.
4. If conservative therapy is ineffective after 4 to 6 weeks, one can consider an incision and drainage procedure or standard chalazion excision (Fig. 10–3). However, with lesions near the lacrimal drainage system, steroid (triamcinolone) injection may be tried.

Procedure: Chalazion Excision, Posterior Approach

1. Infiltrate tissue around chalazion with 2% lidocaine with epinephrine.
2. Apply small chalazion clamp over chalazion and tighten.
3. Evert eyelid with the clamp (17).
4. Vertical incision into chalazion with a no. 11 Bard-Parker blade (Fig. 10–3*A*).
5. Chalazion cavity is evacuated using a curette (Fig. 10–3*B*).
6. Careful sharp excision of excess fibrous tissue may be necessary (Fig. 10–3*C*).
7. Slowly loosen clamp. Firm pressure is used for hemostasis. Coagulation of bleeding points is rarely needed.
8. Instill antibiotic (e.g., Polytrim or erythromycin).

Preseptal Cellulitis

Preseptal cellulitis refers to infection of the soft tissue of the eyelids and periorbital region anterior to the orbital septum. Preseptal cellulitis may be caused by

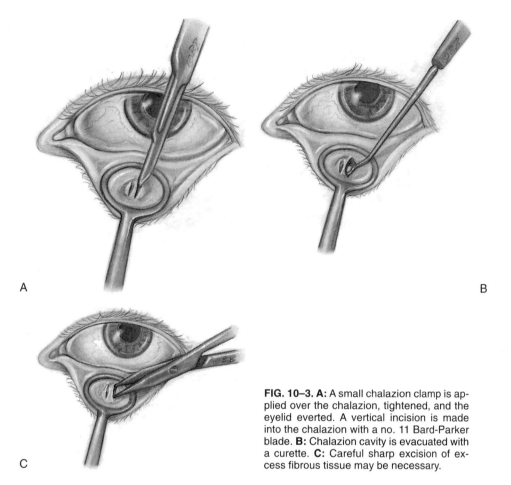

A

B

C

FIG. 10–3. A: A small chalazion clamp is applied over the chalazion, tightened, and the eyelid everted. A vertical incision is made into the chalazion with a no. 11 Bard-Parker blade. **B:** Chalazion cavity is evacuated with a curette. **C:** Careful sharp excision of excess fibrous tissue may be necessary.

eyelid trauma, extraocular infections (of skin), and upper respiratory tract and sinus infections (18).

Differential diagnosis includes orbital cellulitis, cavernous sinus thrombosis, chalazion, dacryocystitis, dacryoadenitis, viral conjunctivitis with lid swelling, angioneurotic edema, and allergic eyelid swelling.

Etiology/Microbiology

1. *Staphylococcus aureus* or *Streptococcus pyogenes* are the usual causes in cases of trauma, with anaerobes and polymicrobial infections being less common.
2. Preseptal cellulitis from associated skin infections may be seen with impetigo (pyoderma due to *S. aureus* or *S. pyogenes* group A), HSV, VZV, and erysipelas (also due to *S. pyogenes* group A) (18). In infants under 9 months of age, a sup-

purative preseptal cellulitis due to *S. aureus* can occur from the contiguous spread of facial cellulitis (usually beginning as infection of the infant's gums, often after contact with a mother with mastitis).

3. Nonsuppurative preseptal cellulitis in children without previous skin infection or trauma is believed to develop from spread from the upper respiratory tract, sinuses, or middle ear and is usually due to *Hemophilus influenzae* type b and *Streptococcus pneumoniae* (18). (Other streptococci and *Staphylococcus aureus* are less common).

Diagnosis

1. Symptoms and signs depend on the etiologic mechanism:
   - Usual features include eyelid edema (may be severe enough to produce ptosis), warmth, erythema, and tenderness (Fig. 10–4A).
   - Distinctive signs may suggest specific etiology. Foul-smelling discharge or necrosis may indicate anaerobic infection. Staphylococcal infection usually produces purulent discharge, whereas *Hemophilus* infection is typically nonpurulent (nonsuppurative), with a bluish purple discoloration of the lid. Sharply demarcated, bright red elevated plaque is typical of erysipelas. Characteristic vesicles of HSV and VZV may be seen. Vesicles and a thick golden or honey-colored crust may suggest impetigo (18).

2. Obtain a careful history, including history of prior trauma, skin infection, upper respiratory infection, or sinusitis. Also, inquire whether there is any pain with eye movements, diplopia, or loss of vision.

3. Complete ophthalmic examination, including visual acuity, color vision, pupillary responses, visual fields, ocular motility, exophthalmometry, slit-lamp examination, intraocular pressure, and ophthalmoscopy, is critical and can eliminate the other entities in the differential. Absence of the critical signs of orbital cellulitis is an important finding. In preseptal cellulitis due to erysipelas, the soft tissues of the orbit may become inflamed from diffusion of bacterial toxins

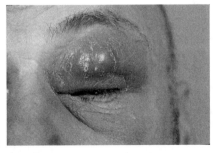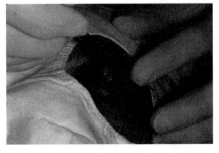

A   B

FIG. 10–4. A: Preseptal cellulitis with abscess (courtesy of Dr. K. Packo). **B:** Surgical drainage of abscess (courtesy of Dr. K. Packo).

(and not invasion of the organism), thus producing chemosis, mild proptosis, and limitation of motion (which can mimic orbital cellulitis).

4. Consider a CT scan to exclude orbital involvement, particularly when examination of the globe is limited by severe lid edema, or there is a possibility of penetration of the orbital septum (especially in cases of trauma).

5. Culture and Gram stain all potential infectious sources:
   - Wound discharge (if present) in cases of eyelid trauma
   - Suppurative material from incision and drainage
   - Culture nose, oropharynx, and conjunctiva in preseptal cellulitis associated with upper respiratory tract infections
   - Blood cultures in febrile patients
   - Culture/smear vesicular fluid or vesicle base (including Tzank smear or viral culture if appropriate) in cases of suspected impetigo or herpes simplex

Management

1. Tetanus prophylaxis should be administered in cases of trauma, if indicated (see Table 4–2).

2. Incision and drainage may be required in suppurative cases (Fig. 10–4*B*) (18):
   - This can be performed in the minor procedure room; general anesthesia may be required in children.
   - Local infiltrative anesthesia should be avoided because this may spread infection.
   - The incision should be kept as small as possible while still allowing adequate drainage. Usually a 1- to 3-cm (depending on the size of the suppurative area) incision through the skin over the fluctuant area is sufficient. Alternatively, in cases of trauma, the wound site can be widened. Penetration of the septum must be avoided.
   - Purulent material should be directly inoculated onto appropriate media (including anaerobic medium, chocolate agar, blood agar) for culture, and slides for Gram stain.
   - After drainage, one can consider packing the cavity with an iodoform wick for 24 hours. The end of the wick should be trimmed to allow a 1- to 2-cm tail to extend out of the wound to facilitate drainage.

3. In cases of (a) moderate to severe preseptal cellulitis, (b) a toxic-appearing patient, (c) a child less than 5 years of age, or (d) an immunocompromised patient, admission to the hospital for i.v. antibiotic therapy is recommended. Otherwise, cases of mild preseptal cellulitis in an immunocompetent patient over the age of 5 years can be managed with oral antibiotics as an outpatient.

4. Antibiotics are chosen based on Gram stain findings (18):
   - Gram positive: i.v. oxacillin (or other penicillinase-resistant penicillin). Vancomycin can be substituted in penicillin-allergic patients. In cases of erysipelas, i.v. penicillin G for 3 days followed by oral penicillin for an additional week is sufficient therapy.

- Gram negative: i.v. aminoglycoside (e.g., tobramycin) or oral ciprofloxacin is usually sufficient therapy. For *Hemophilus* infection (most commonly in children), cefuroxime (or other second-generation cephalosporin), or ceftazidime (or other third-generation cephalosporin) is recommended.
- Empirical therapy with broad-spectrum antibiotics is necessary when Gram stain is unavailable or inconclusive. One suggested regimen consists of clindamycin 600 mg i.v. every 8 hours and ceftazidime 2 g i.v. every 12 hours for adults, and clindamycin 25 to 40 mg/kg/day i.v. divided every 6 to 8 hours and 100 to 150 mg/kg/day i.v. divided every 8 hours (maximum dosage 6 g/day) for children. This regimen will cover most Gram positives, Gram negatives, and anaerobes; vancomycin may be added if there is suspicion for methicillin-resistant *S. aureus* (consult hospital pharmacy for neonatal dosages). Once clear, consistent improvement is demonstrated, one can switch to oral therapy to complete a total 10- to 14-day course of antibiotics. One suggested empiric oral antibiotic choice is Augmentin (SmithKline Beecham) 250 to 500 mg orally three times daily in adults and 20 to 40 mg/kg/day divided every 8 hours in children.

5. Consider infectious disease consultation for immunocompromised patients and patients who fail to improve with therapy.
6. For VZV/HZV-associated preseptal cellulitis in adults: if the patient presents within 72 hours of symptom onset, they should be treated with oral acyclovir (400 to 800 mg) five times daily for 10 days. In immunocompromised patients, i.v. therapy is recommended. Although controversial, there may be a role for steroids in HZV infection.
7. For HSV-associated preseptal cellulitis, efficacy of oral acyclovir therapy is uncertain. Topical acyclovir 5% ointment four times daily may be used.
8. Add bacitracin ointment three times daily to skin lesions in cases of impetigo. This also can be used prophylactically in cases of HSV/VZV to prevent bacterial superinfection.
9. Follow-up: When treated as an outpatient, the patient is observed daily (and watched for signs of orbital involvement) until consistent improvement is evident. Then the patient is followed every 2 to 7 days (depending on severity) until the infection is completely resolved.

ORBITAL CELLULITIS

Orbital cellulitis is an infection of the soft tissue within the orbit, posterior to the orbital septum characterized by infiltration of the orbital tissues by the causative organism(s), inflammatory cells, and edema. Although uncommon, when compared with preseptal cellulitis, its identification is critical given its various ocular and systemic complications, which include exposure keratopathy due to proptosis, neurotrophic keratitis, central retinal artery occlusion, optic neuritis or atrophy, subperiosteal or orbital abscess, cavernous sinus thrombosis, meningitis, brain abscess, and sepsis (18,19).

Orbital cellulitis is most commonly seen in association with sinusitis (in over 90% of cases), particularly ethmoidal disease. The orbital tissues are more susceptible to infection for two reasons: (a) their close proximity to the paranasal sinuses and (b) interconnection between the venous system of the orbit and face (the valveless nature of the orbital venous system compounds this risk). Less common causes of orbital cellulitis include penetrating orbital trauma (especially with retained foreign body), dental infections, dacryocystitis, extraocular or retinal surgery, and hematogenous spread during a systemic infection.

The differential diagnosis includes cavernous sinus thrombosis, orbital pseudotumor, orbital myositis, dysthyroid ophthalmopathy, rhabdomyosarcoma, retinoblastoma, metastatic carcinoma, and infiltrative disorders (leukemia, lymphoma, histiocytosis X, Wegener's granulomatosis) (18).

Etiology/Microbiology

The most common agents in orbital cellulitis associated with sinusitis include *S. pneumoniae*, other streptococci, *S. aureus*, and *H. influenzae* (especially in children); anaerobes are less common.

Staphylococcus aureus is the usual cause in posttraumatic and postsurgical cases, with anaerobes again less common. Polymicrobial infections may occur in all settings. Fungal infections (mucormycosis [species of *Absidia, Rhizopus, Mucor*] and aspergillosis) are rare and are mainly seen in diabetics (in ketoacidosis), children with severe dehydration and metabolic acidosis due to vomiting and diarrhea, and immunocompromised patients (18).

Diagnosis

1. Symptoms: lid edema, erythema, orbital pain, pain on eye movement, diplopia, decreased vision, fever, headache, symptoms of sinusitis (rhinorrhea, sinus pressure)
2. History of sinusitis, trauma, surgery, and dental infections should be ascertained.
3. Signs: conjunctival chemosis and injection, lid edema and erythema, proptosis, and limited ocular motility (Fig. 10–5); may have afferent pupillary defect, reduced color vision, elevated intraocular pressure, diminished sensation in V_1 distribution, resistance to retropulsion, and retinal venous congestion.
4. Typical signs usually appear within 2 to 3 days in cases secondary to trauma but may be delayed for weeks or months in the setting of retained foreign body (18). Signs of postsurgical orbital cellulitis are usually apparent by postoperative day 2 or 3.
5. Complete ophthalmic examination, including visual acuity, color vision, pupillary responses, visual fields, ocular motility, cranial nerve examination (especially V_1, V_2), exophthalmometry, slit-lamp examination, intraocular pressure, and ophthalmoscopy, is required in these patients.
6. Check vital signs, and obtain complete blood count with differential (fever and leukocytosis are commonly present) and blood cultures. Gram stain and culture any discharge (e.g., from nose in patients with sinusitis).

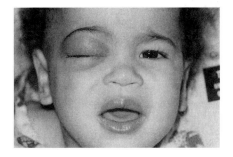

FIG. 10–5. Orbital cellulitis with SPA secondary to ethmoiditis (courtesy of Dr. K. Packo).

7. CT scan of orbits (and brain), including axial and coronal cuts, is required to look for intraorbital or subperiosteal abscess (SPA).
8. Fungal infections (particularly mucormycosis) should be considered in patients with diabetes mellitus (and ketoacidosis), immunosuppression, or children with dehydration and metabolic acidosis.
9. Cavernous sinus thrombosis (CST) should be considered in patients with rapid progression of signs/symptoms. Also, contralateral orbital congestion may develop in patients with CST.
10. Ear, nose, and throat (ENT) consultation is suggested in cases likely related to sinusitis. Aspiration of sinus material for culture may be helpful. Needle aspiration of the orbit is contraindicated.
11. Pediatric consultation is recommended in children.
12. Neurology consultation and lumbar puncture is suggested when symptoms (altered mental status, neurologic deficits) or signs (nuchal rigidity) of meningitis are present.

Management

1. Admit to the hospital.
2. Tetanus prophylaxis should be administered in posttraumatic cases, if indicated (see Table 4–2).
3. Intravenous antibiotics are initiated empirically or based on Gram stain results of any available discharge/infectious material. One suggested regimen includes clindamycin 600 mg i.v. every 8 hours and ceftazidime 2 g i.v. every 12 hours in adults, and 25 to 40 mg/kg/day i.v. divided every 6 to 8 hours and 30 to 50 mg/kg i.v. every 8 hours in children (maximum dosage 6 g/day). This regimen will cover Gram positives, Gram negatives, and anaerobes; vancomycin may be added if there is suspicion for methicillin-resistant *S. aureus* (consult hospital pharmacy for neonatal doses).
   • Fungal infections will require i.v. amphotericin B.
   • Antibiotics should be adjusted based on results of cultures (blood and any discharge).

4. Closely monitor vital signs, complete blood count, and ophthalmic examination for improvement.

5. ENT consultation is suggested for management of significant sinus disease and for surgical drainage of sinuses. Drainage of sinuses is recommended in patients who fail to improve or worsen after 2 to 3 days of antibiotics (18). Intraorbital abscesses, although rare, also should be drained. Management of SPAs is more controversial (see special considerations below).

6. Once clear improvement is seen, the patient may be switched to oral antibiotics to complete a total 14-day course of antibiotics. The antibiotic should be chosen based on cultures, but if cultures are negative, a suggested empiric choice is Augmentin 500 mg orally three times daily in adults and 40 mg/kg/day divided every 8 hours in children.

7. Consider infectious disease consultation for atypical presentations, immuno-compromised patients, or failure to improve with empirical antibiotic therapy.

8. Failure to improve may suggest alternative diagnosis (see differential diagnosis above), including cavernous sinus thrombosis, orbital abscess, and pseudotumor. Repeat orbital imaging should be considered and orbital exploration may become necessary.

9. Neurology/neurosurgery and infectious disease consultation will be required in cases of cavernous sinus thrombosis. Use of anticoagulants and antifibrinolytics may be considered, although efficacy is unknown.

Special considerations for fungal orbital cellulitis (18,19):

1. Acute cases are usually due to mucormycosis (species of *Absidia, Mucor, Rhizopus*)

2. Diagnosed by histopathology (difficult to culture): broad, nonseptate, randomly branching hyphae. Unlike other fungi, they stain more intensely with hematoxylin than with special stains (such as periodic acid-Schiff). Biopsy or smear from necrotic skin or mucous membranes, or nasopharyngeal biopsy and maxillary sinus irrigation (if no visible lesions are present) by ENT is required.

3. Organisms grow intraluminally, producing a thrombosing vasculitis and ischemic necrosis.

4. Patients initially present with unilateral headache, periorbital pain, fever, chemosis, lid edema, and proptosis. Subsequently, with spread to the orbital apex, cranial neuropathies (II, III, IV, V_1, VI) develop and central retinal artery occlusion can occur. Later, involvement of the intracranial portion of cranial nerve VII can produce ipsilateral facial weakness (this distinguishes mucormycosis from other causes of orbital cellulitis) (18).

5. Treatment is often unsatisfactory. Infectious disease and ENT consultation is required. Treatment should include i.v. amphotericin B, debridement of necrotic tissue, and control of metabolic acidosis (20). Hyperbaric oxygen may be considered as an adjunctive measure in patients responding poorly to conventional therapy.

6. Exenteration may be required for severe, refractory infections.

Special considerations for SPAs:

1. SPA is characterized by accumulation of purulent material between the periorbita and the bony walls of the orbit. It is almost always due to associated sinusitis, most commonly ethmoidal sinusitis with resultant medial wall SPA.
2. Microbiology varies considerably, depending on the patient's age. In children, common organisms include *Streptococcus pneuomoniae, Streptococcus pyogenes,* and *Hemophilus influenzae* (21). Although anaerobic and complicated/mixed infections are frequent in adults, they are rare in children. Thus, more conservative management may be appropriate in children.
3. CT scan can aid in differentiation of SPA from orbital cellulitis (22,23). Ultrasound also may be useful in finding SPAs, particularly so in observing patients after drainage of SPA to look for evidence of reaccumulation (24). SPA typically appears as a signal of low to medium reflectivity on echography.
4. Consultation with ENT is required to plan surgical intervention: three different approaches have been suggested by Harris (25):
   a. Emergency drainage: in any patient with optic nerve compromise
   b. Urgent drainage:
      * in large SPAs causing significant discomfort (but not affecting vision)
      * in superior or inferior SPAs extending large distances from ethmoid sinuses (because they are less likely to resolve with medical therapy)
      * in patients with intracranial complications or frontal sinusitis
      * in cases highly suspicious for complex infections with anaerobes (i.e., in patients more than 9 years of age and in all patients with a dental source for infection)
   c. Expectant observation (medical therapy only with the patient hospitalized for careful monitoring for the development of a relative afferent pupillary defect [RAPD] at least every 6 hours) in patients less than 9 years of age (simple infection is predicted), with no visual compromise, a medial SPA of small to moderate size, and no intracranial or frontal sinus involvement (25% of patients with SPA will fit these criteria). Surgical intervention should be undertaken in these patient's if
      * RAPD develops
      * fever does not resolve within 36 hours of appropriate i.v. antibiotics
      * clinical deterioration occurs despite 48 hours of antibiotics
      * no improvement is observed after 72 hours of therapy (22)
5. Antibiotic therapy and follow-up will be similar to uncomplicated orbital cellulitis, although duration of required therapy may be longer.

REFERENCES

1. Boruchoff SA, Boruchoff SE. Infections of the lacrimal system. *Infect Dis Clin North Am* 1992; 6:925–932.
2. Baum JL. Antibiotic use in ophthalmology. In: Tasman W, Jaeger EA, eds. *Duane's Clinical Ophthalmology.* Vol. 4. Philadelphia: Lippincott-Raven; 1990:9–10.

3. Iliff NT. Infections of the lacrimal excretory system. In: Pepose JS, Wilhelmus KR, Holland GN, eds. *Ocular Infections and Immunity.* St. Louis: Mosby-Year Book; 1996:1346–1356.

4. Demant E, Hurwitz JJ. Canaliculitis: review of 12 cases. *Can J Ophthalmol* 1980;15:73–75.

5. Pavilack MA, Frueh BR. Thorough curettage in the treatment of chronic canaliculitis. *Arch Ophthalmol* 1991;110:200–202.

6. Bale RN. Dacryocystits. Bacteriological study and its relation with nasal pathology. *Ind J Ophthalmol* 1987;35:178–182.

7. Hurwitz JJ, Rogers KJ. Management of acquired dacryocystitis. *Ophthalmology* 1983;18:213–216.

8. Huber-Spitzy V, Steinkogler FJ, Huber E, et al. Acquired dacryocstitis: microbiology and conservative therapy. *Acta Opthalmol* 1992;70:745–749.

9. Zolli CL, Shannon GM. Dacryocystorhinostomy: a review of 119 cases. *Ophthalmic Surg* 1982; 13:905–910.

10. Pollard Z. Treatment of acute dacryocystitis in neonates. *J Ophthalmol Strabismus* 1991;29: 341–343.

11. Gordon RA, Schaeffer A, Sood S. Bacteremia following nasolacrimal duct probing. *Opthalmology* 1990;97(suppl):149.

12. McCulley JP, Dougherty JM, Deneau DG. Classification of chronic blepharitis. *Ophthalmology* 1982;89:1173.

13. Groden LR, Murphy B, Rodnite J, Genvert GI. Lid flora in blepharitis. *Cornea* 1991;10:50–53.

14. Ostler HB. Blepharitis. In: Tasman W, Jaeger EA, eds. *Duane's Clinical Ophthalmology.* Vol. 4. Philadelphia: Lippincott-Raven; 1989:1–7.

15. Raskin EM, Speaker MG, Laibson PR. Blepharitis. *Infect Dis Clin North Am* 1992;6:777–787.

16. Seal DV, Wright P, Ficker L, Hagan K, Troski M, Menday P. Placebo controlled trial of fusidic gel and oxytetracycline for recurrent blepharitis and rosacea. *Br J Ophthalmol* 1995;79:42–45.

17. Leone CR, Hollsten DA. Management of conjunctival diseases and chalazion. In: Stewart WB, ed. *Surgery of the Eyelid, Orbit, and Lacrimal System.* Vol. 1. San Francisco: American Academy of Ophthalmology; 1993.

18. Jones DB, Steinkuller PG. Microbial presptal and orbital cellulitis. In: Tasman W, Jaeger EA, eds. *Duane's Clinical Ophthalmology.* Vol. 4. Philadelphia: Lippincott-Raven; 1989:1–24.

19. Moore A. Preseptal and orbital cellulitis. In: Taylor D, ed. *Pediatric Ophthalmology.* Boston: Blackwell Scientific; 1990:107–113.

20. Lessner A, Stern GA. Preseptal and orbital cellulitis. *Infect Dis Clin North Am* 1992;6:933–952.

21. Skedros DG, Haddad J, Bluestone CD, Curtin HD. Subperiosteal orbital abscess in children: diagnosis, microbiology, and management. *Laryngoscope* 1993;103:28–32.

22. Handler LC, Davey IC, Hill JC, Lauryssen C. The acute orbit: differentiation of orbital cellulitis from subperiosteal abscess by computerized tomography. *Neuroradiology* 1991;33:15–18.

23. Andrews TM, Myer CM. The role of computed tomography in the diagnosis of subperiostal abscess fo the orbit. *Clin Pediatr* 1992;31:37–43.

24. Wulc AE. Orbital infections. In: Tasman W, Jaeger EA, eds. *Duane's Clinical Ophthalmology.* Vol. 2. Philadelphia: Lippincott-Raven; 1994:1–24.

25. Harris GJ. Subperiosteal abscess if the orbit: age as a factor in bacteriology and response to treatment. *Ophthalmology* 1994;101:585–595.

Management of Ocular Injuries and Emergencies,
edited by Mathew W. MacCumber.
Lippincott–Raven Publishers, Philadelphia ©1998.

11

Ocular and Periocular Inflammatory Syndromes

Srinivas R. Sadda, Arman K. Fard, and Daniel A. Johnson

*Department of Ophthalmology, Wilmer Eye Institute, The John Hopkins University
School of Medicine, Baltimore, Maryland 21287*

Uveitis 137
    Basic Considerations 137 · Anterior Uveitis 137 · Intermediate Uveitis
    142 · Posterior Uveitis 144 · Panuveitis 148
Episcleritis 150
    Basic Considerations 150 · Etiology 151 · Diagnosis 151 · Manage-
    ment 151
Scleritis 152
    Basic Considerations 152 · Etiology 152 · Diagnosis 152 · Manage-
    ment 154
Orbital Inflammatory Syndrome (Orbital Pseudotumor) 155
    Basic Considerations 155 · Differential Diagnosis 156 · Laboratory Test-
    ing 157 · Diagnosis 157 · Management 159

UVEITIS

Basic Considerations

Uveitis is defined as inflammation of the uveal tract. It may be a phenomenon of the eye alone or the manifestation of more widespread systemic pathology. It may be infectious or sterile, acute (lasting less than 3 months) or chronic (lasting longer than 3 months). The proper diagnosis requires a detailed history, review of systems, ophthalmic examination, and directed workup. The proper management requires regular follow-up, monitoring for drug side effects, and, frequently, coordination of care with internal medicine, rheumatology, or infectious disease specialists.

Anterior Uveitis

Description

Anterior uveitis is characterized by inflammation within the anterior chamber (iritis) or anterior and posterior chambers (iridocyclitis) of the eye. Its prevalence in the United States is 110 per 100,000 (1), and its frequency among cases of general uveitis ranges from 28% to 91% depending upon type of ophthalmology practice (2–4). Presenting symptoms often include pain, photophobia, decreased visual acuity, and redness; however, it may be asymptomatic. Ophthalmic signs often include perilimbal flush, miosis, keratic precipitates, posterior synechiae, increased or decreased intraocular pressure, and decreased visual acuity. Less commonly, hypopyon or hyphema may be present. Complications of anterior uveitis may include permanent decrease in visual acuity, band keratopathy, peripheral anterior synechiae, iris bombe, glaucoma, hypotony, cataract, cyclitic membrane, or cystoid macular edema. The ocular complications are related to the number of attacks of inflammation (5).

Etiology (Frequency Among Cases of Anterior Uveitis)

Idiopathic (31% to 63%) (2–8): no systemic association identified by review of systems, ophthalmic examination, or medical evaluation.

HLA-B27 or spondyloarthropathy (17-41%) (2–4,6,7,9,10): nongranulomatous acute or acute-recurrent anterior uveitis, often with a fibrinous anterior chamber reaction. It is usually unilateral, and attacks may alternate between eyes (bilateral-alternating). Posterior synechiae are common and hypopyon may develop. Chronic disease and posterior segment involvement are uncommon. Systemic associations include ankylosing spondylitis (low back stiffness that is not improved by rest but improves with exercise, decreased chest expansion, decreased lumbar mobility, costochondritis, and sacroiliitis), Reiter's syndrome (constellation of nongonococcal urethritis, arthritis, conjunctivitis and uveitis; may also have oral ulcerations, penile rash, plantar fasciitis, sacroiliitis, low back pain), inflammatory bowel disease (crampy abdominal pain, alternating constipation and diarrhea, arthritis), psoriatic arthropathy (erythematous rash with silver scales on extensor surfaces, associated with nail pits, arthritis of small joints of the hands and feet, neck and back pain from spinal syndesmophytes and sacroiliitis), gastroenteritis associated with *Salmonella, Shigella, Yersinia,* or *Campylobacter.*

Traumatic (2% to 18%) (2,5): history and evidence of trauma.

Herpes simplex virus (HSV) (4% to 12%) (2,11) and varicella-zoster virus (VZV) (3% to 6%) (2,5): acute, acute-recurrent, or chronic granulomatous or nongranulomatous anterior uveitis. History of stromal keratitis common. May have corneal hypoesthesia, corneal scarring, iris atrophy, hyphema, elevated intraocular pressure. Oral acyclovir for HSV iridocyclitis in patients receiving topical corticosteroids and trifluridine may be beneficial (11).

Juvenile rheumatoid arthritis (JRA) (0.2% to 11%) (2–4,7,12,13): insidious-onset chronic nongranulomatous anterior uveitis often associated with band keratopathy, cataracts, glaucoma, posterior synechiae, and cystoid macular edema. There is often minimal external evidence of inflammation (white eye uveitis). Systemic involvement includes arthritis lasting longer than 3 months in a child less than 16 years of age without other cause of the arthritis. Several subtypes of JRA have been identified; however, young girls with pauciarticular arthritis (fewer than five joints involved) who are antinuclear antibody (ANA) positive are at the highest risk of developing uveitis. Older boys who are HLA-B27 positive have ocular and systemic disorders more similar to those described for HLA-B27 above.

Fuchs' heterochromic iridocyclitis (1% to 11%) (2–5,7): chronic unilateral nongranulomatous iritis or iridocyclitis associated with posterior subcapsular cataract, iris heterochromia, absence of posterior synechiae, and fine vessels crossing the trabecular meshwork. There is usually no external evidence of ocular inflammation. Glaucoma is common. The diffusely distributed small stellate keratic precipitates are characteristic. Topical corticosteroids are usually not helpful and may exacerbate cataract and glaucoma.

Sarcoidosis (1% to 6%) (2–4,7,14,15): acute, acute-recurrent, or chronic granulomatous or nongranulomatous intraocular inflammation. May be associated with dry eyes, enlarged lacrimal glands, conjunctival or iris nodules, episcleritis, band keratopathy, posterior synechiae, posterior segment inflammation (retinal periphlebitis, granulomata), and seventh nerve palsy. Systemic involvement includes hilar adenopathy, parenchymal pulmonary involvement, erythema nodosum, and granulomata of many organ systems, including the central nervous system.

Intraocular lens associated (1% to 4%) (2,3): chronic, intraocular lens present and no other etiology of the inflammation identified. Delayed postoperative endophthalmitis with *Staphylococcus epidermidis, Propionibacterium acnes,* and other fungal or bacterial pathogens should be considered and excluded by culture if necessary. Inflammation due to iris chafing from an intraocular lens may respond to topical corticosteroids and cycloplegic agents.

Syphilis (0.5% to 3%) (2,3,7,16): acute or chronic, granulomatous or nongranulomatous, may involve any portion of the eye. Systemic involvement includes palmar rash, genital chancre, or lymphadenopathy in a patient who has been sexually active. Human immunodeficiency virus (HIV) status should be confirmed. Treatment for tertiary syphilis recommended (Table 11–1) (16).

Scleritis with secondary uveitis (2% to 3%) (2): evidence of active scleritis present. Systemic involvement depends on etiology (see Scleritis).

Posner-Schlossman/glaucomatocyclitic crisis (1% to 2%) (3,7): acute or acute-recurrent nongranulomatous anterior uveitis with minimal symptoms and minimal anterior chamber reaction but markedly elevated intraocular pressure. Topical corticosteroids and medical treatment for glaucoma required.

Other etiologies (2–5,7,8): systemic lupus erythematosus, rheumatoid arthritis, Wegener's granulomatosis, relapsing polychondritis, Kawasaki's syndrome/mucocutaneous lymph node syndrome, multiple sclerosis, Lyme disease, tuberculosis, leprosy, coccidiomycosis, chronic granulomatous hepatitis, paraproteinemia, leukemia, corneal graft rejection, metipranolol, rifabutin.

TABLE 11–1. *Treatment of infectious uveitis*

Acute retinal necrosis (ARN) (13)

Acyclovir 500 mg/m^2 intravenously every 8 h for 10–14 days followed by oral acyclovir 800 mg five times per day for 6 wk

Oral corticosteroids may be added after 24–48 h of antiviral therapy in the absence of immunosuppression

Maintenance therapy with acyclovir 800 mg orally five times per day is necessary for patients who are immunosuppressed

Cytomegalovirus (CMV) retinitis

Ganciclovir 5 mg/kg intravenously every 12 h for 2 wk followed by ganciclovir 5 mg/kg/day intravenously for life, or

Ganciclovir 5 mg/kg intravenously every 12 h for 2–3 wk followed by oral ganciclovir 1,000 mg every 8 h for life, or

Foscarnet 90 mg/kg intravenously every 12 h for 2 wk followed by foscarnet 90 mg/kg/day intravenously for life, or

Regimens utilizing cidofovir (HPMPC), the ganciclovir intraocular device (Vitrasert), or intravitreal injections of antiviral medication. Patients with temporary immunosuppression, such as following organ transplantation, generally do not need life-long maintenance therapy.

Lyme disease

Adults

Tetracycline 250 mg orally every 6 h for 10–30 days, or

Doxycycline 100 mg orally every 12 h for 10–30 days, or

Amoxicillin 500 mg orally every 6 h for 10–30 days

Children

Penicillin V 250 mg orally every 8 h or 20 mg/kg/day in divided doses for 10–30 days, or

Amoxicillin 250 mg orally every 8 h or 20 mg/kg/day in divided doses for 10–30 days, or

Erythromycin 250 mg orally every 8 h or 30 mg/kg/day in divided doses for 10–30 days

Severe uveitis or neurologic abnormalities

Ceftriaxone 2 g/day intravenously for 14 days, or

Penicillin G 20–24 million units/day intravenously for 10–14 days

Some patients may respond to oral medication; however, patients with severe involvement of posterior segment involvement may require intravenous therapy. (Modified from Nussenblatt RB, Whitcup SM, Palestine AG: *Uveitis: Fundamentals and Clinical Practice.* Baltimore: CV Mosby, 1996)

Progressive outer retinal necrosis (19)

Acyclovir 500 mg/m^2 intravenously every 8 h, and

Foscarnet 90 mg/kg intravenously every 12 h for 14 days followed by maintenance therapy of acyclovir 800 mg orally five times per day and Foscarnet 120 mg/kg/day for life

Syphilis (16)

Penicillin G (aqueous crystalline) 2.0–4.0 million units intravenously every 4 h for 10–14 days

In patients with concurrent HIV infection, the intravenous regimen should be followed by 2.4 million units of intramuscular benzathine penicillin G weekly for 3 weeks

Response to therapy should be confirmed serologically

Toxoplasmosis

Small, peripheral lesions may not require treatment.

Pyrimethamine (Daraprim) 50 mg orally every 12 h for two doses followed by 25 mg orally every 12 h. Folinic acid (Leucovorin) should be given concurrently at a dose of 3–5 mg orally three times per week to reduce the risk of marrow toxicity, and

Sulfadiazine 2-g loading dose followed by 1 g every 6 h

Clindamycin 300 mg orally every 6 h may be added to the above regimen or substituted for pyrimethamine

Other agents include atovaquone (Mepron), minocycline, tetracycline, sulfisoxasole, and trimethoprim-sulfamethoxazole.

Prednisone 20–40 mg orally per day may be considered 12–24 h after instituting antimicrobial therapy but should *never* be used alone and should be avoided in patients with concurrent HIV infection. Corticosteroids should be discontinued before the antimicrobial therapy is discontinued.

The duration of therapy is generally 4–6 wk. Patients with concurrent HIV infection require maintenance therapy for life (pyrimethamine, sulfadiazine, and clindamycin in different combinations have been used).

Note: Drug monitoring and side effects should be reviewed before administration.

Diagnosis

1. The character of the anterior uveitis (acute, chronic, recurrent, alternating, response to prior therapy, specific features) and the review of systems (with emphasis on symptoms associated with the etiologies above) are important in directing the diagnostic evaluation.
2. All patients with intraocular inflammation should have a chest x-ray and syphilis serology. Some investigators (13) also routinely order a complete blood count with differential and urinalysis because asymptomatic abnormalities may require treatment.
3. Other studies to consider, depending on clinical suspicion, include ANA (children), HLA-B27 (acute, acute-recurrent, bilateral-alternating anterior uveitis, spondyloarthropathy, back pain), serum angiotensin converting enzyme (ACE) and serum lysozyme [recommended by some investigators (7,15) for sarcoidosis], Lyme serology (enzyme-linked immunosorbent assay [ELISA], immunofluorescent assay [IFA], Western blot), sacroiliac spine films (to evaluate for sacroiliitis), purified protein derivative skin test, gallium scan (sarcoidosis) or conjunctival/ lacrimal gland/minor salivary gland/transbronchial biopsy (sarcoidosis). Indiscriminate use of diagnostic tests (shotgun approach) may lead to inappropriate treatment for a false-positive test result.

Management

1. Topical corticosteriods (prednisolone acetate 1%, prednisolone sodium phosphate 1%, rimexolone 1%) are usually effective for noninfectious anterior uveitis. They should be administered frequently (preferably every 1 to 2 hours) until the inflammation is controlled and then gradually tapered. Rapid tapering may lead to recurrent inflammation. If there is a flare of inflammation, the dose should be increased high enough to suppress the inflammation and a more gradual taper begun. Tapering over several months may be necessary. Side effects of topical corticosteroids include glaucoma, cataract, and infection. Steroid-induced glaucoma should be treated medically; however, miotics (pilocarpine) should be avoided because they may worsen the inflammation.
2. Cycloplegia with a strong agent (atropine 1%, scopolamine 0.25%) should be administered one to four times daily for patient comfort and to reduce the risk of posterior synechiae formation.
3. Periocular corticosteroids (posterior subtenons injections of triamcinolone or methylprednisolone) or systemic corticosteroids may be necessary for recalcitrant inflammation.
4. Infectious uveitis requires treatment with appropriate antimicrobial agents (Table 11–1).

Intermediate Uveitis

Description

Intermediate uveitis is characterized by inflammation of the peripheral retina, pars plana, or vitreous. Its prevalence in the United States is estimated between three and 30 cases per 100,000, and its frequency among cases of general uveitis ranges from 1.4% to 15% depending on type of ophthalmology practice (1–3,6,7). Presenting symptoms often include decreased vision and floaters. Pain and redness are uncommon. Ophthalmic signs include minimal anterior chamber reaction, moderate or prominent vitritis, clumps of vitreous debris ("snowballs"), peripheral vascular sheathing and often a pars plana exudate ("snowbank"). Complications may include a permanent decrease in visual acuity, cataract, cyclitic membrane, epiretinal membrane, chronic cystoid macular edema, retinal detachment, vitreous hemorrhage, and phthisis.

Etiology (Frequency Among Cases of Intermediate Uveitis)

Idiopathic (0% to 72%) (2,3,6,7) *and pars planitis* (67% to 100%) (2,7): no systemic systemic association identified by review of systems, ophthalmic examination, or medical evaluation. Some investigators use the term "pars planitis" synonymously with "intermediate uveitis"; however, others reserve the term "pars planitis" to describe an idiopathic condition associated with a snowbank, vitreous snowballs, and cystoid macular edema.

Multiple sclerosis (0% to 33%) (2,3,7): may be associated with a granulomatous anterior uveitis. Retinal perivasculitis common. May have history of optic neuritis or cranial neuropathy. Systemic involvement includes episodes of paresthesias or weakness, gait instability, problems with genitourinary control. Central nervous system plaques present by neuroimaging.

Sarcoidosis (0% to 22%) (3,6,7,14,15): see description under Anterior Uveitis.

Lyme disease (0.6%) (3,13,17): may have history of granulomatous anterior uveitis, retinal vasculitis, neuroretinitis, choroiditis, exudative retinal detachment, orbital myositis, or cranial neuropathies (especially seventh nerve palsy). Systemic involvement includes a history of a tick bite (50% of patients), erythema migrans rash, arthritis, cardiac abnormalities, and meningitis. Exposure and travel to an endemic area (especially northeastern and upper mid-western United States) helpful for the diagnosis. Antimicrobial agents required.

Other etiologies (6,12,13,16,17): amyloidosis, HLA-B27 or spondyloarthropathy, inflammatory bowel disease, juvenile rheumatoid arthritis, systemic lupus erythematosus, Whipple's disease, interstitial nephritis, intraocular lymphoma, human T-lymphotropic virus type 1 (HTLV-1), syphilis, tuberculosis, adenovirus, leptospirosis, toxocariasis.

Diagnosis

1. The associated ophthalmic features and the review of systems (with emphasis on symptoms associated with the etiologies above) are important in directing the diagnostic evaluation.
2. All patients with intraocular inflammation should have a chest x-ray and syphilis serology. Some investigators (13) also routinely order a complete blood count with differential and urinalysis because asymptomatic abnormalities may require treatment.
3. Other studies to consider, depending upon clinical suspicion, include Lyme serology (ELISA, IFA, Western blot), serum ACE and serum lysozyme [recommended by some investigators (7,15) for sarcoidosis], gallium scan (sarcoidosis), neuroimaging and neurology referral (multiple sclerosis, Lyme encephalitis, central nervous system sarcoidosis), or conjunctival/lacrimal gland/minor salivary gland/transbronchial biopsy (sarcoidosis) or vitreous biopsy.

Management

1. Intermediate uveitis of an infectious etiology (syphilis, Lyme disease) requires appropriate antimicrobial agents, often with the assistance of an infectious disease specialist (Table 11–1).
2. Noninfectious intermediate uveitis and pars planitis with good visual acuity (generally 20/40 or better) may not require treatment. When therapy is deemed necessary, periocular and/or systemic corticosteroids may be indicated. Neither should be initiated without a full discussion of the risks, benefits, and side effects.

Periocular Therapy

Triamcinolone (40 mg) or methylprednisolone (80 mg) in 1 ml, given via a posterior subtenons approach (13) after obtaining written informed consent. Other agents and routes have been described (17). The injection may be repeated monthly. Side effects include uncontrolled glaucoma (requiring surgical excision of the injected material), globe penetration, ptosis, proptosis, orbital fibrosis, diplopia, retrobulbar hemorrhage, and central retinal artery occlusion. This treatment should be avoided in cases associated with scleritis or active infection.

Oral Corticosteroids

Prednisone 1 mg/kg/day orally until the eye is quiet followed by a gradual taper. Side effects include hypertension, diabetes, aseptic necrosis of the femoral and humeral heads, osteoporosis, increased susceptibility to infection, neuropsychiatric effects, metabolic alterations, fluid retention, lipid abnormalities, muscle weakness/myopathy, gastrointestinal upset, peptic ulcer disease, easy bruisability, poor wound healing, growth suppression in children, weight gain, adrenocortical suppression, thromboembolism, and others. The patient's internist should be involved in monitoring for side effects. Prophylaxis for gastrointestinal upset or ulceration is often prescribed (ranitidine or others). If the duration of therapy is protracted or the side effects intolerable, a steroid-sparing or systemic immunosuppressive agent should be considered if, and only if, the benefits outweigh the potential risks.

Topical corticosteroids alone are not effective for intermediate uveitis but may be used if there is an associated anterior uveitis. A cycloplegic should be prescribed if there is the potential for posterior synechiae formation or if the patient reports photophobia.

Posterior Uveitis

Description

Posterior uveitis is characterized by inflammation of the posterior segment of the eye. Its prevalence in the United States is 30 per 100,000, and its frequency among cases of general uveitis ranges from 5% to 38%, depending on type of ophthalmology practice (1–4,6,7). Presenting symptoms often include decreased vision, floaters, and photopsia. Pain and redness are uncommon. Ophthalmic signs may include retinal vascular sheathing, vitritis, retinitis, choroiditis, cystoid macular edema, and retinal detachment. Complications may include permanent decrease in visual acuity, cataract, cyclitic membrane, epiretinal membrane, chronic cystoid macular edema, retinal detachment, vitreous hemorrhage, retinal and choroidal neovascularization, and phthisis.

Etiology (Frequency Among Cases of Posterior Uveitis)

Idiopathic (10% to 33%) (3,4,6,7): systemic association not identified by review of systems, ophthalmic examination, or laboratory or radiologic testing.

Toxoplasmosis (18% to 90%) (2–4,6,18,19): granulomatous or nongranulomatous infectious necrotizing retinitis often described as a headlight in the fog due to the prominent vitreous reaction. The white-yellow retinal lesion is often adjacent to a scar from prior involvement. May have associated glaucoma, papillitis, or neuroretinitis. A multifocal outer retinal form (punctate outer retinal toxoplasmosis) may occur that has minimal vitreous reaction. A high incidence of concurrent central nervous system toxoplasmosis exists in patients with the acquired immunodeficiency syndrome (AIDS) and ocular toxoplasmosis. There is generally no systemic involvement due from reactivation of congenitally acquired ocular infection in an immunocompetent patient; however, patients with acquired disease may have a flulike illness, malaise, and pharyngitis. Antimicrobial agents (sulfadiazine, pyrimethamine, and clindamycin, alone or in combination) are recommended for large lesions or those near the optic nerve or macula. Folinic acid is used while patients are taking pyrimethamine. Prednisone may be used concurrently, but it

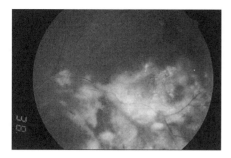

FIG. 11–1. Active fulminant cytomegalovirus (CMV) retinitis in a patient with AIDS. Note the hemorrhage and full-thickness retinal involvement. (Courtesy of Drs. D.A. Jabs and J.P. Dunn, Baltimore, MD.) *For a color representation of this figure, please see the color insert facing p. 256.*

should not be used alone. Periocular corticosteroids should not be used. Chronic suppressive therapy is indicated for patients with HIV infection.

Behcet's disease (0.7% to 14%) (3,4,7,20): inflammatory uveitis that may involve the anterior, posterior, or both segments of the eye often present as a bilateral nongranulomatous anterior uveitis with hypopyon, posterior synechiae, vitritis and retinal vascular occlusive disease. Systemic involvement includes oral ulcers, genital ulcers, skin lesions (erythema nodosum, thrombophlebitis, folliculitis, evidence of cutaneous hypersensitivity by pustule formation after trauma), and arthritis. Association with HLA-B5 or HLA-Bw51. Corticosteroids and/or immunosuppressives are often required.

Cytomegalovirus (CMV) retinitis (2% to 12%) (3,19): infectious white necrotizing retinitis and perivasculitis that may be associated with hemorrhage (fulminant, Fig. 11–1) or without hemorrhage (indolent, Fig. 11–2). Both forms have granular borders. Usually occurs in patients who are immunosuppressed, especially in those with AIDS and concomitant CD4+ T cell counts of less than 50 cells/μl. Iatrogenically immunosuppressed organ transplant patients are also at risk. May have associated gastrointestinal and central nervous system involvement. Life-long antiviral agents required (or for duration of iatrogenic immunosuppression if not associated with HIV infection) (Table 11–1).

Presumed ocular histoplasmosis syndrome (POHS) (0% to 9%) (2,3): multiple punched-out lesions involving the retina, retinal pigment epithelium, and choroid.

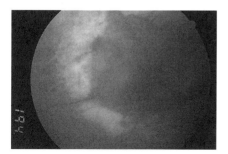

FIG. 11–2. Active indolent cytomegalovirus (CMV) retinitis in a patient with AIDS. Absence of hemorrhage distinguishes this form of CMV retinitis from fulminant CMV retinitis. Both forms are treated identically. (Courtesy of Drs. D.A. Jabs and J.P. Dunn, Baltimore, MD.) *For a color representation of this figure, please see the color insert facing p. 256.*

Peripapillary atrophy is common. Choroidal neovascular membranes may occur, but vitritis is not present. HLA-B7 associated with macular involvement. Patients are often from the midwestern and mid-Atlantic United States. Clinical diagnosis. No treatment required other than routine monitoring for the development of choriodal neovascular membranes.

Serpiginous choroidopathy (0% to 8%) (2,3,6,8,13): condition of unknown etiology generally affecting healthy middle-aged patients of either sex, characterized by bilateral geographic lesions involving retina, retinal pigment epithelium, and choroid that often progress outward from the optic disk. May have associated choroidal neovascularization, perivasculitis, and vitritis. Clinical diagnosis. Corticosteroids and immunosuprrssive agents have been used therapeutically.

Birdshot chorioretinopathy (0% to 8%) (2,3,6): condition of unknown etiology characterized by scattered yellow-white lesions at the level of the retinal pigment epithelium bilaterally. Middle-aged white women of northern European descent are typically affected. There is usually no anterior uveitis, although vitritis, retinal vascular leakage, and cystoid macular edema are common. There is a high association with HLA-A29. Diminished night and color vision not uncommon. Corticosteriods and/or cyclosporine have been used therapeutically.

Multifocal choroiditis (0% to 6%) (2,13,17): condition of unknown etiology characterized by multiple punched-out lesions involving inner choroid and retinal pigment epithelium associated with vitritis and, at times, mild disk edema and cystoid macular edema. It occurs most commonly in young to middle-aged women. Choroidal neovascularization may develop. May have peripheral chorioretinal streaks. Clinical diagnosis. Corticosteroids and/or immunosuppressive agents have been used therapeutically.

Sarcoidosis (2% to 8%) (3,4,6,7,15): see description under Anterior Uveitis. Posterior segment manifestations include vitritis, phlebitis, *taches de bougie* ("candle wax dripping"), venous occlusive disease, retinal and optic nerve neovascularization, choroidal and optic nerve granulomata, Dalen-Fuchs–like lesions, and exudative retinal detachment. Usually corticosteroid responsive.

Toxocariasis (2% to 7%) (3,6,13,17): predominantly in young children, characterized by peripheral or macular granulomata, vitritis, and anterior uveitis. May have hypopyon, serous retinal detachment, and optic neuritis; vitreous abscess may be present. Fever, eosinophilia, hepatosplenomegaly, and pneumonitis suggestive of visceral larva migrans rare with ocular involvement. Corticosteroids with or without antihelminthics have been used.

Progressive outer retinal necrosis (0% to 16%) (2,19): rapidly progressive infectious white outer retinitis occurring in patients with AIDS (Fig. 11–3). There is usually minimal or no vitritis. Retinal detachment common. Often have history of cutaneous varicella-zoster. Life-long antiviral agents required (Table 11–1).

Acute retinal necrosis (3% to 5%) (2,3,6,19): infectious necrotizing retinitis associated with vasculitis and dense vitritis occurring in immunocompetent or immunocompromised patients. Retinal detachment so common that prophylactic barrier laser often used. Antiviral agents required (Table 11–1).

Acute posterior multifocal placoid pigment epitheliopathy (APMPPE) (2% to 5%) (3,6): condition of unknown etiology characterized by discrete yellow-white

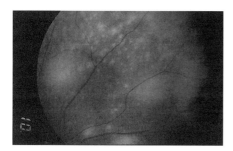

FIG. 11–3. Progressive outer retinal necrosis in a patient with AIDS. The deep retinal appearance of the lesions helps to distinguish the process from CMV retinitis, and the absence of prominent vitritis and vasculitis helps to distinguish it from acute retinal necrosis. (Courtesy of Drs. D.A. Jabs and J.P. Dunn, Baltimore, MD.) *For a color representation of this figure, please see the color insert facing p. 256.*

nummular lesions at the level of the retinal pigment epithelium bilaterally. It usually affects young adults and generally does not recur. There may be a mild nongranulomatous anterior uveitis and vitritis. May follow upper respiratory infection. A cerebral vasculitis may occur. Spontaneous recovery with improvement in visual function toward normal is common.

Syphilis (1% to 2%) (3,4,16): see description under anterior uveitis. Posterior involvement includes vitritis, chorioretinitis, perivasculitis, neuroretinitis, and papillitis.

Punctate inner choroidopathy (1%) (3,13): condition of unknown etiology characterized by small lesions of the outer retina associated with photopsia, blurry vision, and scotomata occurring generally in young myopic women. It may be a variant of multifocal choroiditis.

Multiple evanescent white dot syndrome (MEWDS) (1%) (3,13): condition of unknown etiology characterized by an acute decrease in visual acuity associated with unilateral discrete white deep retinal lesions. Vitreous cells, retinal periphlebitis, macular granularity, an afferent pupillary defect and reversible electroretinogram (ERG) abnormalities may occur. The disease generally occurs in young women, and does not recur and resolves without treatment. Clinical diagnosis.

Other etiologies (2–4,6,7,13,17): tuberculosis, Epstein-Barr chorioretinitis, Lyme disease, congenital rubella, systemic lupus erythematosus, polyarteritis nodosa, Wegener's granulomatosis, subretinal fibrosis and uveitis syndrome, multiple sclerosis, temporal arteritis, intraocular lymphoma, leukemia.

Diagnosis

1. The associated ophthalmic features and the review of systems (with emphasis on symptoms associated with the etiologies above) are important in directing the diagnostic evaluation. Many of the diagnoses are based on clinical criteria. Some of the conditions can be diagnosed by clinical appearance; however, vitreous, retinal, or choroidal biopsy may confirm a diagnosis in certain instances (atypical CMV retinitis, necrotizing herpetic retinopathy, toxoplasmosis, toxocariasis).
2. All patients with intraocular inflammation should have a chest x-ray and syphilis serology. Some investigators (13) also order a complete blood count with differential and urinalysis because asymptomatic abnormalities may require treatment.

3. HIV testing should be offered to patients with disease suggestive of underlying immunosuppression (CMV retinitis, necrotizing herpetic retinopathy, etc.).

4. Other studies to consider, depending on clinical suspicion, include toxoplasma ELISA or Western blot (helpful to rule out the diagnosis of toxoplasma retinochoroiditis if negative; however, a positive test does not confirm the diagnosis), HLA-B5 or HLA-Bw51 (Behcet's syndrome; however, the diagnosis is based on clinical criteria alone), HLA-A29 (birdshot chorioretinopathy; however, the diagnosis is based on clinical criteria), toxocara ELISA, serum ACE and serum lysozyme [recommended by some investigators (7,15) for sarcoidosis], neuroimaging and neurology referral (multiple sclerosis, Lyme encephalitis, central nervous system sarcoidosis), gallium scan (sarcoidosis), biopsy of ulceration (Behcet's syndrome), conjunctival/lacrimal gland/minor salivary gland/transbronchial biopsy (sarcoidosis), test for cutaneous hypersensitivity (Behcet's syndrome) or vitreous/retinal/choroidal biopsy.

Management

Many of the causes of posterior uveitis are infectious and require specific antimicrobial therapy such as CMV retinitis, toxoplasma retinochoroiditis, necrotizing herpetic retinopathy (acute retinal necrosis and progressive outer retinal necrosis), and syphilis (Table 11–1). Some of the causes require no treatment or have no effective treatment (APMPPE, MEWDS, POHS), whereas others may be treated with immunosuppressive agents early (Behcet's syndrome, serpiginous choroiditis). For those causes that are corticosteroid sensitive, periocular or systemic treatment may be considered. Periocular and systemic corticosteroids are discussed in the previous section.

Panuveitis

Description

Panuveitis is characterized by inflammation of the anterior and posterior segments. Its prevalence in the United States is 30 per 100,000, and its frequency among cases of general uveitis ranges from 1% to 24% depending on type of ophthalmology practice (2–4,6). Presenting symptoms often include decreased vision, pain, redness, and floaters. Ophthalmic signs may include anterior uveitis, elevated intraocular pressure, retinal vascular sheathing, vitritis, retinitis, choroiditis, cystoid macular edema, and retinal detachment. Complications may include permanent decrease in visual acuity, cataract, cyclitic membrane, epiretinal membrane, chronic cystoid macular edema, retinal detachment, vitreous hemorrhage, retinal and choroidal neovascularization, and phthisis.

Etiology (Frequency Among Cases of Panuveitis)

Idiopathic (27% to 92%) (2–4,6,7): systemic association not identified by review of systems, ophthalmic examination, laboratory, or radiologic testing.

Sarcoidosis (0% to 28%) (2–4,6,7,15): see descriptions under anterior and posterior uveitis.

Vogt-Koyanagi-Harada (VKH) syndrome (3% to 33%) (2,3,6,8,13): clinical diagnosis based on bilateral granulomatous or nongranulomatous panuveitis with serous or exudative detachments, Dalen-Fuchs–like lesions, and disk edema. May have choroidal or retinal neovascularization. Systemic involvement includes perilimbal vitiligo (Sugiura's sign), tinnitus, poliosis, headache, dysacousis, and stiff neck. Most common in Asians, American Indians, African-Americans, and Latin Americans. Corticosteroids commonly used.

Behcet's disease (0% to 18%) (2,3,6–8,20): see description under Posterior Uveitis.

Sympathetic ophthalmia (0% to 9%) (2,3,8): clinical diagnosis based on bilateral granulomatous inflammation after ocular trauma (usually penetrating). Vitritis, papillitis, and Dalen-Fuch nodules are often present. Exudative retinal detachment may develop. Poor accommodation is an early symptom. Dysacousis, alopecia, and vitiligo may be present but are less common than with VKH. Corticosteroids and immunosuppressive agents have been used. (see Chapter 28).

Toxocariasis (3% to 28%) (4,13,17): see description under Posterior Uveitis.

Toxoplasmosis (8% to 13%) (7,13,17–19): see description under Posterior Uveitis.

Multifocal choroiditis and panuveitis syndrome (12%) (1): see description under Posterior Uveitis.

Bacterial endophthalmitis (2.5%) (2,3): hypopyon, anterior uveitis, vitritis, may have recent history of penetrating trauma or underlying medical condition predisposing to metastatic foci of infection (endocarditis, indwelling catheters, immunosuppression). Antimicrobial agents required (see Chapter 19).

Syphilis (0% to 6%) (2–4,6,7): see descriptions under Anterior and Posterior Uveitis.

Retained intraocular foreign body (0% to 5%) (2): history of penetrating trauma, known or suspected intraocular foreign body, may have iris heterochromia. Degree of damage related to composition of material and size of intraocular fragment. Some material is inert and may be well tolerated (sand, stone, glass, plastic, porcelain, cilia); however, pure copper and iron are toxic. Zinc and aluminum may become encapsulated and cause minimal damage. Surgical removal may be required.

HLA-B27 or spondyloarthropathy associated (2% to 4%) (3,7): see description under anterior uveitis. Posterior segment manifestations are uncommon but can include vitritis, retinal vasculitis, vascular occlusive disease, and pars plana exudate.

Other etiologies (3,4,7,8,13): systemic lupus erythematosus, polyarteritis nodosa, relapsing polychondritis, juvenile rheumatoid arthritis, multiple sclerosis, brucellosis, leprosy, fungal endophthalmitis, tuberculosis, intraocular lymphoma, phacogenic uveitis, retinal detachment.

Diagnosis

1. The associated ophthalmic features and the review of systems (with emphasis on symptoms associated with the etiologies above) are important to tailor the diagnostic evaluation.
2. All patients with intraocular inflammation should have a chest x-ray and syphilis serology. Some investigators (13) also routinely order a complete blood count with differential and urinalysis because asymptomatic abnormalities may require treatment.
3. Other studies to consider, depending on clinical suspicion, include toxoplasma ELISA or Western blot (helpful to rule out the diagnosis of toxoplasma retinochoroiditis if negative; however, a positive test does not confirm the diagnosis), HLA-B5 or HLA-Bw51 (Behcet's syndrome; however, the diagnosis is based on clinical criteria alone), toxocara ELISA, serum ACE and serum lysozyme (recommended by some authors (7,15) for sarcoidosis), neuroimaging and neurology referral (multiple sclerosis, Lyme encephalitis, central nervous system sarcoidosis), gallium scan (sarcoidosis), biopsy of ulceration (Behcet's syndrome), conjunctival/lacrimal gland/minor salivary gland/transbronchial biopsy (sarcoidosis), test for cutaneous hypersensitivity (Behcet's syndrome), vitreous biopsy (lymphoma), or vitreous culture (infectious endophthalmitis)

Management

1. Many of the causes of panuveitis are infectious and require antimicrobial therapy such as toxoplasmosis, syphilis (Table 11–1), and bacterial endophthalmitis (see Chapter 19). Some are treated with immunosuppressive agents (Behcet's syndrome) or radiation therapy and/or chemotherapy (lymphoma). Others often require surgical management (retained intraocular foreign body, retinal detachment, phacogenic uveitis). For those causes that are corticosteroid sensitive, periocular or systemic treatment, which has been discussed earlier, may be required.
2. Topical corticosteroids and cycloplegics are recommended for anterior segment inflammation.

EPISCLERITIS

Basic Considerations

Episcleritis is a typically benign, self-limited inflammatory condition occurring in all ages, but most commonly in young adults. The condition may be unilateral or bilateral. A history of recurrent episodes is common. Episcleritis is divided into simple or nodular forms.

Differential diagnosis includes those conditions that cause a red eye such as conjunctivitis and scleritis.

Etiology

In 70% of cases, no cause can be identified. In the remainder, some associated condition is found, including collagen vascular disease, herpes zoster, gout, or syphilis (21).

Diagnosis

1. History/symptoms: typically there is an acute onset of symptoms with redness (can be sectorial or diffuse) and discomfort. The discomfort or pain is typically localized to the eye, and is never severe and boring as in scleritis (21). The patient may complain of tearing, foreign body sensation, or a feeling of warmth, but photophobia is unusual and suggests an alternative or accompanying condition. Visual acuity is usually not affected.
2. The history also should include a thorough review of systems with questions directed to identify any of the associated conditions listed above: e.g., history of syphilis, rashes, arthritis, or other features of collagen vascular disease
3. Ophthalmologic examination should at least include visual acuity, pupils, extraocular motility, confrontational visual fields, tonometry, external examination, slit-lamp biomicroscopy, and fundoscopy. On examination, in cases of simple episcleritis, there is a diffuse edema of the episcleral tissues with a redness (of varying intensity, but no bluish tinge) that may be sectorial or diffuse. The eye is not tender and there is typically no anterior chamber reaction. In nodular episcleritis, the edema and infiltration is localized, producing a nodule (or nodules). A drop of 10% phenylephrine may help establish the diagnosis because with episcleritis the redness will branch, whereas in scleritis it will not.
4. Any further diagnostic workup to determine the etiology of episcleritis should be based on the history and examination (e.g., rapid plasma reagin (RPR)/fluorescent treponemal antibody-absorption (FTA-Abs) in cases of suspected syphilis, rheumatologic evaluation for suspected collagen vascular disease).

Management

1. Simple episcleritis is self-limited and will resolve spontaneously (usually within 3 to 4 weeks). Nodular scleritis is usually slower to resolve (may take 2 months), and treatment may be considered.
2. For mild cases, reassurance and observation is recommended. Artificial tears four to five times daily may provide some symptomatic relief.
3. For more severe cases with significant patient discomfort, topical corticosteroids (e.g., fluorometholone 0.1% four times daily or prednisolone acetate 1% four times daily depending on severity) may be tried. However, because this condition is self-limited, steroid therapy should be initiated only after a thorough discussion with the patient regarding potential side effects and complications (e.g., cataract, elevated intraocular pressure). Topical corticosteroids

should be tapered off over several weeks after the inflammation subsides. Long-term steroid therapy should be avoided, but such therapy may be necessary in some patients. For recurrent episcleritis, a slower taper is recommended. Also, for patients with significant discomfort, the possibility of an alternative diagnosis, such as scleritis, should be considered.

SCLERITIS

Basic Considerations

Scleritis, unlike episcleritis, is a potentially severe and destructive disease and scleritis may be associated with life-threatening systemic disorders, which should be considered in the evaluation of patients with this condition (22). Scleritis can be divided into anterior and posterior types. Anterior scleritis is further subdivided into diffuse, nodular, or necrotizing (with or without inflammation). Scleritis most commonly occurs in the fourth to sixth decades of life (the necrotizing form occurs later), has a female predilection, and is bilateral in 52% (beginning simultaneously in half of these) (21).

The differential diagnosis includes those diseases that can produce a red eye, such as episcleritis, conjunctivitis, iritis, carotid-cavernous fistula, and orbital pseudotumor (in cases of posterior scleritis).

Etiology

Approximately 50% of patients with scleritis will have a causally related condition (23). Most of these will be related to a systemic vasculitic disease such as rheumatoid arthritis, Wegener's granulomatosis, systemic lupus erythematosus (SLE), relapsing polychondritis, or inflammatory bowel disease. Other associations with scleritis include certain dermatologic diseases such as rosacea and metabolic diseases such as gout. Scleritis also can occur with ocular foreign bodies and chemical injuries, as well as after ocular surgery in susceptible individuals (surgically induced necrotizing scleritis). Infectious scleritis may be caused by bacteria (e.g., *Pseudomonas*), viruses (e.g., herpes zoster), parasites, fungi, spirochetes (e.g., syphilis, Lyme disease), and mycobacteria (e.g., tuberculosis).

Diagnosis

1. *History/symptoms:* Pain is the main symptom (except in scleromalacia perforans). The pain may be localized to the globe but is commonly diffuse, radiating to the forehead, temple, and jaw. The pain is usually boring and severe (especially in the necrotizing form with inflammation). Redness is also a dominant feature. The patient also may complain of tearing and photophobia.
2. Because some systemic conditions are commonly associated with scleritis, a detailed history including a thorough review of systems is essential. Questions

should include history of rash, arthritis, anemia, gastrointestinal problems, sexually transmitted diseases, sinus problems, hemoptysis, and hematuria. A history of previous episodes should be sought.

3. A complete ophthalmologic examination is required, including visual acuity, color vision, pupils, extraocular motility, exophthalmometry, confrontational visual fields, external examination, tonometry, slit-lamp biomicroscopy, and fundoscopy. The external examination should be performed in natural light to best visualize the bluish red hue of the sclera in these patients. Also the use of a drop of 10% phenylephrine to blanch overlying episcleral vessels is a useful adjunct to allow better visualization of the scleral edema and congestion.

4. The presentation will vary depending on the type (21):

   Diffuse anterior scleritis: widespread intense inflammation with scleral edema and maximum congestion at the level of the deep episcleral plexus (best illustrated by blanching (as described above) the overlying superficial plexus and conjunctival vessels that are also congested).

   Nodular anterior scleritis: intense inflammation as above, but with an immovable, tender nodule(s) of scleral tissue.

   Necrotizing anterior scleritis with inflammation: extremely painful with necrotic areas appearing as yellowish white discolorations of the sclera with absence of vessels (detection of avascular areas can be enhanced by use of the red-free filter on the slit lamp). Subsequently, the necrotic areas become transparent (underlying choroidal pigment becomes visible). Areas of necrosis spread and coalesce if the disease is not controlled.

   Scleromalacia perforans: almost total absence of symptoms. Typically occurs in females with long-standing rheumatoid arthritis. An area of yellow-white necrotic slough appears and eventually disappears leaving choroid covered by conjunctiva or nothing at all.

   Posterior scleritis: may or may not be associated with an anterior scleritis, which can make diagnosis difficult. Exudative retinal detachments, choroidal folds or detachments, choroidal "masses," and disk swelling may be seen. Other signs may include proptosis, limitation of ocular motility, and retraction of the lower lid on attempted elevation of the globe (21). Ultrasound is helpful in establishing the diagnosis (24).

5. Numerous complications or associated ocular conditions may occur with scleritis and must be sought during examination. These include scleral thinning or perforation, uveitis (rarely may be granulomatous), glaucoma, cataract, retinal detachment (often associated with underlying sclerochoroidal granuloma), increasing hypermetropia (due to scleral edema), optic disk edema, and characteristic corneal changes (seen in 37%, including acute stromal keratitis, sclerosing keratitis, limbal guttering with lipid deposition, and keratolysis in severe necrotizing disease) (21,25).

6. Workup should include basic chemistries (particularly blood urea nitrogen [BUN] and creatinine), urinalysis (to rule out hematuria from Wegener's), chest x-ray, syphilis serology. We also often include antinuclear antibodies (ANA), serum antineutrophilic cytoplasmic antibody for Wegener's disease or periar-

teritis nodosa, erythrocyte sedimentation rate (ESR), and complete blood count with differential (as a baseline for patients in whom immunosuppressive therapy is being considered). A more extensive workup should be directed by the patient's history and examination and may include internal medicine (or rheumatology) evaluation, serum uric acid (for suspected gout), or anti-double-stranded DNA (for suspected systemic lupus erythematosus).

7. Ancillary studies:

   - B-scan ultrasonography can determine the extent and severity of inflammation and can aid in diagnosing posterior scleritis.
   - Anterior segment fluorescein angiography is not required but can help distinguish non-necrotizing (rapid-flow) from necrotizing (hypo- and nonperfusion) forms, and may guide therapy.

Management

In general, nonsteroidal anti-inflammatory drugs (NSAIDs) are the starting point for treatment of noninfectious scleritis. Medications with greater potential toxicities (systemic steroids and then immunosuppressives) are considered for unresponsive cases. The patient's internist should be involved in monitoring for side effects when these agents are used. As with other inflammatory diseases, therapy should be tapered and not stopped abruptly. Potential side effects of medications (for systemic steroids see Intermediate Uveitis; for NSAIDS, side effects and complications include gastrointestinal discomfort, peptic ulcer disease, and interstitial nephritis) must be discussed with the patient before beginning treatment.

1. NSAIDs are sufficient therapy in most patients with diffuse or nodular scleritis. Not all of the NSAIDs are equally effective. We recommend indomethacin 25 to 50 mg three times daily depending on the severity of the disease. Pain and tenderness, scleral injection, and corneal and intraocular involvement can be followed to assess response to therapy. Pain often improves before the redness. Therapy should be continued at these doses as long as the patient is improving. If there is no response, alternative agents may be needed.

2. Systemic steroids are generally required in necrotizing scleritis, severe refractory non-necrotizing cases, or if areas of vascular closure are seen (by slit-lamp examination or by fluorescein angiography). Sufficiently high doses (usually 1 mg/kg/day) should be given initially to suppress the disease and then gradually tapered. If the disease flares, the dosage is increased to suppress the inflammation, and then tapered to the lowest dose at which the eye remains quiet (the maintenance dose). After continuing therapy at this maintenance level for several weeks, another taper may be attempted. The rate of the taper will be determined by the occurrence of additional flares. Some patients may require chronic low-dose steroids to maintain quiescence; however, the potential for severe side effects is great, and steroid-sparing agents should be considered. Occasionally, high-dose intravenous pulse steroid therapy (e.g., methylprednisolone 1 g/day for 3 days)

and/or immunosuppressive therapy may be considered. Topical steroids are generally ineffective in scleritis. Subconjunctival steroids historically have been avoided in scleritis for fear of potential scleral thinning and perforation. Recently, however, the safety and efficacy of subconjunctival triamcinolone as an adjunctive agent for treating non-necrotizing anterior scleritis has been reported (26).

3. Immunosuppressive agents useful for scleritis include azathioprine, methotrexate, cyclosporine, cyclophosphamide, and chlorambucil. Some investigators have suggested that immunosuppressives should be first-line therapy in necrotizing cases and in cases associated with potentially life-threatening vasculitis (Wegener's granulomatosis) (27). However, immunosuppressive therapy should be initiated only by someone experienced in the use of these agents. A thorough discussion of the side effects and assessment of the patient's likelihood of compliance (with follow-up and laboratory monitoring) is crucial before beginning therapy given the potential life-threatening toxicities of these agents. Topical cyclosporine recently has been reported to be of benefit in some cases and also may be considered (28).

4. Infectious scleritis should be treated with the appropriate antimicrobial therapy, rather than with steroids or immunosuppressives.

5. Surgery may be necessary acutely in cases of persistent scleritis due to a foreign body. Otherwise, surgery to cover scleral or corneal defects (with grafts) should be delayed until systemic disease and ocular inflammation is controlled. Cyanoacrylate glue has been used by some as a temporizing measure to seal perforations until control of inflammation is achieved.

6. Frequency of follow-up will depend on the severity of disease, presence of associated complications, medication requirement (e.g., patients on immunosuppressives will require frequent laboratory studies to monitor for toxicity), and the patient's response to therapy.

7. Patients should be monitored carefully for drug toxicity. Prophylaxis for gastrointestinal upset or ulceration is often prescribed (misoprostol or a histamine H2-antagonist) in patients being treated with NSAIDs or oral steroids.

ORBITAL INFLAMMATORY SYNDROME (ORBITAL PSEUDOTUMOR)

Basic Considerations

Orbital pseudotumor is defined as an idiopathic, nonspecific, benign inflammation with a hypocellular polymorphic lymphoid infiltrate and varying amounts of fibrosis (29). The disease can present at any age but is most commonly seen in middle-aged adults. It is most often unilateral in adults, although more often bilateral in children. Males and females are affected with equal frequency. The inflammation can have diffuse or localized forms (30). The localized forms can be classified as myositis, dacryoadenitits, periscleritis, and perineuritis. The clinical course can be acute, subacute, or chronic.

Patients with orbital pseudotumor often present with acute onset of painful proptosis, lid erythema and edema, conjunctival chemosis and hyperemia, and limitation of eye movement (31). Some of these findings may be seen with other inflammatory or infectious conditions (32).

Differential Diagnosis

Before one assigns the diagnosis of idiopathic orbital inflammatory syndrome to the patient's symptoms, other causes of orbital inflammation must be excluded (33). Careful history and examination in addition to selected laboratory and radiographic studies are essential to differentiate pseudotumor from the disorders listed in Table 11–2.

Orbital cellulitis may be difficult to distinguish from orbital pseudotumor. The patient with orbital cellulitis may appear more ill and often has a history of sinusitis or trauma.

Thyroid eye disease, in contrast to pseudotumor, tends to have a more gradual and painless onset. Thyroid ophthalmopathy is more commonly bilateral. Thyroid eye disease preferentially involves inferior and medial recti, whereas orbital pseudotumor has a predilection for superior and medial recti. The tendons of the extraocular muscles are generally spared with thyroid eye disease and involved with pseudotumor.

Lymphoma may present with a painless salmon-colored conjunctival mass. Orbital lymphoma preferentially involves the superior and retrobulbar areas and tends to spread along the outline of the globe.

Vasculitic disorders (e.g., Wegener's granulomatosis, periarteritis nodosa) often have concomitant pulmonary, renal, or cutaneous manifestations.

An arteriovenous fistula of the cavernous sinus should be considered when there are dilated, tortuous corkscrew conjunctival vessels and an audible bruit. Intraocular pressure is commonly elevated due to congested venous outflow. Elevated intraocular pressure is seen less often with orbital pseudotumor. Patients with carotid-cavernous sinus fistula frequently have a history of trauma, hypertension, or atherosclerosis.

TABLE 11–2. *Differential diagnosis of orbital pseudotumor*

Orbital cellulitis
Thyroid ophthalmopathy
Lymphoma
Vasculitis
Wegener's granulomatosis
Periarteritis nodosa
Arteriovenous fistula
Primary or secondary orbital tumor
Other causes of inflammation
Sarcoidosis
Retained foreign body
Orbital hemorrhage
Ruptured dermoid cyst

Lung and breast carcinomas may metastasize to the orbit and present as an orbital mass. Rhabdomyosarcoma needs to be considered in children with rapidly progressing orbital swelling. Neuroblastoma, metastatic, and invasive cancers may cause bony erosion that is not seen with orbital pseudotumor.

Laboratory Testing

There are no specific laboratory abnormalities associated with orbital pseudotumor. Hematologic and radiologic testing are of value in excluding other conditions entertained in the differential diagnosis. The history and presentation of the patient help narrow the focus of laboratory investigation.

1. Complete blood count with differential to help rule out an infectious process.
2. Thyroid function studies to screen for thyroid dysfunction.
3. Antinuclear cytoplasmic antibody may be positive with Wegener's granulomatosis.
4. ESR or ANA may be elevated in patients with vasculitis.
5. Serum chemistry including BUN and creatinine may show renal dysfunction in patients with vasculitis.
6. Chest radiograph is helpful in evaluating suspected cases of sarcoidosis, tuberculosis, Wegener's granulomatosis, or lung carcinoma.
7. ACE level, gallium scan, serum calcium, and urine calcium may be useful when investigating for sarcoidosis; however, the diagnosis is based on histopathology.
8. Tissue biopsy should be considered in cases with an atypical clinical presentation or a history of malignancy.
9. Orbital imaging with contrast-enhanced orbital CT scan or ultrasound is essential in establishing the diagnosis. The typical findings in these studies are discussed below.

Diagnosis

Each of the subcategories of idiopathic orbital inflammation has a distinctive clinical presentation (32), with characteristic features on orbital imaging (34,35).

Diffuse Form

1. Severe orbital pain, eyelid erythema and edema, proptosis, conjunctival chemosis, restricted ocular motility, and diplopia are the main features.
2. Orbital inflammation also may induce uveitis.
3. Posterior involvement may cause papillitis, optic neuropathy, cystoid macular edema, and exudative detachment of the retina and choroid.
4. Characteristic radiographic findings:
   - CT scan: irregularly circumscribed enhancing orbital mass that follows the contours of the globe and spares the sinuses. There may or may not be extraocular muscle enlargement.

- Ultrasound: B-scan shows mottling with moderate sound absorption in the fat pad. A-scan shows low acoustic reflectivity. A mass with low internal reflectivity suggests a cellular mass, and is also seen with bacterial cellulitis and lymphoma.

Periscleritis (Anterior Orbital Inflammation)

1. Orbital pain, blurred vision, erythema of the eyelid, conjunctival chemosis, hyperemia, iritis, and choroiditis are the main features.
2. Periscleral tissues and tenons capsule are the areas primarily involved. However, when the posterior sclera is affected, distinguishing periscleritis from posterior scleritis may be difficult.
3. Increased intraocular pressure may occur due to angle closure from forward rotation of the lens-iris diaphragm, or from obstruction of the trabecular meshwork by inflammatory cells.
4. Posterior involvement may result in choroidal detachment, choroidal striae, exudative retinal detachment, and cystoid macular edema.
5. Characteristic radiographic findings:

   - CT scan: irregularly circumscribed enhancing orbital mass following contour of the globe without sinus involvement, with or without extraocular muscle enlargement.
   - Ultrasound: thickening of the sclerouveal coat on B-scan. If present, retinal or choroidal detachments also may be detected. With posterior scleral involvement there is perineural and subtenons effusion at the neuro-ocular junction (T-sign).

Myositis

1. Pain on eye movement, proptosis, diplopia, blepharoptosis, and chemosis are the main features.
2. There is infiltration of one or more of the extraocular muscles with an inflammatory process.
3. Hyperemia and chemosis of the conjunctiva over the involved muscle insertion is common.
4. Ocular movement is restricted in the field of action of the affected muscle. Medial and superior recti are the muscles more commonly involved.
5. Characteristic radiographic findings:

   - CT scan: diffuse enlargement of the extraocular muscle with irregular borders. Single or multiple muscles may be involved. In contrast to thyroid eye disease, the tendons are involved in pseudotumor.
   - Ultrasound: extraocular muscle enlargement with involvement of the tendon. Internal reflectivity is low in myositis.

Dacryoadenitis

1. Pain and tenderness in the region of the lacrimal gland, S-shaped deformity and erythema of the upper eyelid, with mild conjunctival chemosis are the main features.
2. Vision and ocular motility are usually unaffected; however, involvement of the lateral rectus muscle may result in diplopia.
3. The enlarged lacrimal gland will be tender and its palpebral lobe may be seen as an erythematous mass in the superotemporal conjunctival fornix.
4. Characteristic radiographic findings:
   CT scan: contrast-enhancing mass in the region of the lacrimal gland occasionally with edema extending into tenons space and the lateral rectus muscle.
   Ultrasound: mass in the lacrimal fossa with homogeneous internal acoustics and thickening of the adjacent muscle.

Perineuritis (Posterior Orbital Inflammation)

1. Pain, decreased vision, visual field defects, dyschromatopsia, and pain on eye movement are the main features. Optic disk edema and a relative afferent pupillary defect are also seen.
2. Inflammation involves the perineural orbital fat, optic nerve sheath, and extraocular muscles in the orbital apex.
3. Clinical features may be similar to optic neuritis; however, in contrast to optic neuritis, mild proptosis and pain on retropulsion may be present.
4. Characteristic radiographic findings:
   • CT scan: enlargement of the optic nerve sheath with contrast enhancement. There is infiltration of the perineural orbital fat and the extraocular muscles in the orbital apex.
   • Ultrasound: although the optic nerve may be enlarged, ultrasound is less useful in evaluating the posterior orbital tissues.

Management

In cases in which the diagnosis is questionable, a biopsy should be performed to rule out malignancy (36). A discrete orbital mass, isolated lacrimal gland involvement, or bony erosion raises the suspicion of a neoplasm or other systemic disorders, which warrants confirmation by tissue biopsy. An infectious etiology also must be excluded. Otherwise, patients who present with typical history and characteristic findings on physical examination and orbital imaging studies are often treated empirically.

1. Begin prednisone at 1 to 1.5 mg/kg/day.
2. Medical contraindications for steroids should be considered and the risks of systemic steroids explained to the patient.

3. In severe cases and those with optic neuropathy consider initiating treatment with intravenous methylprednisolone 1 g/day and switching to oral prednisone (1 mg/kg/day) after 2 to 3 days.

4. Topical corticosteroids can be added for the treatment of anterior uveitis.

5. Topical beta-blockers, dorzolamide hydrochloride, or apraclonidine hydrochloride may be needed to reduce aqueous formation in cases with elevated intraocular pressure.

6. Acute cases commonly respond to treatment within 48 to 72 hours.

7. High dosages of corticosteroids should be maintained for 3 weeks and gradually tapered.

8. If the condition does not respond to systemic steroids, a biopsy should be performed (37).

9. In recurrent and refractory cases, cyclosporine (38) and/or orbital irradiation (39) may be necessary.

REFERENCES

1. Darrell RW, Wagner HP, Kurland LT. Epidemiology of uveitis: incidence and prevalence in a small urban community. *Arch Ophthalmol* 1962;68:502–14.

2. McCannel CA, Holland GN, Helm CJ, Cornell PJ, et al. Causes of uveitis in the general practice of ophthalmology. *Am J Ophthalmol* 1996;121:35–46.

3. Rodriguez A, Calonge M, Pedroza-Seres M, et al. Referral patterns of uveitis in a tertiary eye care center. *Arch Ophthalmol* 1996;114:593–9.

4. Perkins ES, Folk J. Uveitis in London and Iowa. *Ophthalmologica* 1984;189:36–40.

5. Rothova A, van Veenendaal WG, Linssen A, Glasius E, Kijlstra A, de Jong PTVM. Clinical features of acute anterior uveitis. *Am J Ophthalmol* 1987;103:137–45.

6. Smit RL, Baarsma GS, de Vries J. Classification of 750 consecutive uveitis patients in the Rotterdam Eye Hospital. *Int Ophthalmol* 1993;17:71–6.

7. Rothova A, Buitenhuis HJ, Meeken C, et al. Uveitis and systemic disease. *Br J Ophthalmol* 1992;60:137–41.

8. Chung YM, Yeh TS, Liu JH. Endogenous uveitis in Chinese—an analysis of 240 cases in a uveitis clinic. *Jpn J Ophthalmol* 1988;32:64–9.

9. Rosenbaum JT. Characterization of uveitis associated with spondyloarthritis. *J Rheumatol* 1989;16:792–6.

10. Tay-Kearney ML, Schwam BL, Lowder C, et al. Clinical features and associated systemic disease of HLA-B27 uveitis. *Am J Ophthalmol* 1996;121:47–56.

11. The Herpetic Eye Disease Study Group. A controlled clinical trial of oral acyclovir for iridocyclitis caused by herpes simplex virus. *Arch Ophthalmol* 1996;114:1065–72.

12. Jabs DA. Ocular manifestations of rheumatic diseases. In: Tasman W, Jaeger EA, eds. *Duane's Clinical Ophthalmology*. Philadelphia: JB Lippincott; 1992.

13. Nussenblatt RB, Whitcup SM, Palestine AG. *Uveitis: Fundamentals and Clinical* Practice. Baltimore: CV Mosby; 1996.

14. Karma A, Huhti E, Poukkula A. Course and outcome of ocular sarcoidosis. *Am J Ophthalmol* 1988;106:467–72.

15. Baarsma GS, La Hey E, Glasius E, de Vries J, Kijlstra A. The predictive value of serum angiotensin converting enzyme and lysozyme levels in the diagnosis of ocular sarcoidosis. *Am J Ophthalmol* 1987;104:211–7.

16. Ho AC, Guyer DR, Yannuzzi LA, Brown GC. Ocular syphilis: classic manifestations and recent observations. *Semin Ophthalmol* 1993;8:53–60.

17. Opremcak EM. *Uveitis: A Clinical Manual for Ocular Inflammation*. New York: Springer-Verlag; 1994.

18. Engstrom RE, Holland GN, Nussenblatt RB, Jabs DA. Current practices in the management of toxoplasmosis. *Am J Ophthalmol* 1991;111:601–10.

19. Jabs DA. Ocular manifestations of HIV infection. *Trans Am Ophthalmol Soc* 1995;93:623–83.
20. Mishima S, Masuda K, Izawa Y, Mochizuki M, Namba K. The eighth Frederick H. Verhoeff lecture: Behcet's disease in Japan: ophthalmologic aspects. *Trans Am Opthalmol Soc* 1979;77:225–79.
21. Watson P. Diseases of the Sclera and Episclera. In: Tasman W, Jaeger EA, eds. *Duane's Clinical Ophthalmology*. Vol. 4. Philadelphia: JB Lippincott; 1995.
22. de la Maza MS, Foster CS, Jabbur NS. Scleritis associated with systemic vasculitic diseases. *Ophthalmology* 1995;102:687–92.
23. Hakin KN, Watson PG. Systemic associations of scleritis. *Int Ophthalmol Clin* 1991;31:111–29.
24. Rosenbaum JT, Robertson JE. Recognition of posterior scleritis and its treatment with indomethacin. *Retina* 1993;13:17–21.
25. de la Maza MS, Jabbur NS, Foster CS. Severity of scleritis and episcleritis. *Ophthalmology* 1994;101:389–96.
26. Tu EY, Culbertson WW, Pflugfelder SC, Huang A, Chodosh JC. Therapy of nonnecrotizing anterior scleritis with subconjunctival corticosteroid injection. *Ophthalmology* 1995;102:718–24.
27. de la Maza MS, Foster CS, Jabbur NS. An analysis of therapeutic decision for scleritis. *Ophthalmology* 1994;100:389–96.
28. Rosenfeld SI, Kronish JW, Schweitzer WA, Siegal JE. Topical cyclosporine for treating necrotizing scleritis. *Arch Ophthalmol* 1995;113:20–1.
29. Kennerdell JS, Dresner SC. The nonspecific orbital inflammatory syndromes. *Surv Ophthalmol* 1984;29:93–103.
30. Mombaerts I, Goldschmeding R, Schlingemann RO, et al. What is orbital pseudotumor? *Surv Ophthalmol* 1996;41:66–78.
31. Snebold NG. Noninfectious orbital inflammation and vasculitis. In: Albert DM, Jackobiec FA, eds. *Principles and Practices of Ophthalmology*. Vol. 3. Philadelphia: WB Saunders; 1994:1923–42.
32. Rootman J, Nugent R, The classification and management of acute orbital pseudotumors. *Ophthalmology* 1982;89:1040–8.
33. Mauriello JA, Flanagan JC. Management of orbital inflammatory disease. A protocol. *Surv Ophthalmol* 1984;29:104–16.
34. McNicholas MM, Power WJ, Griffin JF. Idiopathic Inflammatory pseudotumor of the orbit: CT features correlated with clinical outcome. *Clin Radiol* 1991;44:3–7.
35. Byrne SF, Green RL. *Ultrasound of the Eye and Orbit*. St. Louis: Mosby-Year Book; 1992:283–8.
36. Kennerdell JS. Management of nonspecific inflammatory and lymphoid orbital lesions. *Int Ophthalmol Clin* 1991;31:7–15.
37. Char DH, Miller T. Orbital pseudotumor. Fine-needle aspiration biopsy and response to therapy. *Ophthalmology* 1993;100:1702–10.
38. Diaz-Llopis M, Menezo JL. Idiopathic inflammatory orbital pseudotumor and low-dose cyclosporine. *Am J Ophthalmol* 1989;107:547–8.
39. Lanciano R, Fowble B, Sergott RC, et al. The results of the radiotherapy for orbital pseudotumor. *Int J Radiat Oncol Biol Phys* 1990;18:407–11.

Management of Ocular Injuries and Emergencies,
edited by Mathew W. MacCumber.
Lippincott–Raven Publishers, Philadelphia © 1998.

12

Ocular Burns

Julie S. Yu, Robert A. Ralph, and Jonathan B. Rubenstein

Department of Ophthalmology, Rush-Presbyterian St. Lukes Medical Center, Chicago, Illinois 60612 and Department of Ophthalmology, Wilmer Eye Institute, The Johns Hopkins University School of Medicine, Baltimore, Maryland 21287

Chemical Burns   163
    Basic Considerations   163 · Diagnosis   163 · Initial Management   165
    Other Initial Management Options   167 · Intermediate Treatment   168
    Rehabilitation   169
Thermal Burns   170
    Basic Considerations   170 · Diagnosis   170 · Management   171

CHEMICAL BURNS

Basic Considerations

Chemical burns are the one type of ocular emergency in which every minute counts. Prognosis depends on rapidity of treatment, duration of exposure, concentration of solution, and the pH of the solution. Alkali burns result in worse injury because they penetrate the eye rapidly, saponifying cell membranes, denaturing collagen, and thrombosing vessels. Acids generally cause less damage because the hydrogen ion precipitates protein and forms a barrier to additional penetration. The anterior cornea may become cloudy, but the stroma underneath may remain intact and clear. Treatment and potential complications are similar regardless of the offending agent.

Diagnosis

Once a history of chemical burn is obtained, immediate irrigation should be initiated as described below. The examiner should then elicit the patient's history, including the time elapsed since exposure, the duration of exposure, the type of chemical (Table 12–1), the time and duration of irrigation, and whether safety glasses were worn at the time of exposure.

Ocular burns do not always occur in isolation. Those occurring simultaneously with blast injury, as in exploding car batteries, may be overshadowed by structural

TABLE 12–1. *Common causes of chemical injury*

Class	Compound	Common sources/uses	Comments
Alkali	Ammonia [NH₃]	Fertilizers Refrigerants Cleaning agents (7% solution)	Combines with water to form NH₄OH fumes Very rapid penetration (in aqueous solutions)
	Lye [NaOH]	Drain cleaners	Penetrates almost as rapidly as ammonia
	Potassium hydroxide [KOH]	Caustic potash	Severity similar to that of lye
	Magnesium hydroxide [Mg(OH)₂]	Sparklers	Produces combined thermal and alkali injury
	Lime [CA(OH)₂]	Plaster Mortar Cement Whitewash	Most common cause of chemical injury in work place Poor penetration Toxicity increased by retained particulate matter
Acid	Sulfuric acid [H₂SO₄]	Industrial cleaner Battery acid	Combines with water to produce corneal thermal injury May have associated foreign body or laceration from battery acid
	Sulfurous acid [H₂SO₃]	Formed from sulfur dioxide (SO₂)by combination with corneal water Fruit and vegetable preservative Bleach Refrigerant	Penetrates more easily than other acids
	Hydrofluoric acid [HF]	Glass polishing Glass frosting Mineral refining Gasoline alkylation Silicone production	Penetrates easily Produces severe injury
	Acetic acid [CH₃COOH]	Vinegar—4–10% Essence of vinegar—80% Glacial acetic acid–90%	Mild injury with less than 10% contamination Severe injury with higher concentration
	Chromic acid [Cr₂O₃]	Used in the chrome plating industry	Chronic exposure produces chronic conjunctivitis with brown discoloration
	Hydrochloric acid [HCl]	Used as a 32–38% solution	Severe injury only with high concentration and prolonged exposure

Courtesy of Wagoner and Kenyon (2).

tissue damage resulting from the explosion or from shrapnel. Patients with pulmonary and/or cutaneous involvement may have other more life-threatening problems. These, of course, should be addressed first or concomitantly.

The appearance of chemical burns can range from superficial punctate keratopathy and subconjunctival hemorrhage to complete marbleization of the cornea. Injuries are usually more severe at the inferior limbus as the eyes close and the Bell phenomenon occurs.

The examiner should direct special attention to the following:

- presence and site of epithelial defect
- conjunctiva, especially limbus (white eye is bad)
- corneal clarity (iris details)
- inflammation
- increased intraocular pressure (IOP)—immediate increase usually is due to collagen shrinkage
- cloudy lens suggests intraocular penetration

Local necrotic retinopathy corresponding to the region of scleral damage also has been reported. Several classification schemes exist to predict prognosis. The Thoft's scale is a helpful and easy one to remember (Table 12–2 and Fig. 12–1).

Initial Management

1. Irrigate the injured eye immediately at the site of injury with any neutral solution (Fig. 12–2*A*). When the patient arrives at the emergency room, instill proparacaine and place a lid speculum. Continue flushing the eye with any available neutral solution, including water or normal saline, for a minimum of 30 minutes. Intravenous (i.v.) delivery systems are available that consist of tubing attached to a contact lens (e.g., Mediflow lens (Mor-Tan, Inc.) or percutaneous irrigating tube [Fig. 12–2*B*]) (1). Apply litmus paper into the fornices to check the pH. If the eye is not neutral, then continue irrigation.
2. Perform a thorough examination for any retained particles and debride. Instill proparacaine and doubly evert the lid. Swab the fornices with a moistened cotton tip and remove any foreign bodies with a fine forceps or by scraping with a no. 15 Bard-Parker blade. Cotton tips moistened with 0.01 mol/L to 0.05 mol/L solution of 10% EDTA can make sticky CaOH easier to remove (1).

TABLE 12–2. *Thoft's classification of chemical injury*

Grade I	Corneal epithelial damage, no ischemia (good prognosis)
Grade II	Cornea hazy but iris details seen, ischemia less than one third of limbus (good prognosis)
Grade III	Total loss of corneal epithelium, Stromal haze blurring iris details, ischemia of one third to one half of limbus (guarded prognosis)
Grade IV	Cornea opaque obscuring view of iris or pupil, ischemia of more than one half of limbus (poor prognosis)

Courtesy of Wagoner and Kenyon (2).

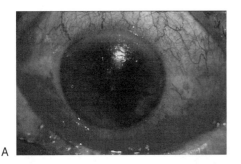

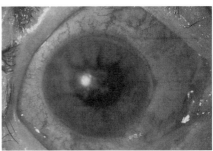

A

B

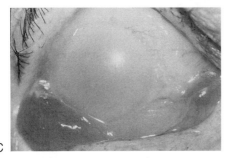

C

FIG. 12–1. Thoft's classification. **A:** Grade I. **B:** Grade II. **C:** Grade IV. *For a color representation of (A) and (B) please see the color insert facing p. 256.*

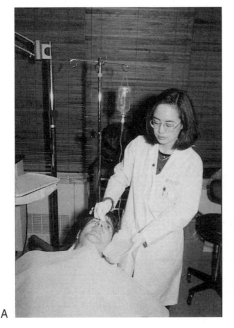

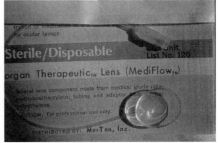

A

B

FIG. 12–2. A: Ocular irrigation using a neutral solution. **B:** Mediflow lens for ocular irrigation.

3. Use antibiotics to decrease the chance of secondary infection of a necrotic and inflamed eye. We recommend erythromycin ointment four times daily or any other broad-spectrum antibiotic.

4. Cycloplege the eye to relieve ciliary spasm, decrease posterior synechiae, and decrease inflammation by strengthening the blood aqueous barrier; examples include scopolamine 0.25% four times daily, homatropine 5% three times daily, or atropine 1% three times daily. Avoid mydriatics, such as phenylephrine, which can contribute further to anterior segment ischemia.

5. The use of topical steroids decreases the inflammatory response that will delay epithelial migration. However, steroids also potentiate collagenase after the first week, which can lead to corneal thinning. Therefore, use prednisolone acetate 1% four times daily (1) to every hour (2) for the first 7 to 10 days only. If an epithelial defect is still present at this time, begin tapering the steroids to decrease the risk of perforation. One can also consider switching to medroxyprogesterone, which is a progestational steroid with less anti-inflammatory action but also with less suppression of stromal collagen repair (3). Use a 1% suspension topically every 1 to 2 hours (2).

6. Intraocular pressure in a chemically injured eye can be high or low. Hypotony is usually secondary to ciliary body damage. A high IOP is caused by collagen shrinkage, inflammatory debris obstructing the trabecular meshwork, trabecular meshwork damage, or increased episcleral venous pressure. Control of IOP may require suppression of aqueous production by topical β-adrenergic antagonists (betaxolol, carteolol, levobunolol, metopranolol, or timolol) twice daily, α-adrenergic agonists (apraclonidine or brimonidine) three times daily, or carbonic anhydrase inhibitors (acetazolamide 250 mg orally or i.v. four times daily or dorzolamide topically three times daily).

Other Initial Management Options

1. In severe injuries consider anterior chamber paracentesis with aqueous removal/irrigation to modulate severe pH changes in the anterior chamber. This is only useful if performed within 2 hours of the injury. It is not universally recommended because of the high rate of complications, including lens injury, iris prolapse, and hemorrhage. Instill tetracaine or proparacaine and use a 27- or 30-gauge needle on a tuberculin syringe. A no. 11 Bard-Parker blade can facilitate the needle entrance (see Chapter 23, under Retinal Artery Occlusion) (4).

2. Topical citrate is thought to inhibit corneal ulceration by chelating extracellular calcium, which results in decreased polymorphonuclear activity and chemotaxis (4). Use 10% citrate in artificial tear solution every 30 to 60 minutes while awake. Topical 10% citrate is probably more effective in promoting re-epithelialization than ascorbic acid (5).

3. Ascorbic acid is an essential cofactor in the synthesis of collagen. Decreased aqueous levels are thought to be associated with corneal perforation (2). Use

topical 10% ascorbic acid in artificial tears every hour for 14 hours/day for 1 week, then decrease to four times daily. Use sodium ascorbate (2 g) orally four times daily to keep the aqueous level at greater than 15 mg/dl. Continue both until complete re-epithelialization occurs. Again, citrate is probably more effective than ascorbic acid (5). Topical ascorbic acid and topical citrate are not commonly used because of poor patient compliance with their hourly dosing.

4. Tetracycline 250 mg orally every 6 hours chelates the calcium necessary for collagenase to function, thereby inhibiting collagenase.

Intermediate Treatment

The goal is to prevent stromal ulceration, which usually starts 2 to 3 weeks after injury (Fig. 12–3), especially by promoting re-epithelialization.

1. Intense lubrication with nonpreserved tears is essential. Lid surgery may be necessary to decrease corneal exposure from entropion, trichiasis, or inadequate lid closure.
2. A therapeutic soft contact lens, patching, and/or temporary tarsorrhaphy may contribute to re-epithelialization.
3. Prevent symblepharon by sweeping fornices with a glass rod to lyse adhesions.
4. Consider collagenase inhibitors in severe cases. N-acetylcysteine chelates calcium and reduces a critical disulfide bond in the collagenase molecule (6). EDTA works as a calcium chelator. Use topical N-acetylcysteine 10% every 2 hours beginning 7 days after the injury (4) or topical 0.05 to 0.10 mol/L disodium EDTA four times daily (7).
5. Topical vitamin A has been shown to improve goblet cell function. Use all trans retinoic acid 0.01% ointment every hour (2).
6. If corneal perforation occurs (Fig. 12–4A), use cyanoacrylate glue to seal the defect, although it is not currently approved by the U.S. Food and Drug Administration for this application.
7. If the glue is not successful, an emergent corneal transplant or patch graft (Fig. 12–4B) may be necessary to restore the anterior chamber.

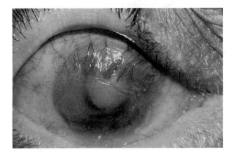

FIG. 12–3. Severe alkali burn at 16 weeks. Note pannus and stromal thinning.

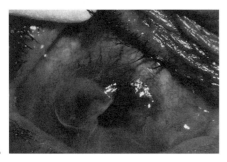 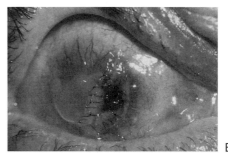

A   B

FIG. 12–4. A: Severe alkali injury with corneal perforation at 20 weeks. **B:** Same eye with patch graft after perforation.

Rehabilitation

1. The primary goal is to restore the ocular surface.
   - In unilateral burns, a conjunctival-limbal autograft, in which conjunctiva from the uninjured eye is transplanted to the traumatized eye, will repopulate limbal stem cells to re-epithelialize the cornea (8).
   - In cases of bilateral injury, three surgical options are available to restore the stem cell population, thus improving the ocular surface. These include cadaver conjunctival-limbal allograft, living related conjunctival-limbal allograft, or keratolimbal allograft (8).
   - In severe cases, a mucous membrane transplant from the buccal mucosa may be necessary. The mucosal graft stimulates neovascularization and scar tissue formation that is resistant to collagenase and therefore to perforation (6).
2. The final step is the attempt to restore corneal integrity and optical clarity.
   - Lamellar keratoplasty provides tectonic structure.
   - Corneal transplant surgery is most successful 18 to 24 months after injury in an eye without ulceration, perforation, or glaucoma. When necessary, conjuncti-

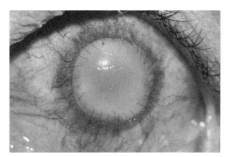

FIG. 12–5. Penetrating keratoplasty after ammonia burn with early opacification.

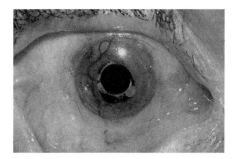

FIG. 12–6. Keratoprosthesis after severe alkali burn. Note melting around central optical post.

val and limbal stem cell transplantation should be performed at least 6 months before penetrating keratoplasty to increase the long-term chance of graft survival. Because of the numerous complications and high failure rates, penetrating keratoplasty is only recommended in cases where both eyes have poor vision (Fig. 12–5).

• Consider keratoprosthesis only in the most severe cases (Fig. 12–6).

THERMAL BURNS

Basic Considerations

Direct thermal injury to the eye is rare; however, ocular damage does occur in burn patients. Burn patients, especially those with facial involvement, often require life-saving measures, and the ophthalmologist is usually consulted after the patient is stabilized. Diagnosis, treatment, and prevention of ocular damage is imperative to retain good visual acuity.

Diagnosis

Despite the fact that burn patients may be critically ill, a thorough ocular examination must be performed.

1. Ocular injury primarily involves the eyelids. A first-degree burn involves the epidermis only, as in a sunburn. The skin has a blanching erythema and heals in 3 to 6 days. A second-degree burn involves the epidermis and dermis and can destroy skin appendages. Blisters form, and the erythematous skin is painful. These burns generally heal within 10 to 21 days. Third-degree burns are the most serious, resulting in necrosis of all skin layers and destruction of all skin appendages. They cause coagulation of the subdermal plexus and thrombosis of dermal vessels and heal into dry, hard, pearly white scars. Ocular surface damage secondary to lid burns usually occurs after eyelid scarring has caused cicatricial changes. Ectropion, entropion, and trichiasis can all result in corneal damage. These lid deformities are usually repaired secondarily, often with skin grafts.

2. Corneal injury from thermal burns is rare (9,10). The burn has a gray opaque appearance with raised irregular edges of epithelium and is usually located in the inferior or central cornea.
3. Ocular perforation is usually associated with missile injury (see Chapters 15 and 21).
4. Canalicular injury is associated with epiphora and medial lid burn. The puncta are cauterized or stenotic.

Management

1. Use gauze and saline to remove lid crusting. Topical antibiotic ointment (e.g., erythromycin two to four times daily) should be applied to the cornea and conjunctiva. Frequent lubrication with artificial tears and ointments is often required. Apply skin antiseptics such as silver nitrate 0.5% or providone-iodine 5%, but be sure to avoid corneal contact (11).
2. Treat a corneal burn as a corneal abrasion. Monitor closely for the development of corneal ulcers (see Chapter 14).
3. Evaluate the canalicular system if there are adjacent burns. If the puncta are identified and probed without resistance, re-evaluate with the dye disappearance test and repeat probing every 1 to 2 days for 7 to 10 days. If the puncta cannot be identified and/or probed, consider surgical debridement with punctoplasty, canaliculoplasty, and silicone intubation (12).

REFERENCES

1. Arffa RC. *Granson's diseases of the cornea.* 3rd ed. St. Louis: CV Mosby; 1991:649–665.
2. Wagoner MD, Kenyon KR. Chemical injuries of the eye. In: Albert DM, Jakobiec FA, eds. *Principles and Practice of Ophthalmology—Clinical Practice.* Philadelphia: WB Saunders; 1994:234–45.
3. Newsome DA, Gross J. Prevention by medroxyprogesterone of perforation in the alkali-burned rabbit cornea: inhibition of collagenolytic activity. *Invest Ophthalmol Vis Sci* 1977;16:21–31.
4. Pfister RR. Chemical injuries of the eye. *Ophthalmology* 1983;90:1246–53.
5. Pfister RR, Nicalaro ML, Paterson CA. Sodium citrate reduces the incidence of corneal ulcerations and perforations in extreme alkali-burned eyes—acetylcysteine and ascorbate have no favorable effect. *Invest Ophthalmol Vis Sci* 1981;21:486–490.
6. Ralph RA. Chemical burns of the eye. In: Tasman W, Jaeger EA, eds. *Duane's Clinical Ophthalmology.* Vol. 4. Philadelphia: JB Lippincott; 1990:1–24.
7. Brown SI, Weller CA. Collagenase inhibitors in prevention of ulcers of alkali-burned corneas. *Arch Ophthalmol* 1970;83:352–3.
8. Holland EJ, Schwartz GS. The evolution of epithelial transplantation for severe ocular surface disease and a proposed classification system. *Cornea* 1996;15:549–56.
9. Sloan DF, Huang TT, Larson DL, Lewis SR. Reconstruction of eyelids and eyebrows in burned patients. *Plast Reconstr Surg* 1976;58:340–6.
10. Asch MJ, Moylan JA, Bruch HM, Pruitt BA. Ocular complications associated with burns; review of a 5-year experience including 104 patients. *J Trauma* 1971;11:857–61.
11. Burns CL, Chyback LT. Thermal burns; the management of thermal burns of the lids and globes. *Ann Ophthalmol* 1979;11:1358–68.
12. Meyer DR, Kersten RC, Kulwin DR, Paskowski JR, Selkin RP. Management of canalicular injury associated with eyelid burns. *Arch Ophthalmol* 1995;113:900–3.

Management of Ocular Injuries and Emergencies,
edited by Mathew W. MacCumber.
Lippincott–Raven Publishers, Philadelphia © 1998.

13

Noninfectious Disorders of the Conjunctiva and Cornea

Laura L. Harris, Jonathan B. Rubenstein, Walter J. Stark, and Dimitri Azar

Wilmer Eye Institute, The Johns Hopkins University School of Medicine, Baltimore, Maryland 21287; Cornea Service, Department of Ophthalmology, Rush Medical College, Chicago, Illinois 60612; and Cornea Service, Massachusetts Eye and Ear Hospital, Boston, Massachusetts 02114

Basic Considerations   174
Patient Evaluation   174
  History   174
Ocular Examination   174
Conjunctival Blunt Injury   175
Subconjunctival Hemorrhage   175
  Diagnosis   175 · Management   175
Conjunctival Foreign Body   176
  Diagnosis   176 · Management   176
Conjunctival Lacerations   176
  Diagnosis   176 · Management   176
Allergic Conjunctivitis   177
  Diagnosis   177 · Management   177
Toxic Conjunctivitis   178
  Diagnosis   178 · Management   178
Corneal Blunt Trauma   178
  Diagnosis   178 · Management   178
Corneal Abrasion   179
  Diagnosis   179 · Management   179
Corneal Recurrent Erosion   180
  Diagnosis   180 · Management   181
Corneal Foreign Body   181
  Diagnosis   181 · Management   182
Ultraviolet Radiation and Electrical Injury   182
  Diagnosis   182 · Management   183

BASIC CONSIDERATIONS

Superficial injuries of the eye and the ocular response to foreign substances (e.g., allergies, drugs, toxins) are associated with symptoms of pain, tearing, and foreign body sensation. A history of trauma may be reported. Careful examination to eliminate the diagnosis of an occult ruptured globe or intraocular foreign body is critical.

PATIENT EVALUATION

History

1. If a history of chemical injury is given or suspected, immediate, copious sterile irrigation should be started. All other emergent ocular injuries should be approached in a step-wise evaluation to assess the potential of globe perforation (1).
2. Mechanism of injury: The physician should obtain complete information about the place, time, and events of the injury. Note if an object was involved, i.e., fist, metal, nails, missile objects, explosives, vegetative material, or contaminated material.
3. Ask if safety glasses were worn and if the injury was job related.
4. Obtain status of tetanus immunization (see Table 4–2).
5. Also include complete past medical, ocular, family, and social history. Include ocular history such as prior trauma, amblyopia, refractive error, or use of contact lenses.
6. Include time of recent food intake, then prohibit the patient from taking anything by mouth until the need for surgical repair has been decided.

OCULAR EXAMINATION

A detailed clinical evaluation is required (see Chapter 3), including visual acuity, pupillary examination, and visual fields.

Special considerations are listed as follows:

1. Slit-lamp examination with eversion of the upper lid. This may demonstrate a foreign body on the palpebral conjunctiva. Look for linear, vertical scratches on the corneal epithelium that stain positively with fluorescein, suggestive of a retained foreign body under the lid.
2. Subconjunctival foreign body may be observed under conjunctival laceration. Hemorrhage also may be present.
3. Look for the possibility of an open globe in patients with high-velocity foreign body injuries (see Chapter 15) (2).
4. Retroillumination through the pupil to detect any transillumination defects in the iris should be performed.
5. Gonioscopy may reveal the presence of an intraocular foreign body in the angle that may not be seen on slit-lamp examination alone (see Fig. 15–2).

6. After an open globe is ruled out, check intraocular pressure (IOP).
7. A dilated funduscopic examination must be performed, especially if the examination results showed the presence of a subconjunctival foreign body with hemorrhage. B-scan is often useful if the posterior view is obscured. Computed tomography scanning can also be diagnostic on an open globe injury or intraocular foreign body.

CONJUNCTIVAL BLUNT INJURY

Signs and symptoms of conjunctival blunt injury range from mild tearing, hyperemia, and irritation to more severe complications of pain, subconjunctival hemorrhage, chemosis, and conjunctival laceration. The spectrum of injury can range from minor trauma, scleral rupture, retained intraocular foreign body, and orbital fracture. Therefore, a systematic, detailed inspection is required for even the most minor appearing injury.

SUBCONJUNCTIVAL HEMORRHAGE

Diagnosis

1. Examination should begin with inspection of the lower palpebral and anterior bulbar conjunctiva. Delay eversion of the lid until occult rupture of the globe is ruled out.
2. If dark subconjunctival hemorrhagic chemosis is present, consider the possibility of occult rupture (Fig. 13-1). Other suspicious signs include ocular hypotony, deep anterior chamber, hyphema, and vitreous hemorrhage (see Table 15–1) (2).

Management

1. Generally, no long-term consequence to patient.
2. Condition clears gradually in 1 to 2 weeks.

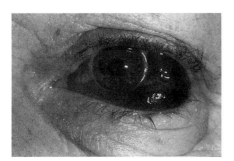

FIG. 13–1. Subconjunctival hemorrhagic chemosis with no evidence of conjunctival laceration in a patient who was hit in the left eye with a hammer. Surgical exploration showed 8-mm scleral rupture and complete expulsion of the crystalline lens.

3. For persistent, bilateral, or recurrent spontaneous subconjunctival hemorrhage, refer patient to internist for bleeding dyscrasia workup.

CONJUNCTIVAL FOREIGN BODY

Diagnosis

Foreign bodies may become embedded in the bulbar or palpebral conjunctiva. These are common after explosive injuries. Linear, vertical scratches on the cornea may be seen. Eversion of the lid may show embedded foreign material in the tarsal conjunctiva. It is important to find and remove particles to prevent corneal damage (3).

Certain animal fibers (i.e., spider or insect hairs) or vegetable matter may be inflammatory and/or carry high risk of infection.

Management

1. Careful examination under topical anesthesia (e.g., proparacaine). In children, conscious sedation or general anesthesia may be required (see Chapter 4).
2. Evert the lid, sometimes requiring Desmarres lid retractors for double eversion.
3. Remove superficial subconjunctival foreign body by saline irrigation, sweeping with soaked cotton tip applicator, fornice sweep, or spud remover.
4. Embedded foreign body can be removed with a jeweler's forceps or the tip of a 25-gauge, 1/2-inch needle.
5. Topical prophylactic antibiotic drops or ointment can be prescribed, e.g., erythromycin ointment twice daily, bacitracin ointment twice daily, or polymyxin-B/trimethoprim (Polytrim, Allergan) drops four times daily. Ointment will result in blurring of vision.

CONJUNCTIVAL LACERATIONS

Diagnosis

1. Symptoms include ocular irritation and foreign body sensation. There is usually history of trauma.
2. Signs include chemosis, subconjunctival hemorrhage, torn and rolled conjunctiva.
3. There is positive fluorescein staining of the conjunctiva.
4. Subconjunctival chemosis and hemorrhage may obscure vitreous, uveal, or retinal prolapse.

Management

1. Careful examination under topical anesthesia (proparacaine) or general anesthesia in the case of uncooperative patient or children.
2. Dissection of conjunctiva and tenons fascia off the sclera with blunt forceps to assess extent of laceration, puncture, or rupture (Fig. 13-2).
3. Look for occult foreign body.

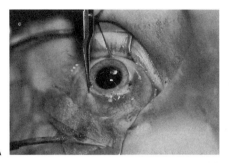
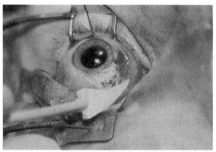

A   B

FIG. 13–2. A: Initial slit-lamp examination of subconjunctival hemorrhage and laceration did not show scleral rupture. **B:** Surgical exploration with partial conjunctival peritomy down to bare sclera showed a full-thickness rupture.

4. Test for open globe with Siedel test, 2% fluorescein followed by gentle pressure on the globe using a cotton tip applicator or finger.
5. Nonsurgical management is appropriate for conjunctival lacerations measuring less than 10 to 12 mm.
6. For surgical repair, use interrupted or continuous closure with 7-0 or 8-0 Vicryl (Ethicon) or collagen sutures (3,4).
7. Topical prophylactic antibiotic drops of ointment:

   1. Erythromycin or bacitracin ointments twice daily.
   2. Polymyxin-B/trimethoprim, tobramycin, or ofloxacin drops four times daily.

Late complications include inclusion cysts, tenons fascia incorporation into wound, and disruption of the plica semilunaris.

ALLERGIC CONJUNCTIVITIS

Diagnosis

1. Symptoms of watery, itchy eyes. May present seasonally.
2. Signs of hyperemia, chemosis, Trantas dots (eosinophils of limbus), tarsal papillae, without palpable preauricular nodes.
3. Types include hay fever, atopic, vernal, phlyctenular, and giant papillary.

Management

1. Use topical agents, e.g., Livostin (Ciba) or NSAID drops (Allergan) two to four times daily for acute relief of symptoms. Do not use Livostin in pregnant women because it is a reported teratogen.
2. Mast cell stabilizers, e.g., cromolyn sodium 4% or Alomide™ four times daily, can be used in conjunction with above, particularly with vernal conjunctivitis. It may take up to 2 weeks to see a clinical response.

3. For severe swelling, topical steroids, e.g., prednisolone acetate 1% four times daily, should be given. Make sure regular monitoring of IOP is performed while on these drops (i.e., return 4–6 weeks after beginning drops).
4. Oral antihistimines can be prescribed: asterizole (Hismanol, Janssen) 10 mg daily, terfendaine (Seldane, Hoescht) 60 mg daily, or ioratadine (Claritin, Schering) 10 mg daily.
5. Cool compresses for symptomatic relief two to four times daily are helpful.
6. Referral to allergist if systemic symptoms and chronic rhinitis are present.

TOXIC CONJUNCTIVITIS

Toxic conjunctivitis can occur after exposure to miotics, aminoglycosides, atropine, idoxuridine, apraclonidine, antiviral drops and contact lens solutions.

Diagnosis

1. There is follicular response and hyperemia, especially in the inferior palpebral conjunctiva and may be accompanying superficial puritate keratopathy.
2. Obtain detailed history of topical drug use and history of any known drug allergies.

Management

1. Stop application of offending drug or solutions.
2. Cool compresses and artificial preservative free tears two to four times daily.

CORNEAL BLUNT TRAUMA

Diagnosis

1. Symptoms include acute blurred vision, photophobia, foreign body sensation.
2. Direct blunt injury to the cornea can cause mild trauma with findings of epithelial edema and no evidence of stromal or endothelial damage. In severe trauma a focal concussive force can cause a mechanical deformation injury resulting in endothelial damage causing a ring of cornea edema, or breaks in Descemet's membrane, with acute edema (Fig. 13–3). An example is seen in association with forceps delivery injury, where there are vertical Haabs striae and unilateral corneal edema.
3. Direct blunt trauma rarely ruptures the cornea unless it is already thinned, as seen in inflammatory peripheral corneal thinning; corneal ectasias such as Terriens marginal degenereation, keratoconus or pellucid degeneration; previous keratoplasty; radial keratotomy; or poorly healed corneal ulcerations (5).

Management

1. Semi-pressure patch for 24 hours, or bandage contact lens if epithelial defect is present (see Corneal Abrasion).

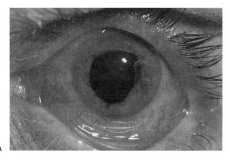 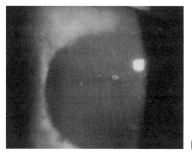

A   B

FIG. 13–3. A: Iris sphincter tears, corneal edema, traumatic mydriasis, and traumatic cataract are present, caused by an explosion of a hand-held, ether-fueled potato spud launcher. **B:** Vertical breaks in Descemet's are seen on high magnification. There was no rupture of the globe.

2. Topical antibiotic if epithelial defect is present.
3. Topical steroids, fluoromethalone (FML, Allergan) 0.1% or prednisolone/acetate 1% two to four times daily, only if significant anterior chamber inflammatory response is present.
4. Pressure-lowering agents if necessary.
5. Hypertonic saline preparations, Muro 128 ointment twice daily or drops four times daily.
6. Good visual recovery is usually reported within 3 months.

CORNEAL ABRASION

Diagnosis

1. Most common sources are direct or tangential impact with paper, fingernail, tree branches, twigs, mascara brush, curling irons, and contact lenses.
2. Symptoms of acute pain, blurred vision, photophobia, and foreign body sensation
3. Epithelial defect is seen by positive fluorescein staining where the epithelium is missing (Fig. 13-4A).

Management

1. Document size of abrasion.
2. Look for associated stromal infiltrate or anterior chamber inflammation; if present, culture the cornea.
3. Evert lid and look for foreign body.
4. If a deeper wound is suspected, a Siedel's test with 2% fluorescein is indicated.
5. Standard current treatment includes:
   • Cycloplegics, homatropine 5% twice daily.
   • Application of topical antibiotics, erythromycin or bacitracin ointments, before patching and continued after patching three times daily.

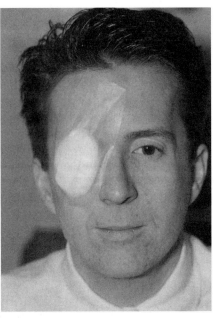

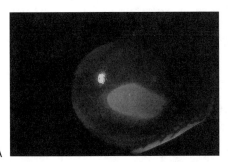

A   B

FIG. 13–4. A: Epithelial defect from a corneal abrasion stained positively with fluorescein. **B:** Proper placement of a semi-pressure patch. Two eye pads are used; the inner one is folded in half.

- Semi-pressure patch may be considered for 24 hours (Fig. 13–4*B*); withhold if causative agent vegetative matter and fingernail (precaution against fungal contaminate) or if related to wearing of contact lenses (concern of *Pseudomonas* infection).
6. Alternative treatments for corneal abrasions include:
   - Use of a bandaged contact lens and topical NSAID, Acular (Allergan) or Voltaren (Ciba) (6).
   - No patching and use of antibiotic ointment (7).
   - Although patients usually heal quickly, generally within 24 hours they should be monitored daily, especially if diabetic.
7. For contact lens–related injury, antibiotics with good Gram-negative coverage (polymyxin-B/trimethoprim, tobramycin, or ofloxacin drops) should be used four times daily.

CORNEAL RECURRENT EROSION

Diagnosis

1. Similar signs and symptoms of corneal abrasion are present, including pain, tearing, and foreign body sensation (Fig. 13–5).
2. A history of previous corneal abrasion is often obtained. These cases are generally unilateral.

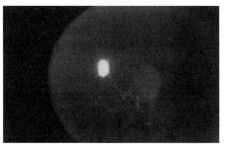
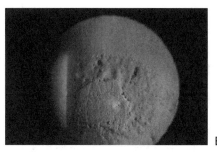

A   B

FIG. 13–5. A: Recurrent erosion with epithelial irregularity staining with fluorescein stain. **B:** Retro-illumination of irregular epithelium in area of recurrent erosion.

3. Classically these symptoms occur spontaneously without additional trauma.
4. Irritation usually starts after awaking from sleep, and symptoms improve throughout the day.
5. Also seen in corneal dystrophies, i.e., epithelial basement membrane dystrophy, Reis-Bucklers, and stromal dystrophies (lattice, macular, and granular). These cases are usually bilateral.
6. Believed to be caused by a defect in the healing between the hemidesmosome of the corneal epithelium and the basement membrane. Diagnosed by detailed examination of the fellow eye.

Management

1. As above (see Corneal Abrasion).
2. If persistent erosion add hypertonic saline, Muro 128 drops, or ointment before sleep.
3. Additional treatment for frequent or persistent erosions might include anterior stromal puncture with a needle (8) or YAG laser (9), epithelial debridement, or excimer laser phototherapeutic keratectomy.

CORNEAL FOREIGN BODY

Diagnosis

1. Slit-lamp evaluation for foreign body; if metallic, look for presence of rust ring (Fig. 13–6*A*).
2. If present more than 24 hours, look for stromal infiltrate.
3. Obtain history of trauma with vegetative matter which could have higher risk of secondary bacterial or fungal keratitis. Certain animal fibers (i.e., spider or insect hairs) may be inflammatory and may cause associated conjunctivitis.
4. Look for anterior chamber inflammatory reaction or hypopyon.
5. Be suspicious of penetrating injury, endophthalmitis, and or retained intraocular foreign body.

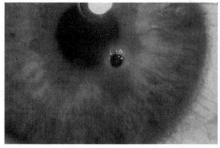

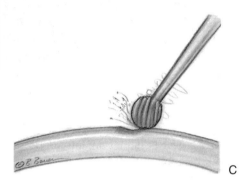

FIG. 13–6. A: Corneal metallic foreign body with corneal edema. Rust ring was present after removal. **B:** Removal of surface epithelial foreign body with a 25-gauge needle. **C:** Debridement of rust ring using mechanical burr.

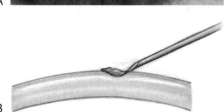

A

B

C

Management

1. Topical anesthesia, proparacaine drops. General anesthesia or conscious sedation may be required (see Chapter 4).
2. Extract corneal foreign body at the slit lamp, with a 25-gauge needle, spud, or burr (Fig. 13–6*B*).
3. Remove rust ring with burr (Fig. 13–6*C*). If penetrating injury is suspected, perform a Seidel test (2% fluoroscein) with cautious digital pressure of the eye. Extraction of deep stromal foreign bodies may require controlled repair in the operating room (10–12).
4. Consider semi-pressure patch for 24 hours, no patch for vegetative causative agents.
5. Daily follow-up.
6. Cycloplegic homatropine 5% three times daily.
7. Topical antibiotics (e.g., erythromycin ointment twice daily, bacitracin ointment twice daily, or polymyxin-B/trimethoprim four times daily) after patch is removed for 3 to 5 days until epithelium is healed.

ULTRAVIOLET RADIATION AND ELECTRICAL INJURY

Diagnosis

1. History of exposure to welder's arc, sun lamps and beds, or laboratory ultraviolet lamps.
2. Pain, photophobia, sunburned skin in exposure areas, 6 to 24 hours from time of insult.
3. Slit-lamp examination shows superficial punctate keratopathy (Fig. 13-7).

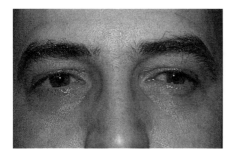

FIG. 13–7. Laboratory worker who suffered epithelial superficial punctate keratitis from observing an agarose gel on a UV light source without protective goggles.

Management

1. Cycloplegics, e.g., homatropine 5% three times daily.
2. Lubrication with artificial tears or ointments.
3. Erythromycin ointment twice daily or bacitracin ointment twice daily.
4. Semi-pressure patch for 24 hours.
5. Analgesics, aspirin or NSAIDS.

Similar occurrences have been reported from unshielded radiation therapy to the orbit, electrocution, and lightening (3).

REFERENCES

1. Whitwell J. Treatment of nonperforating ocular injuries. *Trans Ophthalmol Soc* 1959;79:49.
2. Werner MS, Dana MR, Vianna MA, et al. Predictors of occult scleral rupture. *Ophthalmology* 1994; 101:1941.
3. Kenyon K, Wagner M. Conjunctival and corneal injuries. In: Shingleton BJ, Hersh PS, Kenyon KR, eds. *Eye Trauma.* St. Louis: Mosby-Year Book; 1991:95.
4. Hamill MB, Hoover JA. Ocular trauma. In: Jay B, Kirkness CM, eds. *Recent Advances in Ophthalmology.* New York: Churchill Livingstone; 1996:117.
5. Sambursky D, Azar D. Corneal and anterior segment trauma and reconstruction. *Issues Ocular Trauma* 1995;8:609.
6. Donnenfeld ED, Selkin BA, Perry HD, et al. Controlled evaluation of a bandage contact lens and a topical non-steroidal anti-inflammatory drug in treating traumatic corneal abrasions. *Ophthalmology* 1995;102:979.
7. Kaiser P, the Corneal Abrasion Patching Study Group. A comparison of pressure patching versus no patching for corneal abrasions due to trauma or foreign body removal. *Ophthalmology* 1995;102: 1936.
8. McLean EN, Mac Rae SM, Rich LF. Recurrent erosion: treatment by anterior stromal puncture. *Ophthalmology* 1986;93:784.
9. Buxton JN, Fox ML. Superficial epithelial keratectomy in the treatment of epithelial basement membrane dystrophy: a preliminary report. *Arch Ophthalmology* 1983;101:392.
10. Cullom RD, Chang B, eds. Trauma. In: *The Wills Eye Manual. Office and Emergency Room Diagnois and Treatment of Eye Disease.* 2nd ed. Philadelphia: JB Lippincott; 1994:19.
11. Cullom RD, Chang B, eds. Cornea. In: *The Wills Eye Manual. Office and Emergency Room Diagnosis and Treatment of Eye Disease.* 2nd ed. Philadelphia: JB Lippincott; 1994:51.
12. O'Brien TP, Sangkyung C, Trauma-related ocular infections. *Ophthalmol Clin North Am* 1995;8: 667.

Management of Ocular Injuries and Emergencies,
edited by Mathew W. MacCumber.
Lippincott–Raven Publishers, Philadelphia ©1998.

14

Infectious Conjunctivitis and Keratitis

Laura L. Harris and Terrence P. O'Brien

*Cornea Service, Wilmer Eye Institute, The Johns Hopkins University School of Medicine,
Baltimore, Maryland 21287-9121*

Basic Considerations 185
Signs and Symptoms 186
  Differential Diagnosis Based on Clinical Signs 186
Microbial Conjunctivitis 187
Severe Bacterial Conjunctivitis 187
  Diagnosis 187 · Management 189
Nonsevere Bacterial Conjunctivitis 190
  Diagnosis 190 · Management 190
Viral Conjunctivitis 191
  Adenovirus Conjunctivitis 191 · Herpes Simplex Conjunctivitis 192
  Chlamydia Conjunctivitis 193
Keratitis 194
  Bacterial Keratitis 195 · Viral Keratitis 198 · Fungal Keratitis 201
  Parasitic Keratitis 203 · Interstitial Keratitis (Stromal) 205

BASIC CONSIDERATIONS

Evaluation of the patient presenting with a red eye is frequently required in general medical, pediatric, and ophthalmic practice. Entities resulting in a red eye can be described in many ways: acute versus chronic, with infectious versus noninfectious etiologies, or involvement of the conjunctiva with or without involvement of the cornea. Correct diagnosis is imperative to decrease potential morbidity. This chapter addresses the infectious causes of a red eye, with emphasis on emergent clinical presentation and management. Corneal thinning with perforation may require corneal tissue adhesive or keratoplasty (see Chapter 15).

Noninfectious causes of keratitis include connective tissue disease (e.g., rheumatoid arthritis, relapsing polychondritis, Wegener's granulomatosis, polyarteritis nodosa) and Mooren's ulcer. Management of these causes of keratitis is difficult and may require systemic steroids and immunosuppressive agents as well as corneal tissue adhesive or keratoplasty for perforation (see Chapter 15).

SIGNS AND SYMPTOMS

General symptoms of conjunctivitis and keratitis include redness, discharge, pain, heat, foreign body sensation, photophobia, and blurred vision (Table 14–1).

Differential Diagnosis Based on Clinical Signs

Signs of conjunctivitis include conjunctival hyperemia, tearing, chemosis, hemorrhagic chemosis, and discharge. Serous or clear discharge is associated more frequently with viral infections; stringy, ropy, white discharge with allergic reactions; purulent discharge with bacterial infections; and mucopurulent discharge with chlamydial infections.

Preauricular and submandibular lymph nodes may be enlarged and often tender in viral or gonococcal disease. Nontender regional lymphadenopathy may be associated with chlamydial infections.

Pseudomembranes (easily removed without bleeding) are seen most often in conjunctivitis caused by severe adenoviral infection, gonococci, *Staphylococcus, Chlamydia,* or Stevens-Johnson's syndrome.

True membranes involve the epithelium (and often bleed when removed). These may be present with adenovirus, pyogenic *Streptococcus, Corynebacterium diphtheriae,* herpes simplex, erythema multiforme, chemical injuries, and ligneous and vernal conjunctivitis.

Follicles represent focal lymphoid hyperplasia of the conjunctiva. They are rounded avascular whitish structures predominantly observed with adenovirus, primary herpes simplex virus (HSV), trichiasis, molluscum contagiosum, eye drops, chalazion, and masquerade syndrome caused by basal cell carcinoma in patients in their 50s to 70s.

Papillae are small elevations with a central vascular core of vessels surrounded by a small amount of fluid accumulation (usually ≤1 mm). Papillae are a less specific sign than follicles but may be observed in bacterial and allergic diseases.

Superficial punctate keratopathy manifests as punctate erosions of the epithelium or punctate focal inflammation within the epithelium. This may be seen in

TABLE 14–1. *General characteristics of a red eye*

Characteristics	Conjunctivitis	Corneal	Uveitis	Angle-closure glaucoma
Symptoms	Discharge	Tearing, pain	Photophobia	Pain, irritation
Vision	Normal	Blurred	Normal/Decreased	Highly decreased
Hyperemia	Conjunctiva diffuse	Limbal	Perilimbal	Perilimbal generalized
Cornea	Usually clear	Hazy	Keratic precipites	Edematous/cloudy
Pupil	Normal	Normal	Normal/small	Mid-dilated
Intraocular pressure	Normal	Normal	Normal/elevated/low	Highly elevated

keratoconjunctivitis, dry eyes, lagophthalmos, hydrops, blepharitis, contact lens wear, staphylococcal infection, and in antibiotic use, specifically neomycin and gentamicin drops.

Micropannus, superficial vascular invasion of the peripheral cornea, usually greater than 0.5 mm but less than 1.5 mm, is seen after inflammation from rosacea keratitis, trachoma, vernal, staphylococcus, or contact lens overwear.

Peripheral, nonulcerative, infiltrative keratitis usually represents an antigen-antibody reaction (type III, immunologic reaction).

Marginal infiltrates are usually associated with colonization of lid margins with *Staphylococcus* (most common), herpes simplex infection, and antangular blepharitis. Allergic disease, infiltrative infections, drug toxicity, and lid tumors are less common.

Keratoconjunctivitis sicca, vitamin A deficiency (xerophthalmia), ocular cicatricial pemphigoid, and Stevens-Johnson's syndrome can result in changes in the aqueous tear production from alteration of meibomian, Krause, or Wolfring glands, affecting oil and aqueous film production. The loss of goblet cells may result in deficient mucin, loss of surfactant function, instability of the tear film, and chronic dry eye syndrome (1,2).

MICROBIAL CONJUNCTIVITIS

Acute infectious conjunctivitis may be judged clinically as either nonsevere or severe based on the pace of the inflammation and severity of clinical features (3). See Table 14–2 for a listing of etiologic agents of infectious conjunctivitis. Likely organisms differ depending on the age of the host (Table 14–3).

SEVERE BACTERIAL CONJUNCTIVITIS

Principle causes:

- *Neisseria*
- *Hemophilus*
- *Strep. pyogens*
- *Staph. aureus* species

Gonorrheal

Typically severe causative species include *Neisseria gonorrhoeae, N. meningitidis,* and *N. kochii.*

Diagnosis

1. Hyperacute onset of copious, purulent discharge, markedly swollen lids, regional lymphadenopathy, extreme hyperemia, chemosis, and occasional membranes (Fig. 14–1*A* and *B*).

TABLE 14–2. *Etiologic agents of infectious conjunctivitis*

Bacteria
  Streptococcus pneumoniae
  Streptococcus pyogenes
  Streptococci of the viridans group
  Staphylococcus aureus
  Haemophilus influenzae (includes *H. aegyptius*)
  Neisseria gonorrhoeae
  Haemophilus ductreyi
  Neisseria meningitidis
  Proteus vulgaris
  Moraxella lacunata
  Corynebacterium diphtheriae
  Mycobacterium tuberculosis
  Francisella tularensis
  Treponema pallidum
  Moraxella catarrhalis
  Shigella flexneri
  Yersinia enterocolitica
  Staphylococcus epidermidis
  Acinetobacter species
  Aeromonas hydrophila
  Peptostreptococcus
  Bartonella (Rochalimaea) henselae (cat scratch bacillus)
Viruses
  Adenoviruses
  Poxviruses (variola, vaccinia, molluscum contagiosum)
  Herpesviruses (herpes simplex, varicella-zoster, Epstein-Barr virus)
  Papillomaviruses
  Influenza A and B viruses
  Paramyxoviruses (measles, mumps, Newcastle disease virus)
  Picornaviruses (echovirus, enterovirus, coxsackievirus, and poliovirus)
  Chlamydia trachomatis
Fungi
  Candida species
  Sporothrix schenckii
  Rhinosporidum seeberi
Parasites
  Onchocerca volvulus
  Loa loa
  Wuchereria bancrofti
  Oestrus ovis (myiasis)
  Microsporidiosis
  Nosema species
  Encephalitozoon species
  Toxocara canis

2. Rapid diagnosis and aggressive systemic and topical treatment of this infection is required due to intrinsic virulence factors of the organism and the recruitment of a polymorphic neutrophilic infiltrative response with resultant release of lytic enzymes causing destruction of the conjunctiva and cornea. Progressive keratolysis and the risk of frank perforation may occur within 24 to 36 hours. With *N. meningitidis,* septicemia, meningitis, arthritis, and death can occur (4).

TABLE 14–3. *Common etiologic organisms related to patient age*

Age of onset	Organism
Newborn	*Neisseria gonorrhoeae*
	Chlamydia
Children (ages 1–10 yr)	*Haemophilus influenzae*
	Staphylococcus, Streptococcus
Youths	*Chlamydia*
Adults	*Neisseria*
	Chlamydia
	Pseudomonas aeruginosa
	Moraxella
	Proteus, Klebsiella, Serratia, and *Eschericia coli*
Elderly	*Staphylococcus, Streptococcus*

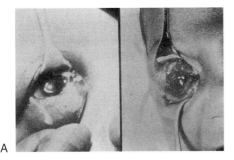
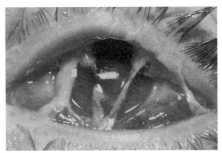

A

B

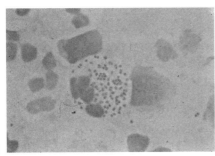

C

FIG. 14–1. A: Ophthalmia neonatorum due to *N. gonnorrhea*. **B:** Hyperacute conjunctivitis with marked lid edema, conjunctival hyperemia, chemosis, and copious purulent discharge due to *N. gonorrhoea*. **C:** Smear with numerous polymorphonuclear cells and Gram-negative intracellular diplococci. (Courtesy American Academy of Ophthalmology)

Management

1. These organisms are fastidious and difficult to grow on standard culture media.
2. Conjunctival scrapings with a sterile spatula should be performed after instillation of topical anesthesia and smears created for Gram and Giemsa staining. Prompt microscopic analysis to look for characteristic Gram-negative intracellular diplococci and polymorphonuclear neutrophil response should be performed (Fig. 14–1*C*).
3. Cotton tip swab for culture and antibiotic susceptibility testing should be performed. Material should be plated on blood agar, chocolate agar (37°C, 10% CO_2), and Thayer martin plate. Also prepare a *Chlamydia* DFA test, geneprobe assay, or culture because the incidence of coinfection is relatively high.
4. Copious irrigation with normal saline is required while discharge is present to reduce the action of toxic virulence factors and enzymes.
5. Current therapy of choice in adults is 1 g Ceftriaxone or Cefotaxime intramuscularly (i.m.) by single dose for adult, plus doxycycline or azithromycin if *Chlamydia* is present.
6. For an adult patient with corneal involvement, if a nonpenicilliase-producing *N. gonorrhoeae* strain is the causative agent, continue 1 g Ceftriaxone or Cefotaxime or use ciprofloxacin or ofloxacin drops intravenously (i.v.) every 12 to 24 hours and penicillin G 100,000 U/ml drops every hour, then taper while patient is awake (5,6).

7. The newborn or pediatric dose is Ceftriaxone or Cefotaxime 50 mg/kg/day i.v. or i.m. with a maximum dose of 125 mg/day (7). Apply topical erythromycin or bacitracin ointment four times daily to cornea.

8. Discharge home medications are as follows:
   - In adults, doxycycline 100 mg orally twice daily for 1 week or erythromycin 250 to 500 mg orally for 2 to 3 weeks to treat possible *Chlamydia* coinfection
   - In children, erythromycin 250 mg orally three times daily

Daily examination is required with observation of the cornea until resolution of symptoms (8). The clinician should be suspicious of sexual abuse in prepubertal children. Sexual contracts should be treated.

NONSEVERE BACTERIAL CONJUNCTIVITIS

Principal causes:

- *Staphylococcus aureus*
- *Streptococcus pneumoniae*
- *Haemophilus influenzae*
- *Moraxella* species

Diagnosis

Signs and symptoms include acute onset, unilateral or bilateral; minimal edema; no preauricular lymphadenopathy; moderate mucopurulent discharge; mild conjunctival hyperemia; and normal cornea.

Management

1. Gram stain and conjunctival swab for bacterial culture. Transport to lab promptly.
2. Topical antibiotic therapy:
   - Gram-positive coverage
     Erythromycin or bacitracin ointment four to six times/day, or
     Trimethoprim/polymyxin B (Polytrim, Allergan Pharmaceuticals) drops four to six times/day
   - Gram-negative coverage:
     Tobramycin ointment or drops four to six times/day or gentamicin
   - Broad-spectrum coverage:
     Ciprofloxacin 0.3% (Ciloxan, Alcon Labs) drops four to six times/day, or
     Ofloxacin 0.3% (Ocuflox, Allergan Pharmaceuticals) drops four to six times/day
3. Continue therapy for 5 days unless otherwise directed by laboratory results.
4. *Haemophilus influenzae* conjunctivitis (Fig. 14–2) may be present with associated pneumonitis and preseptal cellulitis. Some clinicians advocate the addition

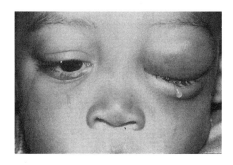

FIG. 14–2. *Haemophilus influenzae* conjunctivitis and preseptal cellulitis in a 3-year-old. (Courtesy of Dr. Dan B. Jones)

of oral amoxicillin/clavulanate 20 to 40 mg/kg/day divided three times daily for children (9).

VIRAL CONJUNCTIVITIS

Viral conjunctivitis is very common, with adenovirus and herpes viruses being the most common etiologic agents (Table 14–2). The majority of cases of adenovirus are self-limiting and need supportive therapy only. A few strains progress to cause major ocular disease with corneal involvement. However, these serotypes are highly contagious, and proper management is critical to prevent epidemic outbreaks in the community or iatrogenic spread in an office setting (8).

Precautions to prevent spread of virus in an office setting:

1. Development of a separate red eye room segregated from the normal examination rooms.
2. Wipe off all instruments after use.
3. Defer elective examination procedures (intraocular pressure measurements).
4. Wash hands with soap and disinfect. Use paper, not cloth, towels.
5. Studies have shown the mechanical effect of wiping with dry gauze is as effective as use of water, isopropanol, iodopine, or H_2O_2.
6. Use Wescodyne or sodium hypochlorite bleach in a 1:10 dilution for soaking the tonometer applanator tip. Avoid tonometry unless necessary. If indicated, use a Tonopen with disposable latex cover.

Additional viral diseases, including influenza, mumps, measles, Newcastle's, rubeola, rubella, and human papilloma virus, have been associated with nonspecific conjunctivitis. No specific antiviral treatment is available. Supportive therapy, including artificial tears, is recommended.

Adenovirus Conjunctivitis

Diagnosis

Adenovirus is the most common cause of viral conjunctivitis. There are over 41 known serotypes that produce mild to severe symptoms. The hallmark diagnostic signs are tarsal conjunctival follicles, serous discharge, and regional lymphade-nopathy with preauricular or submandibular nodes.

Three syndromes of adenovirus are listed as follows:

1. Acute follicular conjunctivitis (endemic serotypes 1 to 4): presents with mild symptoms and follicles (may also be subacute).
2. Epidemic keratoconjunctivitis (serotypes 8, 19, and 37): characterized by se-vere, abrupt onset of large, tender preauricular nodes, serous discharge, hyper-emia, subconjunctival hemorrhage, and follicles. The second eye is typically af-fected within 5 to 7 days. Other sequelea include keratitis (80%), epithelitis seen in the first 7 days, superficial punctate keratopathy at 6 to 20 days, and/or subepithelial infiltrates at 6 to 20 days.
3. Pharyngoconjunctival fever (serotypes 3 and 7): presents with moderate con-junctivitis symptoms along with pharyngitis and fever. Has been associated with outbreaks in summer and occasionally with outbreaks in inadequately chlorinated swimming pools.

Hemorrhagic conjunctivitis is caused by enterovirus 70 or coxsackic A24 virus. This entity is most commonly associated with epidemics in Florida characterized by acute subconjunctival hemorrhage lasting 4 to 5 days. It was the causative factor in an epidemic of the Apollo II mission. It has low morbidity and is self limiting (10).

Management

1. Supportive therapy includes compresses and/or natural tear drops several times per day for comfort and acetaminophen for pain.
2. Stress hand washing, hygiene, and education.
3. Perform viral culture with calcium alginate swab if health care professional, food worker, or questionable diagnosis (low yield).
4. For membrane peel, use topical proparacaine and topical anesthesia and peel off membrane using calcium alginate, cotton tipped swab, or forceps.
5. If corneal involvement is present and occupational demand for improved vision is great, the following judicious topical ocular steroid treatments may be con-sidered: fluorometholone, prednisolone acetate 0.125%, or prednisolone maleate 1% twice daily to four times daily, tapering for 1 to 6 months.
6. Late subepithelial infiltrate can be treated with mild topical steroids, including fluoromethalone 0.1% or rimexolone (Vexol, Alcon Labs) 1% with slow taper, followed by nonsteroidal anti-inflammatory agents such as diclofenac (Voltaren, Cibavision Ophthalmics) or ketorolac (Acular, Allergan Pharmaceuticals).

Herpes Simplex Conjunctivitis

Herpes simplex conjuctivitis may occur as a component of primary or recurrent infection, with or without eyelid vesicles and with or without epithelial keratitis. It is most commonly caused by HSV type I. It may occur in any age group (predomi-nantly 20 to 35 years). Unilateral involvement is most common (80%); attack rate for second eye is approximately 25%. (See diagnosis and management of herpes simplex keratitis below.)

Chlamydia Conjunctivitis

Diagnosis

Chlamydial infections affect 500 million people worldwide and approximately 4 million annually in the United States. Groups 1 to 3 cause hyperendemic blinding trachoma and serogroups D through K result in adult inclusion conjuctivitis (11). (The trachoma biovar include serovars A through K. Lymphogranuloma venereum (LGV) includes serovars L1 to L3.) Conjunctivitis is usually bilateral and can be seen in sexually active young adults and newborns/ neonates. This infection is caused by serotypes D through K. Measurements of IgM antibodies are helpful in the diagnosis of chlamydial pneumonitis in newborns (12).

1. *Adult chlamydial keratoconjunctivitis*
   - Clinical diagnosis:
     Subacute onset; chronic course if untreated
     Unilateral or bilateral
     Mucopurulent discharge
     Prominent lymphoid reaction with limbal and bulbar conjunctival follicles
       and regional lymphadenopathy (nontender preauricular lymph node)
       Micropannus formation
     Coarse, pleomorphic randomly distributed punctate epithelial keratitis and
       subepithelial infiltrates
   - Differential diagnosis:
     Viral keratoconjunctivitis
     Blepharoconjunctivitis
     Allergy
     Contact lens wear
     Bacterial conjunctivitis
     Molluscum contagiosum
     Benign lymphoid hyperplasia
     Floppy eyelid syndrome
     Superior limbic keratoconjunctivitis
2. *Hyperendemic, blinding trachoma* is one of the leading causes of blindness in the world. The affliction is usually bilateral and clinical features include Arlt's line, Herbert's pits, and scarring. This is caused by serotypes A, B, Ba, or C. Usually seen in areas of poor hygiene and sanitation (13).
3. Other clinical signs include nontender preauricular nodes, mucopurulent discharge, lymphoid response, micropannus or more than 1.5 mm macropannus, and punctate epithelial keratopathy.
4. Giemsa stain of conjunctival scrapings may be positive for chlamydial basophilic intracytoplasmic inclusions (Halbstaedter-Prowazek). Sensitivity is

low, with high incidence of false-negative results in adults. Fluorescent anti-body stains (DFA) and enzyme immunoassay (EIA) are widely used. Poly-merase chain reaction (PCR) testing is highly specific.

5. Culturing remains the gold standard. Use chlamydial transport medium and iso-late in cell culture (cycloheximide-treated McCoy cells, HeLa, BHK-21).

Management

1. Design for treatment of adults
   - High index of suspicion; clinical diagnosis
     Perform DFA, DNA probe or other rapid detection test
     Initiate oral doxycycline or alternate agent
     Reexamine in 1 week
     If test result is positive and/or clinical signs are improved, (a) complete the course of tetracycline, (b) initiate topical steroids for keratitis, and (c) pro-vide treatment for sexual partner
   - Low index of suspicion
     Perform DFA or DNA probe
     Defer management pending result
     If test result is positive, initiate treatment as above
     If test result is negative, defer treatment and reevaluate
2. Treatment for adults: Doxycycline 100 mg orally twice daily for 7 days (drug of choice) (be alert for pregnancy or lactation). Alternatives include azithromycin 1 g for one dose, erythromycin ethylsuccinate 250 to 500 mg orally four times daily, or tetracycline 250 to 500 mg orally four times daily for 7 days (con-traindicated in pregnant woman or children under age 8). Also may add ery-thromycin or tetracycline ointment three times daily for 7 days.
3. Treatment indicated for sexual partner as well. Search for other sexually trans-mitted diseases.
4. Treatment for infants
   - Oral erythromycin suspension, 40 mg/kg/day in four divided doses for at least 14 days

Topical antibiotics are usually not necessary, but erythromycin ointment four times daily is optional if abundant discharge is present.

KERATITIS

Keratitis caused by bacterial, viral, fungal or parasitic organisms is often seen in the emergency setting. Symptoms of keratitis include red eye, pain, decreased vi-sion, and photophobia.

Risk factors for keratitis are listed as follows:

- Trauma
- Contact lens wear (20% to 40% of patients developing culture-proven microbial keratitis)

- Systemic illness
- Postsurgery
- Keratitis sicca
- Neurotrophic cornea
- Alcohol abuse

Bacterial Keratitis

Clinical Features

Determinants:

- Strain (virulence) of the responsible organism(s)
- Method of inoculation or introduction
- Time interval from inoculation
- Antecedent status of cornea

Pathogenesis:

- Adherence of bacteria to epithelium
- Microbial invasion
- Derangement of host immune system
- Corneal infection

Diagnosis

The most common agents causing bacterial keratitis are listed in Table 14–4 (14). Keratitis can be divided into a typical, severe or atypical, nonsevere form (Table 14–5).

Gram Positive

Coagulase-negative and coagulase-positive *Staphylococcus epidermidis* and *S. aureus* are the most common causative organisms. The clinical features include an infiltrative keratitis that is characterized by a round or oval ulceration of the epithelium with an associated white or yellow-white distinct border (Fig. 14–3*A*). *Staphylococcus aureus* causes ulcerative keratitis, having well-circumscribed stromal infiltrates, occasionally with hypopyon.

Bacillus cereus is associated with trauma, especially with soil-contaminated injury, and is characterized by rapid progression, severe pain within 24 hours, lid edema, and chemosis. It may produce a characteristic ring ulcer with deep abscess.

Streptococcus pneumoniae is less frequent but may result in a serpiginous ulcerative keratitis with hypopyon.

Gram Negative

Neisseria gonorrhoeae and *N. meningitidis* conjunctivitis can progress to fulminant keratitis, which has the capacity to penetrate intact corneal epithelium and to

TABLE 14–4. *Some infectious agents that cause keratitis*

Bacteria	Mycobacteria
Gram-positive cocci	*Mycobacterium tuberculosis,*
Staphylococcus aureus	*M. fortuitum, M. chelonae,*
Staphylococcus epidermidis	*M. gordonae, M. avium-intracellulare*
Streptococcus pneumoniae	Actinomycetes
Streptococci of the viridans group	*Nocardia* species
Streptococcus pyogenes (group A)	Chlamydia
Enterococcus (Streptococcus) faecalis	*Chlamydia trachomatis*
Peptostreptococcus species	Viruses
Gram-negative bacilli	Herpes simplex virus
Pseudomonas aeruginosa, P. mallei, P.	Adenovirus
fluorescens, P. pseudomallei,	Varicella-zoster virus
P. stutzeri	Epstein-Barr virus
Comamonas (Pseudomonas)	Poxviruses (vaccinia, molluscum
acidovorans	contagiosum)
Proteus mirabilis	Rubeola (measles)
Morganella moragnii	Fungi
Klebsiella pneumoniae	Acremonium species
Serratia marcescens	Fusarium species
Escherichia coli	Bipolaris species
Aeromonas hydrophila	Candida species
Cat-scratch bacillus	Aspergillus species
Gram-negative coccobacilli	Pseudallescheria boydii
Moraxella lacunata, M. nonliquefaciens	Penicillium species
Acinetobacter calcoaceticus	Paecilomyces species
Pasteurella multocida	Neurospora species
Neisseria gonorrhoeae	Phialophora species
Moraxella (Branhamella) catarrhalis	Curvularia species
Gram-positive bacilli	Parasites
Bacillus coagulans, B. laterosporus,	Onchocerca volvulus
B. cereus, B. licheniformis, B. brevis	Acanthamoeba polyphaga, A. castellani
Corynebacterium diphtheriae	Leishmania brasiliensis
Clostridium perfrinens, C. tetani	Trypanosoma species
Spirochetes	Microsporidia
Treponema pallidum	Nosema species
Borrelia burgdorferi	*Encephalitozoon* species

cause stromal keratolysis with acute perforation. Most often occurs in newborns (ophthalmia neonatorum) and in adults with history of sexually transmitted diseases (see section on Gonorrheal Conjunctivitis above) (15,16).

Pseudomonas aeruginosa has rapid onset, forming central, suppurative keratitis (Fig. 14–3B). There is often a history of trauma or contact lens wear. Damage to the epithelium occurs from proteases, lipase, and three exotoxins.

TABLE 14–5. *Corneal signs of typical, severe versus atypical, nonsevere keratitis*

Distinctive corneal signs	Typical, severe	Atypical, nonsevere
Status of epithelium	Ulcerated	Intact
Type of stromal inflammation	Suppurative	Nonsuppurative
Site of inflammation	Focal, diffuse	Multifocal

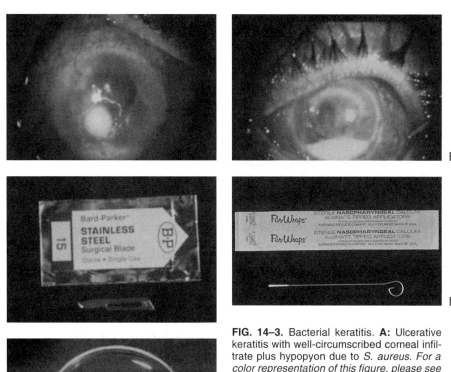

FIG. 14–3. Bacterial keratitis. **A:** Ulcerative keratitis with well-circumscribed corneal infiltrate plus hypopyon due to *S. aureus. For a color representation of this figure, please see the color insert facing p. 256.* **B:** Fulminant keratitis with ring abscess and hypopyon due to *P. aeruginosa.* **C:** Corneal scraping can be performed with a sterile, disposable no. 15 surgical blade. **D:** Culture can be performed by obtaining a deep corneal swabbing with the calcium alginate-tipped applicator. **E:** Material is plated in C streak rows on blood agar and on other selective media.

Moraxella presents as a chronic, indolent keratitis with a peripheral or paracentral infiltrate. Commonly this entity is seen in debilitated patients or after corneal transplants.

Proteus, Klebsiella, Serratia, and Escherichia coli are less common and form ring-shaped ulcers (17).

Atypical mycobacteria, especially *Mycobacterium fortitum* and *Mycobacterium chelonei,* can be agents causing intractable, recalcitrant posttraumatic keratitis (18).

Management

1. Obtain corneal scrapings by use of a Kimura platinum spatula or a no.15 Bard-Parker blade for culture and smears (Fig. 14–3*C*). Culture also can be performed

by obtaining a deep corneal swabbing with the calcium alginate-tipped applicator (Fig. 14–3*D*). Prepare smears on several slides if possible for Gram, Griemsa, and periodic acid-Schiff (PAS), and hematoxylin and eosin stains. More recently acridine orange stain has been found to be useful in screening slides rapidly with high sensitivity using epifluorescent microscopy. Other stains may be useful for certain organisms (Table 14–6).

2. Corneal culture and antimicrobial susceptibility testing are recommended in all cases if resources are available (Fig. 14–3*E*). Culture is mandatory in central, sight-threatening fulminant keratitis before initiating antibiotic therapy. Specimens obtained by use of a calcium algnate swab and blade should be inoculated onto three plates: blood agar, chocolate agar (37°C, 10% CO_2), and thioglycolate and inoculate thiol or other broth.

3. Initiate frequent broad-spectrum antibiotic coverage until organism identification and laboratory susceptibility testing is completed (see Appendix B for fortified antibiotic preparation).

   Start fortified antibiotics:

   • Gentamicin 14 mg/ml, tobramycin 14 mg/ml, ciprofloxacin 0.3%, or ofloxacin 0.3% for Gram-negative coverage and cephalosporin (Cefazolin) 50 mg/ml alternating every 30 minutes to 1 hour, then taper. Cefazolin provides excellent coverage for Gram-positive organisms and is generally well tolerated topically. Alternatively, use single-agent quinolone antibiotic coverage:

   • Ciprofloxacin 0.3% (3 mg/ml) (Ciloxan, Alcon Labs) or ofloxacin 0.3% (3 mg/ml) (Ocuflox, Allergan Pharmaceuticals) drops every 30 minutes to 1 hour can be the first drug initiated for small to moderate size infectious ulcerations (19–22). For methicillin-resistant strains of *Staphylococcus* and penicillin-resistant strains of *Streptococcus, Bacillus, Clostridium,* and *Corynebacterium* use vancomycin 25 mg/ml. Otherwise cefazolin is effective against most Gram-positive aerobic organisms (23,24).

4. Cycloplegic (e.g., homatropine 5% three times daily) is usually used for symptomatic relief of accompanying photophobia.

Viral Keratitis

Herpes Simplex Keratitis

Herpes simplex keratitis is the leading infectious cause of corneal blindness in developed countries. Annual incidence of 500,000 cases estimated per year. The

TABLE 14–6. *Special diagnostic stains for keratitis*

Type of stain	Organism stained
Gram stain	Bacteria
Acridine orange	Bacteria, fungi, acanthamoeba, mycobacteria
Calcofluor white	Fungi, acanthamoeba
Acid fast	Mycobacteria

virus remains latent in neurons of the trigeminal ganglion. Reactivated, it causes the disease spectrum of epethilial and/or stromal keratitis, stromal opacities, corneal vascularizations, and perforations. Newborns, patients with acquired immunodeficiency syndrome, and other immunosuppressed patients such as transplant patients may require hospitalization to prevent possible dissemination.

Diagnosis

1. First distinguish and classify by region of corneal involvement:
   - Epithelial: punctate, linear (dendritiform), or geographic (macroulceration)
   - Stromal: non-necrotizing keratitis (disciform) or necrotizing, suppurative with keratic precipitates
   - Intraocular: uveitis
2. Signs and symptoms include vesicles involving the skin and margins of eyelids, primary follicular hypertrophy, preauricular nodes, conjunctivitis, epithelial keratitis (dendrites usually present), and/or stromal keratitis. Other findings include inflammatory cells, corneal vascularization, tissue necrosis, and inflammation of the corneal endothelium (disciform edema).
3. Usually nonpainful and unilateral 90% of the time.
4. Associated with previous trauma, environmental exposure, stress, and gingivostomatitis.
5. Corneal involvement includes the presence of dendrites, usually with terminal end bulbs that stain positive with rose bengal staining (Fig. 14–4). Stromal scars and in severe cases keratolysis with descemetocele formation can occur (25).

Management

1. Perform viral scraping of skin vesicles, conjunctiva, and cornea, and examine microscopically for characteristic multinucleated giant cells and eosinophilic intranuclear inclusion bodies (Lipschutz bodies, low yield); perform viral culture.

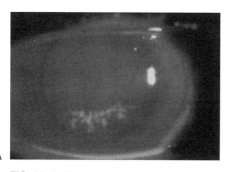 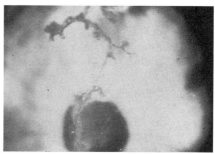

A   B

FIG. 14–4. Herpes simplex keratitis. **A:** Fluorescein sodium staining of dendritic epithelial keratitis. **B:** Rose bengal staining of dendrite. *For a color representation of this figure, please see the color insert facing p. 256.*

2. Additional laboratory tests could include: cytology, immunofluorescent antibody testing, Microtrak-latek agglutination, DNA probe testing, or PCR.
3. Start antiviral therapy as follows:
   - Conjunctivitis only
     Topical vidarabine 3% ointment (Vira-A, Parke-Davis) five times per day, or Idoxuridine 0.5% (Stoxil, Burroughs-Wellcome) drops, five times per day for approximately 5 to 7 days
   - Epithelial keratitis
     Trifluridine 1% (Viroptic, Burroughs-Wellcome) eight times per day after minimal wiping debridement
   - Stromal keratitis (no epithelial involvement present)
     Prednisolone phosphate or acetate 1% six to eight times per day with gradual, slow taper
     Trifluridine 1% (Viroptic) three to four times per day for prophylactic antiviral umbrella
4. Cycloplegic, e.g., homatropine, 5% three times daily, can be helpful for symptomatic relief.
5. Oral acyclovir (Zovirax, Burroughs-Wellcome) 400 mg five times daily for severe skin involvement. The Herpetic Eye Disease Study did not find therapeutic benefit in visual outcomes by the addition of acyclovir during treatment of steroid-treated stromal keratitis (26).
6. Frequent follow-up examination is necessary to identify signs of advancement (26).

Herpes Zoster Ophthalmicus (HZO)

Recurrent infection after latency: zoster (shingles) can lead to epithelial and stromal keratitis or neurotrophic keratopathy.

- HZO is more common over age 60 years
- Increased risk among young people with human immunodeficiency virus infection

Diagnosis

1. Ophthalmic division of trigeminal dermatome affected (often but not always) including the nasociliary branch. Disseminated lesions to other dermatomes are uncommon ($\leq$2% of all cases).
2. Linear epithelial keratitis is present, associated with conjunctivitis and skin rash. Distinguish from noninfectious mucous plaques that are often linear in shape.
3. Stromal keratitis develops in 6% to 54% of individuals with ophthalmic zoster:
   - Nonsuppurative (disciform, subepithelial infiltrative)
   - Suppurative, necrotizing (uncommon)
   - Mixed
     Stromal keratitis is frequently accompanied by iritis and ocular hypertension.

Neurotrophic keratopathy may result in protracted course with corneal scarring, neovascularization, lipid keratopathy, and bullous keratopathy.

Management

1. Laboratory evaluation may include rapid antigen detection (DFA, EIA, DNA probe), viral culture in established cell lines, and serologic tests to detect increase in antibody titer.
2. Topical antiviral or steroid not needed.
3. Oral acyclovir. Adult dose: 800 mg five times per day; initiate within 3 days of onset of skin eruption. Administered for 7- to 10-day course. Parenteral acyclovir for severely immunodeficient individuals over age 60 years.
4. Oral prednisone
   - Consider for immunocompetent individuals over age 60 years
   - 40 to 60 mg every day for average adult weight
   - Taper over approximately 3 weeks
5. See Chapter 10 if secondary preseptal cellulitis is suspected.

Fungal Keratitis

Diagnosis

1. Fungal keratitis is the most common cause of posttraumatic keratitis in adults.
2. It is often seen in plant or soil-contaminated injuries, immunocompromised patients, and in certain geographic locations (27).
3. Characteristically the infiltrates may have feathery borders with gray-white coloration that can be slightly elevated from the corneal border.
4. Satellite lesions and endothelial plaques may be observed.
5. Organisms may be classified as filamentous (septate and nonseptate), yeasts, and dimorphic. Common nonfilamentous yeasts (unicellular) include *Candida albicans, Candida parapsilosis,* and *Candida tropicalis.* Common filamentous fungi (multicellular and hyphae) include *Aspergillus* and *Fusarium.*

Management

1. Steps in management:
   - Identify risk factors
   - Assess distinct corneal signs
   - Construct a differential diagnosis
   - Perform laboratory studies
   - Initiate antifungal therapy
2. Obtain scrapings as for bacterial keratitis (above). Stains useful for fungi include PAS, Giemsa, and acridine orange (28,29).
3. Obtain sample for culture. Corneal biopsy may be required to obtain an adequate sample (Fig. 14–5). A disposable skin punch or small trephine may be

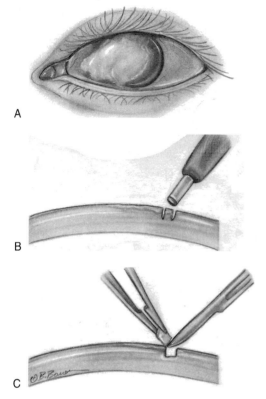

A

B

C

FIG. 14–5. A: Microbial keratitis with inconclusive culture and smear results after corneal scraping. **B:** Corneal punch biopsy. **C:** Punched area is removed with a Bard-Parker blade and forceps.

used. Lamellar dissection is performed using a sharp blade. Biopsy specimen is grasped carefully with fine-toothed forceps and excised.

4. Topical antifungal therapy includes:
   - Polyenes
     Natamycin (Alcon Labs) 5% suspension, first-line therapy for filamentous fungal keratitis
     Amphotericin B 0.1% to 0.5% (see Appendix B for preparation)
     Use one drop every 1 hour while awake, then every 2 hours at night.
     (Natamycin is the only approved antifungal agent currently available in the United States.) Alternatives must be prepared by a pharmacist.
   - Imidazoles (all the following are dosed as above)
     Miconazole 1%
     Ketoconazole 1.5%
     Fluconazole 2 mg/ml (from i.v. solution)
   - Antimetabolites
     Flucytosine 1% or itraconazole (made from i.v. preparation solutions)
5. Oral antifungal therapy
   - Fluconazole 200 mg orally twice daily

- Itraconazole 100 mg orally two to three times daily. Check liver function tests (30).

Parasitic Keratitis

Acanthamoeba

Acanthamoeba is a free-living parasitic amoeba that has worldwide distribution in fresh water, well water, bracking water, sea water, hot tubs, sewage, and soil. The amoeba are capable of existing in two forms, as trophozoites or encapsulated cysts. This tenacious organism can cause a destructive keratitis that can be challenging to diagnose and to treat effectively.

Risk factors include:

1. Contact lens wear (any type)
2. Use of homemade saline
3. Corneal trauma

A high index of suspicion for *Acanthamoeba* should always be present in the setting of a presumed bacterial or herpetic infection that has been resistant to previous treatment (31).

Diagnosis

1. Predominant symptoms include:
   - Foreign body sensation, irritation, and often extreme pain
   - Unilateral, redness, tearing, and photophobia
   - Preauricular nodes
   - Pain out of proportion to the examination
2. Predominant signs include:
   - Early: fine punctate epithelial erosions (PEE), epithelial ulceration, and multifocal stromal keratitis
   - Established: typical ring-shaped corneal infiltrate, coarse granular central infiltrate, biomicroscopically visible cysts, iridocyclitis, and occasionally scleritis (32)
   - Advanced: suppurative, necrotizing keratitis with possible perforation

Management

1. *Acanthamoeba* is difficult to treat because trophozoites tend to encyst and become highly resistant to treatment.
2. The following topical treatments can be used as single-line therapy or in combination, starting in the following order:
   - Polyhexamethylene biguanide 0.02% or chlorhexidine gluconate 0.02%. Treat for 6 to 12 months. First 72 hours, every hour; 4 to 7 days, every hour while awake, every 2 hours at night; 1 to 6 months, taper to four times daily. Monitor for corneal toxicity.

- Propamidine isethionate (Brolene 0.1%) or hexamidine diisethionate 0.1% (Desomedine, Laboratoire Chauvin) (same dosage as above).
- Polymyxin-B-neomycin-gramicidin or paramomycin 10 mg/ml (same dosage as above).
3. Dibromopropamidine ointment every 4 hours can be substituted for drops.
4. Oral azole therapy can be added:
   - Itraconazole (Sporanox) 100 mg orally two to three times daily
   - Fluconazole 200 mg orally twice daily
5. Cycloplegics can be prescribed for photophobia or discomfort. Homatropine 5% or atropine 1% three times daily.
6. Role of steroids is controversial.

Interstitial Keratitis (Stromal)

Interstitial keratitis is much less common than bacterial or viral keratitis. The differential diagnosis includes congenital syphilis, tuberculosis, and Cogan's syndrome (vertigo, tinnitus, hearing loss, and interstitial keratitis). Other causes include Lyme disease, mumps, rubeola (measles), HSV, HZV, lymphogranuloma venereum, leprosy, onchocerciasis, and systemic gold therapy.

Diagnosis

1. Assess and define the distinctive corneal signs
   - Status of epithelium: intact (abnormal or normal)
   - Type of stromal inflammation: simple, nonsuppurative or suppurative (necrotizing)
   - Site of inflammation: focal or diffuse, multifocal, or marginal
2. Search for distinctive corneal signs
3. Analyze the risk factors of microbial keratitis

Management

If infection is suspected:
   - Perform laboratory investigation in all cases
   - Initiate therapy based on clinical impression
   - Modify therapy based on clinical response, results of laboratory testing
   - Terminate therapy
   - Correct residual structural alterations

See Fig. 14–6.

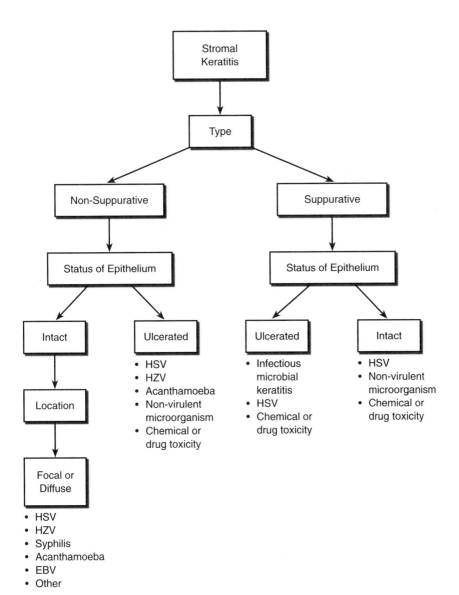

FIG. 14–6. Algorithm for stromal keratitis.

REFERENCES

1. Chandler JW, Sugar J, Edelhauser HF. *External Diseases; Cornea, Conjunctiva, Sclera, Eyelids, and Lacrimal System.* Vol. 8. St. Louis: CV Mosby; 1994:11.1–11.34.
2. Syed MA, Hyndiuk RA. Infectious conjunctivitis. Infectious conjunctivitis. *Infect Dis Clin North Am* 1992;789–805.
3. O'Brien TB, Green WR. Conjunctivitis. In: Mandell GL, Bennett JE, Dolin R, eds. *Principles and Practice of Infectious Diseases.* 4th ed. New York: Churchill Livingstone; 1995:575–583.
4 Barquet, Gasser I, Comingo P, et al. Primary meningococcal conjunctivitis: report of 21 patients and review. *Rev Infect Dis* 1990;12:838–847.
5. Detoledo AR, Chandler JW. Conjunctivitis of the newborn. *Infect Dis Clin North Am* 1992;6: 807–813.
6. Pang R, Teh LE, Rajan VS. Gonococcal ophthalmic neonatorum caused by beta-lactamase–producing *Neisseria gonorrhoeae. Br Med J* 1979;280–380.
7. Laga M, Naamara W, Brunham RC, et al. Single-dose therapy of gonococcal ophthalmia neonatorum with ceftriaxone. *N Engl J Med* 1986;315:1382.
8. Weiss A, Brinser JH, Nazar-Stewart V. Acute conjunctivitis in childhood. *J Pediatr* 1993;122:10–4.
9. Trottier S, Stenberg K, Von Rosen LA, et al. *Haemophilus influenzae* causing conjunctivitis in day-care children. *Infect Dis J* 1991;10:578–584.
10. Epidemiology: acute haemorrhagic conjunctivitis. *Br Med J* 1982;284–833.
11. Schacter J. Chlamydial infections. *N Engl J Med* 1978;298:428.
12. Beem MO, Saon EM. Respiratory-tract colonization and a distinctive pneumonia syndrome in infants infected with *Chlamydia trachomatis. N Engl J Med* 1977;296:306.
13. Holmes KK. The *Chlamydia* epidemic. *JAMA* 1981;245:1718.
14. O'Brien TB, Green WR. Keratitis. In: Mandell GL, Bennett JE, Dolin R, eds. *Principles and Practice of Infectious Diseases.* 4th ed. New York: Churchill Livingstone; 1995:1110–1119.
15. Clinch TE, Palmon FE, Robinson MJ, et al. Microbial keratitis in children. *Am J Ophthalmol* 117; 65:1994.
16. Cruz OA, Sabir SM, Capo H, et al. Microbial keratitis in childhood. *Ophthalmology* 100:192;1993.
17. Jones DB. A plan for antimicrobial therapy in bacterial keratitis. *Trans Am Acad Ophthalmol Otolaryngol* 1975;79:95.
18. Grigg J, Hirst LW, Whitby M, et al. Atypical mycobacterium keratitis. *Aust N Z J Ophthalmol* 1992; 20:257.
19. O'Brien TP, Sawusch MR, Dick JD, et al. Topical ciprofloxacin treatment of *Pseudomonas* keratitis in rabbits. *Arch Ophthalmol* 1988;106:1444.
20. Callegan MC, Engel LS, Hill JM, et al. Ciprofloxacin versus tobramycin for the treatment of staphylococcal keratitis. *Invest Ophthalmol Vis Sci* 1994;35:1033.
21. Gwon A. Ofloxacin vs tobramycin for the treatment of external ocular infection. *Arch Ophthalmol* 1992;110:1234.
22. O'Brien TP, et al. Results from the bacterial keratitis study: topical ofloxacin versus cefazolin and aminoglycoside in therapy for acute bacterial keratitis. *Arch Ophthalmol* 1995;113:1257–1265.
23. Gardner S, Pharm D. *Current Treatment of Bacterial Endophthalmitis and Keratitis.* Vol. 2. Georgia: Ocular Therapeutics and Management; 1991.
24. Gudmundsson OG, Ormerod LD, Kenyon KR, et al. Factors influencing predilection and outcome in bacterial keratitis. *Cornea* 1989;8:115.
25. Jones BR. The management of ocular herpes. *Trans Ophthalmol Soc UK* 1959;79–425.
26. Wilhelmus KR, et al. Herpetic Eye Disease Study: a controlled trial of topical corticosteroids for herpes simplex stromal keratitis. *Ophthalmology* 1994;101:1883–1896.
27. Rosa RH Jr, Miller D, Alfonso ED. The changing spectrum of fungal keratitis in south Florida. *Ophthalmology* 1994;101:1005.
28. Groden LR, Rodnite J, Brinser JH, et al. Acridine orange and Gram stains in infectious keratitis. *Cornea* 1990;9:122.
29. Chandler J, Chakrabarti A, Sharma A, et al. Evaluation of Calcofluor staining the diagnosis of fungal corneal ulcer. *Mycosis* 1993;36:243.
30. Jones DB. Diagnosis and management of fungal keratitis. In: Tasman W, Jaeger EA, eds. *Duanes's Clinical Ophthalmology.* Revised ed. Philadelphia: JB Lippincott; 1994.
31. Dart JKG, Stapleton F, Minassian D. Contact lenses and other risk factors in microbial keratitis. *Lancet* 1991;338:650.
32. Florakis GJ, Folberf R, Krachmer JH, et al. Elevated corneal epithelial lines in *Acanthamoeba* keratitis. 1988;106:1202.

Management of Ocular Injuries and Emergencies,
edited by Mathew W. MacCumber.
Lippincott–Raven Publishers, Philadelphia © 1998.

15

Corneoscleral Lacerations and Ruptures

Martin G. Edwards, Dante J. Pieramici, Sharon Fekrat,
Dimitri T. Azar, Walter J. Stark, and Mathew W. MacCumber

*Department of Ophthalmology, McGuire Air Force Base, New Jersey 08641;
Department of Ophthalmology and Visual Science, Yale University, New Haven,
Connecticut 06520-8061; Cornea Service, Massachusetts Eye and Ear Hospital,
Boston, Massachusetts 02114; Wilmer Eye Institute, The Johns Hopkins University
School of Medicine, Baltimore, Maryland 21287; and Retina Service, Department
of Ophthalmology, Rush Medical College, Chicago, Illinois 60612*

Basic Considerations   207
Definitions   209
Patient Evaluation   209
　　History   209 · Examination   209 · Ancillary Testing   210 · Initial
　　Management   210
Prognostic Factors   211
Medical Management of Isolated Corneal Lacerations   211
　　Patching and Bandage Contact Lens   211
Partial-Thickness Scleral Laceration   212
　　Diagnosis   212 · Management   212
**Surgical Management of Corneal and Corneoscleral Lacerations and
Ruptures   212**
　　Preparations for Surgery   213 · Surgical Management   213 · Postoperative
　　Management   218
Visual Rehabilitation   218
　　Contact Lenses   218 · Penetrating Keratoplasty   219
Occult Scleral Ruptures and Ruptured Cataract Wounds   219
　　Ruptured Cataract Wounds   219 · Diagnosis   220 · Management   221
**Surgical Management of Posterior Full-Thickness Scleral Lacerations
and Ruptures   221**
　　Management   221
Ocular Trauma Classification System   224

BASIC CONSIDERATIONS

Corneoscleral lacerations and ruptures make up a significant portion of ocular
trauma and may result in permanent ocular morbidity. However, a good visual out-

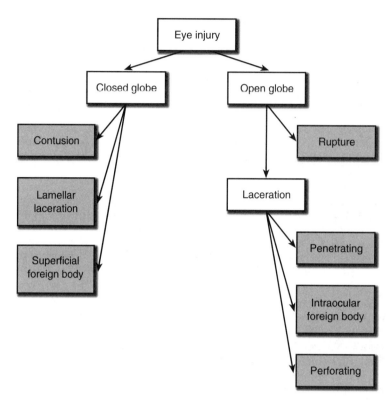

FIG. 15–1. The new ocular classification system.

come can be achieved in many cases by using microsurgical techniques and kerato-refractive principles to minimize postoperative astigmatism and other complications.

The overall goals of managing corneoscleral lacerations and ruptures include reapproximation of wound edges with a water-tight closure, minimization of postoperative astigmatism and scarring, prevention of postoperative complications such as infection, and visual rehabilitation with optical correction.

To clarify technology describing these injuries, the American Academy of Ophthalmology, the International Society of Ocular Trauma, and the Retina and Vitreous Societies have endorsed the use of ocular trauma–specific terminology (1) (Fig. 15–1). This terminology is used throughout this text and should be adopted for every injured patient. Note that the tissue of reference is always the entire globe. If a tissue is specified, it refers to location and not to type of injury (e.g., a corneal penetrating injury is an open globe injury with single laceration located in the cornea). While in press, the Ocular Trauma Classification Group proposed further classification based on four key prognostic indicators at the initial examination. See the end of this chapter for this system.

DEFINITIONS

Eyewall: Sclera and cornea

Closed globe injury: No full-thickness wound of eyewall (contusion), partial-thickness wound (lamellar laceration), or superficial foreign body

Open globe injury: Full-thickness wound of eyewall; intact, prolapsed, or damaged choroid/retina

Rupture: Caused by a blunt object momentarily increasing the intraocular pressure; wound is by an inside-out mechanism and not necessarily at impact site; tissue herniation frequent and potentially substantial

Laceration: Usually caused by a sharp object; wound is by an outside-in mechanism at impact site

Penetrating injury: Single (entrance) laceration

Intraocular foreign body injury: Retained foreign object(s) causing entrance laceration(s) (technically a penetrating injury but grouped separately because of different clinical implications)

Perforating injury: Two (entrance and exit) wounds caused by the same object

PATIENT EVALUATION

History

1. A detailed history and thorough ocular examination is required.
2. Evaluate specifically for the possibility of wound contamination or the presence of a foreign body.
3. In cases involving metallic intraocular foreign bodies, the nature of the material should be identified to determine potential toxicity to the eye. Metals with the highest toxicity are copper and iron. It is also useful to know if the metal is magnetic (see Chapter 21).
4. The status of the eye before injury and any previous medical or surgical ocular history should be noted.

Examination

1. A careful assessment of the extent of the injury is necessary to develop a therapeutic plan. Desmarres retractors may help open the lids without applying pressure to the globe. Examination should be limited so as not to result in iatrogenic injury. The main objective of the initial examination is to determine whether the globe is open or not. When an open globe is diagnosed or suspected, further evaluation can be performed intraoperatively or by using ancillary tests (x-ray, computed tomography [CT] scan).
2. A Seidel test may help when there is uncertainty as to whether a full-thickness corneoscleral wound is present. To perform the Seidel test, administer a drop of sterile 2% fluorescein dye. Under blue light at the slit lamp, carefully look for bright green dye streaming from the site of penetration.

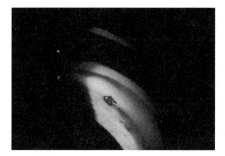

FIG. 15–2. Small metallic foreign body in the inferior angle visualized with gonioscopy (courtesy of Dr. K. Packo).

3. Gonioscopy may aid in identifying an occult foreign body in the anterior chamber angle (Fig. 15–2). This should only be performed if the wound is self-sealing; otherwise, it can be performed intraoperatively following wound closure.
4. Occult scleral rupture should be suspected when there is hemorrhagic chemosis, vitreous hemorrhage, an abnormally shallow or deep anterior chamber, or peaking of the pupil. The intraocular pressure is often low but may be normal or elevated. In general, all eyes with possible occult rupture should undergo ancillary testing and surgical exploration.

Ancillary Testing

Axial and coronal CT of the orbit or ultrasound may be necessary to evaluate for occult intraocular foreign bodies or evidence of occult rupture (see Chapter 5). Ultrasonography is generally not performed on the non-self sealing open globe injury but may be used intraoperatively after wound closure.

Initial Management

Referring physicians should perform the following before transfer to the treating ophthalmologist.

1. Patient is to take nothing by mouth (NPO).
2. Shield is placed over the injured eye(s). If a metallic or plastic shield is unavailable, then a rigid paper cup taped in place may suffice (see Fig. 1–1).
3. Administer tetanus toxin. Persons who have not received a tetanus booster in the past 10 years or are unsure of their booster status should receive 250 U of tetanus antitoxoid intramuscularly.
4. Administer prophylactic intravenous (i.v.) antibiotics. We currently use i.v. clindamycin (600 mg every 8 hours; pediatric dose 25 to 40 mg/kg/day divided every 8 hours) and i.v. ceftazidine (1 g every 12 hours; pediatric dose 100 to 150 mg/kg/day divided every 8 hours).
5. Antiemetic given intramuscularly or i.v. for nausea or vomiting.
6. Protruding foreign bodies should not be disturbed.
7. Transfer patient with copies of ancilliary tests.

PROGNOSTIC FACTORS

The prognosis for useful visual recovery is largely dependent on the severity of the injury. In general, larger wounds tend to do poorly. Predictors of good visual outcome after penetrating corneoscleral injuries include a good initial visual acuity, absence of an afferent pupillary defect, anterior-located wounds, and small wound. Predictors of no light perception and/or enucleation include an initial visual acuity of hand motions or worse, wound length of greater than 4 mm, and the presence of a relative afferent pupillary defect in the injured eye (2).

MEDICAL MANAGEMENT OF ISOLATED CORNEAL LACERATIONS

Small isolated corneal lacerations can occasionally be managed without surgical intervention. The use of patching, bandage soft contact lenses, or tissue adhesives in conjunction with topical and/or systemic antibiotics, cycloplegics, and corticosteroids may be considered (3).

Patching and Bandage Contact Lens

1. Partial thickness corneal lacerations or self-sealing small pinpoint lacerations can sometimes be managed with semi-pressure patching (see Fig. 13-4*B*).
2. Self-sealing (Seidel negative) corneal lacerations less than 2 mm in length and located outside of the visual axis can occasionally be supported by a soft bandage contact lens. In children or uncooperative adults it is advisable to suture even small wounds because eye rubbing can be anticipated.
3. With patching or a bandage lens, initially daily follow-up is necessary in the acute phase to evaluate for infection and wound leakage.
4. Prophylactic topical antibiotics should be used. We typically use ciloxan every 2 hours while awake and erythromycin ointment.
5. Cycloplegics such as Cyclogel four times daily or atropine twice daily can aid in making the eye more comfortable and reduce inflammation.
6. Topical steroids should be used with caution initially and then adjusted to minimize scarring and inflammation once the risk of infection has decreased.
7. Tissue adhesives may be useful in treating small lacerations less than 2 mm in length (4); however, to date none have been approved by the U.S. Food and Drug Administration for ophthalmic use. Tissue adhesives can be applied at the slit lamp with topical anesthesia only. They are applied with a 27-gauge needle after debriding the surrounding epithelium and thoroughly drying the surface with a weck-cel sponge. A therapeutic soft contact lens should be placed over the adhesive for patient comfort and to help prevent the glue from dislodging. Judicious follow-up, prophylactic antibiotic therapy, and a high index of suspicion for infectious complications (5) is warranted because tissue adhesives may predispose the cornea to infectious keratitis and the glue may conceal underlying infections.
8. We generally prescribe prophylactic ciprofloxacin 750 mg orally twice daily for

a 5- to 10-day course (adult dose; systemic ciprofloxicin should not be used in children).

PARTIAL-THICKNESS SCLERAL LACERATION

A partial-thickness scleral laceration is almost always caused by a sharp object.

Diagnosis

1. If there is any question whether the globe is ruptured, a conjunctival peritomy should be performed in the operating room to explore and examine the suspicious area(s). See Occult Scleral Ruptures and Ruptured Cataract Wounds below.
2. The overlying conjunctiva is almost always lacerated when there is a partial-thickness scleral laceration, thus allowing the diagnosis to be made at the slit-lamp.
3. Good exposure of the affected area is necessary to make the diagnosis despite laceration of the overlying conjunctiva. After applying sterile topical anesthesia, careful exploration of this area with a sterile cotton tip and/or 0.12 forceps will show the partial-thickness laceration. One must be certain that the laceration is not full thickness at any point along its extent. Exploration of the area in the operating room under controlled conditions may be preferred in certain cases.
4. By definition, no intraocular contents are visible through or within the laceration.

Management

Medical

1. Topical antibiotic ointment, such as erythromycin, with a semi-pressure patch may be applied to allow for healing of the overlying conjunctiva (see Fig. 13–4B). Subsequent application of the ointment two to three times per day for several days is suggested.
2. The patient should be instructed to refrain from placing pressure on or rubbing the eye.
3. Protective eyewear should be worn because the integrity of the globe has been compromised.

Surgical

1. Surgical intervention to approximate the scleral and/or conjunctival edges is not necessary.
2. Other associated ocular injuries may require surgical intervention.

SURGICAL MANAGEMENT OF CORNEAL AND CORNEOSCLERAL LACERATIONS AND RUPTURES

The vast majority of isolated corneal and corneoscleral wounds and wounds with other associated ocular injuries, such as uveal prolapse, lens injury, intraocular foreign body, or posterior segment involvement, require surgical repair. The primary goal of surgical repair is to obtain a water-tight closure. This should be performed when possible in a manner that allows one to restore normal anatomic relationships, restore functional architecture, prevent postoperative complications, and prepare for secondary procedures (6).

An attempt at a surgical repair should always be made. Even eyes that initially have no light perception can sometimes regain useful vision with proper management. If the globe is markedly disrupted, the patient should be informed that a primary enucleation may be appropriate. However, it may be psychologically easier for the patient to accept loss of the eye if the enucleation is delayed for several days after initial wound closure (see Chapter 28).

Preparations for Surgery

1. The majority of cases require general anesthesia because intraocular contents can be expulsed during injection of retrobulbar anesthetic.
2. Preoperative photographs are advisable in work-related injuries or in cases where litigation is likely.
3. Patients should be advised of the prognosis and potential need of primary enucleation when the consent for surgery is obtained.
4. In severe injuries resulting in a large amount of tissue loss, donor corneal and or scleral tissue should be available should patch grafting be necessary.
5. With lens injury, previous refraction if known, and axial length and ketatometric readings in the uninvolved eye are useful should cataract removal be necessary and intraocular lens (IOL) placement considered.

Surgical Management

1. Lashes should be carefully trimmed, the globe gently irrigated with sterile balanced salt solution, and the skin prepared in a sterile fashion. A fenestrated drape combined with a Jaffe lid speculum results in little pressure exerted on the globe.
2. The extent of the wound should be delineated. If the wound extends beyond the limbus, a conjunctival peritomy should be performed and Tenon's capsule dissected from the wound until the end of the wound is identified (Fig. 15–3A). If the wound extends well beyond the insertion of the rectus muscles, it is advisable to stabilize the globe by closing the anterior portion of the wound before proceeding to removal of a muscle. Protruding foreign bodies are usually removed after good exposure has been achieved. A foreign body with a barbed end (e.g., a fish hook) may need to be cut so additional ocular trauma does not occur during removal.
3. Tissue prolapse is frequently encountered when repairing corneal lacerations. Most would agree that retina, choroid, and ciliary body should be reposited. Vitreous should be excised at the wound margin with a weck-cel and scissors or with vitrectomy instrumentation. The iris presents somewhat of a controversy. The iris is usually excised if exposed for more than 12 hours or if it ap-

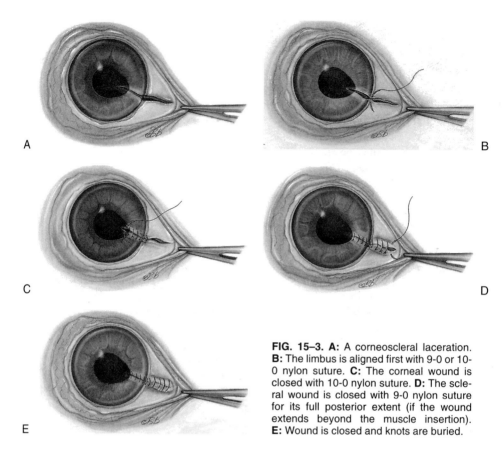

A

B

C

D

E

FIG. 15–3. A: A corneoscleral laceration. B: The limbus is aligned first with 9-0 or 10-0 nylon suture. C: The corneal wound is closed with 10-0 nylon suture. D: The scleral wound is closed with 9-0 nylon suture for its full posterior extent (if the wound extends beyond the muscle insertion). E: Wound is closed and knots are buried.

pears contaminated and nonviable. If the cornea has re-epithelialized over iris prolapsed into the wound, the iris should be excised or the epithelium mechanically or chemically debrided from the iris before repositing the tissue to prevent seeding of the anterior chamber with epithelial cells (7,8). If there is evidence of infection, fluids should be taken for appropriate stains and bacterial and fungal culture.

4. Frequently the anterior chamber is shallow and needs to be reformed before repair. This can be accomplished by creating a separate paracentesis tract and injecting sterile air or viscoelastic into the chamber (Fig. 15–4A). Care should be taken to avoid injuring the lens during this procedure. Viscoelastic (e.g., sodium hyaluronate) when injected will often deepen the chamber and thereby retract the incarcerated iris (9). Viscoelastic also helps maintain the chamber depth during repair. However, if left in the eye it may lead to transient postoperative elevated intraocular pressure. An iris sweep also can be used through the paracentesis tract to help pull iris (and vitreous or fibrin clot) from the

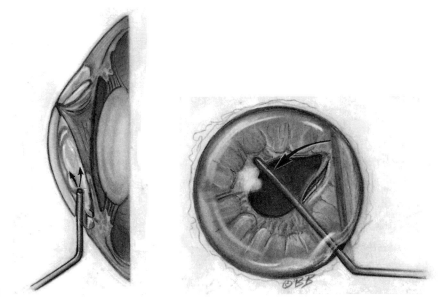

A   B

FIG. 15–4. A: The anterior chamber is deepened with viscoelastic injected via a paracentesis site opposite the wound. **B:** Iris, vitreous, and/or fibrin clot are swept free from wound.

wound before or after the wound is sutured (Fig. 15–4*B*). Use care to avoid angle injury by the iris sweep.

5. To reapproximate wound margins, anatomic landmarks should be identified. The corneal limbus serves as the most useful landmark, and when limbal involvement is present, the limbus should be carefully aligned first using 9-0 or 10-0 monofilament nylon suture (Fig. 15–3*B*).

6. Corneal lacerations are sutured with 10-0 monofilament nylon. Sutures should be placed perpendicular to the wound margin with equal bites taken on both sides and a suture depth of 75% to 90% corneal thickness achieved (Fig. 15–5). Interrupted sutures allow for selective suture removal postoperatively. Slip knots allow the tension to be adjusted, and all knots are trimmed and buried. Stellate lacerations often require several sutures near the central portion of the wound (Fig. 15–6*A*).

7. Astigmatism is a major cause of visual morbidity after corneal wound repair. Wound closure should therefore be performed in a manner that minimizes postoperative astigmatism. The cornea will flatten over any vertical incision or sutured laceration, the center of the cornea will flatten more than the periphery, and the cornea will steepen anterior to a tight peripheral suture (10). Therefore, to minimize postoperative astigmatism the laceration should be sutured from the periphery to the center (Fig. 15–3*C*). Large compressive sutures should be placed in the periphery, and fewer, shorter sutures should be placed

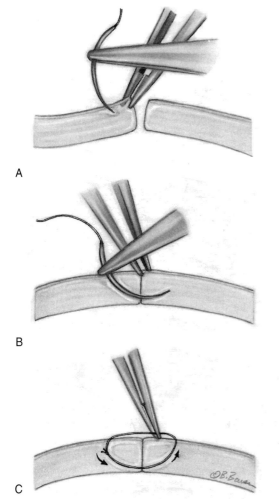

A

B

C

FIG. 15–5. A: Proper placement of a corneoscleral suture. One edge of the wound is grasped with 0.12 forceps. The suture is passed initially perpendicular to the tissue surface to 75% to 90% depth. **B:** The opposite edge of the wound is grasped and the wound is aligned. The suture must be at equal depth on each side of the wound. **C:** The suture is tied and the knot buried. Suture ends should be facing away from the tissue surface so they will not need to cross the wound at the time of removal.

centrally. This theoretically flattens the periphery and lessens central flattening (Fig. 15–6B).

8. Extensive wounds with tissue loss may require lamellar or full-thickness keratoplasty for repair. Lamellar keratoplasty is indicated when irregular wound margins and tissue loss preclude primary repair. Penetrating keratoplasty is rarely indicated acutely and should be delayed if possible to maximize chances of maintaining a clear graft.

9. When the wound extends beyond the limbus, a 360-degree peritomy should be performed and the entire extent of the globe opening identified. A technique of sequentially suturing the sclera (usually with 9-0 or 8-0 monofilament nylon) as conjunctiva and tenons are dissected free allows for wound stabilization

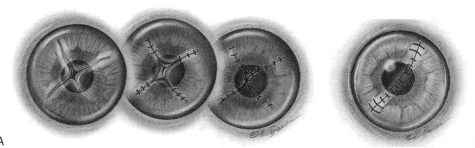

A   B

FIG. 15–6. A: Repair of Steellate corneal laceration. Additional sutures are often required near the central portion of the wound. **B:** Corneal sutures placed to reduce postoperative astigmatism.

while the tissue is manipulated further posteriorly and more of the laceration exposed (Fig. 15–3*D*) (see Surgical Management of Posterior Full-Thickness Scleral Lacerations and Ruptures below).

10. Once the wound is surgically repaired, the area should be carefully inspected to assure that a water-tight closure is present. A Seidel test with 2% fluorescein can help confirm this. Intraoperative keratometry can help in adjusting suture tension to minimize irregularity while maintaining a water-tight closure. Stellate lacerations may require tissue adhesive (see Medical Management of Isolated Corneal Lacerations, above) or keratoplasty if sutures alone cannot create a water-tight closure. Make sure all corneal suture knots are buried. Loose sutures should be removed and replaced if necessary. Scleral suture knots should be buried or trimmed very short (Fig. 15–3*E*).

11. Associated lens injuries can be addressed after repair of the globe opening or deferred. Mild traumatic cataract may stabilize or improve spontaneously. When the lens capsule is clearly violated and flocculent cortex is present, the lens is removed at the time of the initial procedure (see Chapter 18). Placement of an IOL under these circumstances is controversial. A secondary procedure in an uninflamed eye with an accurate axial length and IOL power calculation may be advisable. In select cases of definite rupture of the anterior lens capsule with zonulocapsular integrity and no evidence of posterior segment injury, cataract extraction and posterior chamber IOL implantation can be performed at the time of the initial repair (11) (see Chapter 18).

12. If endophthalmitis is present at the time of surgical repair, samples of intraocular fluids should be taken for appropriate stains, as should samples for bacterial and fungal cultures (see Chapter 19). Performing a pars plana vitrectomy in these eyes at the time of primary repair is controversial, but we recommend that vitrectomy be considered, particularly if the endophthalmitis is severe with significant vitreous involvement (see Chapter 19) .

13. A decision must be made by the surgeon whether further surgery should be performed or deferred (12–16). In general, further surgery can be deferred unless an intraocular foreign body or endophthalmitis is present. Intraocular for-

eign bodies are usually removed primarily to decrease the risk of endophthalmitis and metal toxicity (see Chapter 21).

14. If the risk of endophthalmitis is high based on the clinical history, consideration should be given to the injection of intravitreal antibiotics (see Chapter 19).

15. If more extensive surgery is not performed, Tenon's capsule and conjunctiva should be carefully examined for the presence of foreign bodies. Conjunctiva is closed with 6-0 collagen suture with knots buried or trimmed short. Subconjunctival injections of antibiotics and corticosteroids are usually given. Antibiotic and steroid ointment are applied and the eye is patched and shielded.

Postoperative Management

Postoperative management goals include control of infection, inflammation, and elevated intraocular pressure, minimizing corneal scarring, and stabilizing the ocular surface epithelium.

1. Patients are usually initially hospitalized for close follow-up.

2. Shield is maintained over the injured eye(s) at all times.

3. We routinely prescribe prophylactic intravenous antibiotics for 48 to 120 hours. Typically, we use clindamycin (600 mg every 8 hours; pediatric dose 25 to 40 mg/kg/day divided every 8 hours) and Ceftazidine (1 g every 12 hours; pediatric dose 100 to 150 mg/kg/day divided every 8 hours). For small, clear wounds we substitute ciprofloxacin 750 mg orally twice daily for 5 to 10 days for i.v. antibiotics (adult patients only).

4. Topical broad-spectrum antibiotic is given (e.g., ciprofloxacin every 2 hours). For dirtier wounds or evidence of keratitis we add fortified antibiotics (see Chapter 14).

5. Cycloplegia is desirable. We typically use atropine 1% twice daily.

6. Topical steroids are used cautiously during the early postoperative period (e.g., prednisolone acetate 1% four times daily) and then adjusted accordingly when the risk of infection has subsided and oral corticosteroids may be indicated in severely inflamed eyes.

7. Topical glaucoma medications or systemic carbonic anhydrase inhibitors may be required to lower intraocular pressure.

8. Selected sutures can be moved as early as 3 months postoperatively.

VISUAL REHABILITATION

Contact Lenses

A contact lens can be successfully fit and worn in 73% to 81% of patients after corneoscleral laceration repair to successfully correct aphakia and astigmatism (17).

A contact lens can be prescribed 6 weeks postoperatively, after topical steroids have been discontinued, earlier in children if amblyopia is a risk. Intact sutures usually do not hinder contact lens fitting. Many patients can avoid penetrating keratoplasty or further surgery with contact lens use. However, contact lenses have limited success for larger lacerations and those involving the optical axis.

Penetrating Keratoplasty

Penetrating keratoplasty may be necessary when corneal scarring or irregularity limits visual rehabilitation. Delaying penetrating keratoplasty for 3 months significantly improves the chance of success (18).

OCCULT SCLERAL RUPTURES AND RUPTURED CATARACT WOUNDS

The preoperative diagnosis of scleral rupture after blunt ocular trauma may be difficult, whereas the diagnosis of scleral laceration after penetrating injury is much easier. Marked subconjunctival and/or intraocular hemorrhage may prevent visualization of a scleral rupture site and should raise the examiner's suspicion of the presence of an occult rupture site and prompt surgical exploration. Several studies have examined the clinical characteristics of eyes with scleral rupture caused by blunt trauma (Table 15–1) (19–23).

Ruptured Cataract Wounds

The traumatic rupture or dehiscence of a cataract wound is an uncommon but potentially devastating complication of cataract surgery (24,25). It may occur in the immediate postoperative period or many years after surgery depending on the mechanism of trauma and the healing of the corneal scleral incision. Patients are often elderly; in one series the average age was 73 years (26). Blunt mechanisms account for the majority of cataract wound dehiscence, with a history of a fall being the most common. In one series it accounted for 67% of wound dehiscence (25). Blunt injury results in anterior-posterior compression of the globe, which produces stretching forces along the corneal scleral incision. In theory, smaller incisions created with scleral tunneling should reduce the risk of wound dehiscence;

TABLE 15–1. *Signs suggestive of occult open globe (19,20)*

Hemorrhagic chemosis
Hypotony (IOP <5), although elevated IOP may be present
Abnormally deep (or shallow) anterior chamber
Visual acuity of light perception or less
Vitreous hemorrhage
Peaking of the pupil (which also may be a result of previous cataract surgery)
Choroidal detachment or choroidal congestion on ultrasound (see Chapter 5)
Dislocation/subluxation of an IOL
Vitreous to a preexisting cataract wound

---

however, this has not been substantiated with a prospective clinical trial. Likewise, it has not been determined whether no-stitch surgery will predispose to wound dehiscence.

Cataract wound rupture is associated with other ocular injuries; iris damage, hyphema, vitreous hemorrhage, and retinal detachment. In pseudophakic patients the lens may be expulsed or subluxated, causing associated ocular injuries and complicating the management of these patients. Overall, the prognosis for these injuries is comparable with that for all globe ruptures. Poor prognosis is associated with the presence of an afferent pupillary defect, expulsion of the IOL, poor initial visual acuity, and posterior segment pathology (27). One should always have a high level of suspicion for an occult scleral rupture or wound dehiscence. Use the clinical signs described in Table 15–1 as a guide and have a low threshold for exploration in the operating room with general anesthesia (particularly in children).

Diagnosis

History

Document the mechanism of injury because it will help predict associated ocular injuries and dictate prognosis. It is important to question the patient about a history of cataract surgery and the presence of an IOL. Intraocular hemorrhage may obscure the view of an IOL. Inquire about pretraumatic visual acuity because a poor outcome may be related to pre-existing pathology. In elderly patients, a fall is a common mechanism of injury and may suggest pre-existing or traumatic neurologic or orthopedic pathology that requires consultation.

Examination

Assess clinical signs of occult wound dehiscence, scleral rupture or scleral laceration (Table 15–1 and Fig. 15–7) (19,20).

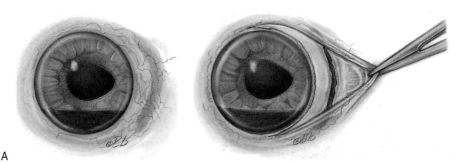

A   B

FIG. 15–7. A: Signs of wound dehiscence or scleral rupture include hemorrhagic chemosis, hyphema, abnormally shallow or deep anterior chamber and peaking of the pupil (usually toward the wound). **B:** The scleral rupture exposed.

Assessment of the status of the IOL is important in cases of wound dehiscence. IOLs are often, but not always, expulsed at the time of the injury. The IOL presence and location may be evident on slit-lamp examination or ophthalmoscopy. If not, then B-scan ultrasonography is performed.

Assessment of associated ocular injuries should include ophthalmoscopy. Ancillary tests including CT scan and ultrasound will help detect associated intraocular and orbital pathology (see Chapter 5).

Management

See Surgical Management of Posterior Full-Thickness Scleral Lacerations and Ruptures below. After wound closure, the management of an IOL still present in the eye can be addressed, keeping the following suggestions in mind:

- If the lens is subluxed with remaining capsule, then it may be rotated with a Sinsky hook to recenter. One should then tap on the optic to test stability. If unstable, then McCannel (variation on repair of radial iris defect) or scleral sutures are placed, securing the haptic to the iris (see Chapter 18).
- Alternatively, the IOL can be removed and a new lens secured with scleral fixation (see Chapter 18).
- In cases of severe associated ocular injuries, one should consider removing the IOL without replacement because this may allow better visualization of the posterior pole and easier postoperative management.
- If the patient has an iris-fixated IOL that has decentered or dislocated, it should be repositioned or replaced with an open-loop haptic anterior chamber IOL or scleral fixated posterior chamber IOL.
- If the IOL has dislocated into the vitreous cavity, then vitrectomy techniques must be used (28). Once the scleral wound has been closed, the IOL can be managed at a second procedure if the primary surgeon is not trained in vitreoretinal techniques.

SURGICAL MANAGEMENT OF POSTERIOR FULL-THICKNESS SCLERAL LACERATIONS AND RUPTURES

Management

1. Follow preparations for surgery and surgical technique under Surgical Management of Corneal and Corneoscleral Lacerations and Ruptures above through surgical technique step 2 if there is no anterior segment involvement and through step 9 if there is anterior segment involvement.
2. Good exposure of all quadrants of the eye must be obtained to determine the full extent of the laceration and to ensure that no other areas of occult rupture are present (Fig. 15–8). In those cases in which the laceration extends posteriorly toward the optic nerve, the full extent of the injury may not be fully appreciated despite adequate exposure. A 360-degree conjunctival peritomy followed by sharp dissection of the conjunctiva and Tenon's from the sclera in all four quad-

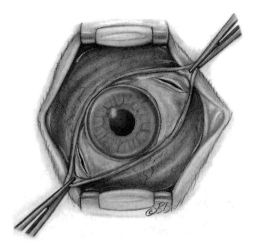

FIG. 15–8. The globe must be thoroughly examined so as not to miss a second scleral rupture or laceration.

rants is performed to provide exposure and to decrease the pressure on the globe during intraoperative manipulation. Do not disturb any prolapsed intraocular tissues during the dissection. Inspection of the area posterior to each of the four rectus muscle insertion sites may be done meticulously and carefully with a muscle hook and a cotton-tipped applicator without removal of the muscles from their insertion site.

3. Scleral lacerations may be repaired with 8-0 or 9-0 nylon suture material on a spatulated needle. Interrupted sutures should be used to close the laceration in almost all cases with partial-thickness bites, beginning anteriorly and continuing posteriorly, with eversion of the edges of the wound. Closure of the laceration should continue posteriorly only to the point at which closure becomes technically difficult or requires undue pressure on the globe. Very posterior lacerations benefit from effective physiologic tamponade by orbital tissue and are best left alone.

4. If vitreous is incarcerated in the laceration site, it may be cut with sharp scissors flush with the sclera without excising any retinal tissue. A vitrectomy instrument should not be used to excise incarcerated vitreous because of the high risk of damaging the retina. Extruded intraocular tissues, such as uvea or retina, may be reposited; extruded uveal tissue may rarely be excised if necrotic and surgical repair occurs more than 24 hours after the injury. If retina is prolapsing into the laceration, it should be carefully reposited without incarcerating it into the wound.

5. If the scleral laceration extends under a rectus muscle (Fig. 15–9A), it may be exposed by carefully passing a muscle hook under the muscle to elevate it out of the way. If this is not adequate, the muscle insertion may be isolated with 6-0 Vicryl suture and removed from the globe (Fig. 15–9B and C). After repair of the wound (Fig. 15–9D) and placement of a prophylactic scleral buckle (Fig. 15–9E), the muscle is resutured to its insertion site (Fig. 15–9F).

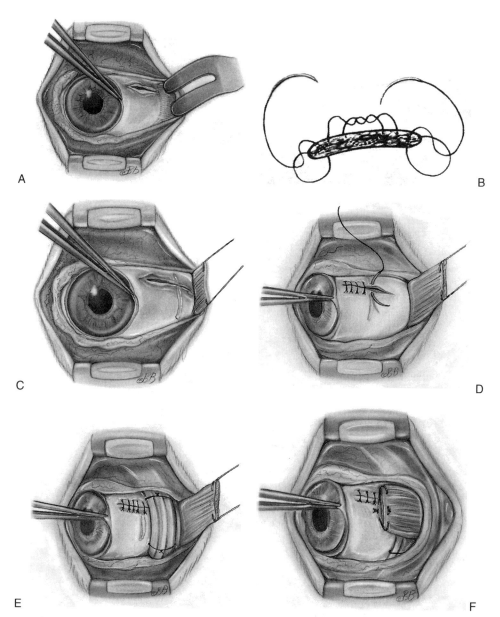

FIG. 15–9. A: The scleral wound is observed to extend through the rectus muscle insertion. **B:** If retraction of the rectus muscle does not permit closure of the wound, then a 6-0 Vicryl suture is passed through the anterior portion of the muscle (technique of Dr. D. Guyton). **C:** The muscle is removed at the insertion site. **D:** The scleral wound is closed. **E:** An encircling scleral buckle (and radial element if necessary) is placed to support the wound and the entire vitreous base. **F:** The rectus muscle is reattached at its insertion.

6. A scleral patch graft may be necessary if extensive loss of scleral tissue occurred.
7. It is often impossible to identify a retinal break upon presentation in these eyes because of associated vitreous hemorrhage. Cryotherapy should not be performed unless a specific break is noted. At Wilmer, a prophylactic encircling buckle (and an additional element to support the wound, if necessary) is placed around these eyes at the time of primary repair if there is vitreous base involvement or extensive loss of vitreous (see Chapter 20 for technique).
8. Continue at step 10 under Surgical Management of Corneal and Corneoscleral Lacerations and Ruptures above.

TRAUMA CLASSIFICATION

Open-globe injury classification
Type
  A. Rupture
  B. Penetrating
  C. Intraocular foreign body
  D. Perforating
  E. Mixed
Grade
  Visual acuity[a]
    1. ≥20/40
    2. 20/50 to 20/100
    3. 19/100 to 5/200
    4. 4/200 to light perception
    5. No light perception[b]
Pupil
  Positive: Relative afferent pupillary defect present in affected eye
  Negative: Relative afferent pupillary defect absent in affected eye
Zone
  I. Isolated to cornea (including the corneoscleral limbus)
  II. Corneoscleral limbus to a point 5 mm posterior into the sclera

Closed-globe injury classification
Type
  A. Contusion
  B. Lamellar laceration
  C. Superficial foreign body
  D. Mixed
Grade
  Visual acuity[a]
    1. ≥20/40
    2. 20/50 to 20/100
    3. 19/100 to 5/200
    4. 4/200 to light perception
    5. No light perception[b]
Pupil
  Positive: Relative afferent pupillary defect present in affected eye
  Negative: Relative afferent pupillary defect absent in affected eye
Zone[c]
  I. External (limited to bulbar conjunctiva, sclera, cornea)

CORNEOSCLERAL LACERATIONS AND RUPTURES 225

III. Posterior to the anterior 5 mm
of sclera

^aMeasured at distance (20 ft, 6 m) using
Snellen chart or Rosenbaum near card, with
correction and pinhole when appropriate.

^bConfirmed with bright light source and fellow
eye well occluded.

Reprinted with permission (29).

II. Anterior segment (involving
structures in anterior
segment internal to the
cornea and including the
posterior lens capsule; also
includes pars plicata but
not pars plana)

III. Posterior segment (all
internal structures posterior
to the posterior lens
capsule)

^aMeasured at distance (20 ft, 6 m) using
Snellen chart or Rosenbaum near card,
with correction and pinhole when appropriate.

^bConfirmed with bright light source and
fellow eye well occluded.

^cRequires B-scan ultrasonography when
media opacity precludes assessment of
more posterior structures.

Reprinted with permission (29).

REFERENCES

1. Kuhn F, Morris R, Witherspoon CD, et al. A standardized classification of ocular trauma. *Ophthalmology* 1996;103:240–243.
2. Barr CC. Prognostic factors in corneoscleral lacerations. *Arch Ophthalmol* 1983;101:919.
3. Linn DT, Webster KRG, Abbott RL. Repair of corneal lacerations and perforations. *Int Ophthalmol Clin* 1988;18:69.
4. Leahey AB, Gottsch JD, Stark WJ. Clinical experience in N-butyl cyanoacrylate (Nexacryl) tissue adhesives. *Ophthalmology* 1993;100:173.
5. Cavanaugh TB, Gottsch JD. Infectious keratitis and cyanoacrylate adhesives. *Am J Ophthalmol* 1991;111:466.
6. Hamill MB, Thompson WS. The evaluation and management of corneal lacerations. *Retina* 1990;10(suppl):1.
7. Orlin SE, Farber MG, Brucker AJ, Frayer WC. The unexpected guest: problem of iris reposition. *Surv Ophthalmol* 1990;35:59.
8. Hamill ME. Repair of the anterior segment. Focal Points, American Academy of Ophthalmology, San Francisco, CA 10:1,1992.
9. Drews RC. Sodium hyaluronate (Healon) in the repair of perforating injuries of the eye. *Ophthalmic Surg* 1986;17:23.
10. Rowsy JJ, Hays JC. Refractive reconstruction for acute eye injuries. *Ophthalmic Surg* 1984;15:659.
11. Lamkin JC, Azar DT, Meade MD, Volpe NJ. Simultaneous corneal laceration repair, cataract removal, and posterior chamber intraocular lens implantation. *Am J Ophthalmol* 1992;113:626.
12. Spalding SC, Sternberg P Jr. Controversies in the management of posterior segment ocular trauma. *Retina* 1990;10(suppl):76.
13. Ryan SJ. Results of pars plana vitrectomy in penetrating ocular trauma. *Int Ophthalmol* 1978;1:5.
14. Ryan SJ. Guidelines in the management of penetrating ocular trauama with emphasis on the role and timing of pars plana vitrectomy. *Int Ophthalmol* 1979;1:105.

15. Stucchi CA, Vignanelli M. Early vitrectomy in the treatment of severe eye injuries. *Klin Monatsbl Augenheilkd* 1990;196:346.
16. Meredith TA, Gordon PA. Pars plana vitrectomy for severe penetrating injury with posterior segment involvement. *Am J Ophthalmol* 1987;103:549.
17. Smiddy WE, Hamburg TR, Kratcher GP, et al. Contact lenses for visual rehabilitation after corneal laceration repair. *Ophthalmology* 1989;96:293.
18. Nobem JR, Moura BT, Robin JB, Smith RE. Results of penetrating keratoplasty for the treatment of corneal perforations. *Arch Ophthalmol* 1990;108:939.
19. Russell SR, Olsen KR, Folk JC. Predictors of scleral rupture and the role of vitrectomy in severe blunt ocular trauma. *Am J Ophthalmol* 1988;105:253–257.
20. Kylstra JA. Management of suspected ocular lacerations or rupture. *Can J Ophthalmol* 1991;26:224–228.
21. Kylstra JA, Lamkin JC, Runyan DK. Clinical predictors of scleral rupture after blunt ocular trauma. *Am J Ophthlamol* 1993;115:530.
22. Cherry PMH. Rupture of the globe. *Arch Ophthalmol* 1972;96:498.
23. Cherry PMH. Indirect traumatic rupture of the globe. *Arch Ophthalmol* 1978;96:252.
24. Lambrou FH, Kozarsky A. Wound dehiscence following cataract surgery. *Ophthalmic Surg* 1987;18:738–740.
25. Assis EI, Blotnik CA, Powers TP, et al. Cliniopathologic study of ocular trauma in eyes with intraocular lenses. *Am J Ophthalmol* 1994;117:30–36.
26. Kass MA, Lahav M, Albert DA. Traumatic rupture o f healed cataract wounds. *Am J Ophthalmol* 1976;81:722–724.
27. Harris LL, Pieramici DJ, MacCumber MW, Humayun ME, Azar D. Traumatic dehiscence of cataract wounds. *Invest Ophthalmol Vis Sci* 1995;36(suppl):793.
28. Campo RV, Chung KD, Oyakawa RT. Pars plana vitrectomy in the management of dislocated posterior chamber lenses. *Am J Ophthalmol* 1987;108:529–534.
29. Pieramici DJ, Sternberg P, Aaberg TM, et al. Perspective: A system for classifying mechanical injuries of the eye (globe). *Am J Ophthalmol* 1997;123:820.

Management of Ocular Injuries and Emergencies,
edited by Mathew W. MacCumber.
Lippincott–Raven Publishers, Philadelphia ©1998.

16

Injuries of the Anterior Segment

Sharath C. Raja and Morton F. Goldberg

Department of Ophthalmology, Walson Airforce Hospital, McGuire Air Force Base, New Jersey 08641 and Wilmer Eye Institute, The Johns Hopkins University School of Medicine, Baltimore, Maryland 21287

Basic Considerations   227
  Traumatic Iritis   228
  Diagnosis   228 · Management   228
Iris Sphincter Tear/Iridodialysis   228
  Diagnosis   228 · Management   229
Angle Recession   229
  Diagnosis   229 · Management   229
Cyclodialysis   230
  Diagnosis   230 · Management   230
Hyphema   231
  Diagnosis   231 · Management   231 · Surgical Procedures   233

BASIC CONSIDERATIONS

Blunt trauma to the globe with compression along the anteroposterior axis and expansion equatorially can result in damage to the anterior segment by two distinct mechanisms:

1. Vascular damage: Scleral expansion of the equatorial zone of the globe after blunt trauma can result in posterior displacement of the lens-iris complex with associated disruption of the major arterial circle of the iris and arterial branches of the ciliary body. This culminates in a damaged blood-aqueous barrier with leakage of blood constituents (e.g., serum, etc.) into the anterior segment. Injuries in this category include traumatic iritis and hyphema.
2. Mechanical damage: Tractional forces induced by the rapid compression and expansion after blunt trauma can cause damage to the structures comprising the anterior segment. Such damage can result in glaucoma or hypotony. This category encompasses iris sphincter tears, iridodialysis, angle recession, and cyclodialysis.

A careful examination by the ophthalmologist is critical in the diagnosis of these injuries. Appropriate therapy, when indicated, and close follow-up are essential to mitigate permanent ocular damage that can occur in the immediate (or remote) period after the precipitating blunt trauma.

For corneal injuries see Chapter 13, and for lens injuries see Chapter 18.

TRAUMATIC IRITIS

Diagnosis

1. A history of blunt trauma to the affected eye during the preceding 72 hours can usually be elicited.
2. Decreased visual acuity in the affected eye with photophobia.
3. In the absence of damage to the outflow tract, reduced intraocular pressure is typically present.
4. A mild inflammation of the anterior segment is apparent on slit-lamp biomicroscopy. Cells within the aqueous humor should be examined carefully with red-free illumination to ensure that no hyphema is present (red blood cells disappear with red-free light).
5. Traumatic mydriasis or miosis is often present in this condition; careful biomicroscopy is essential to exclude the possibility of an iris sphincter tear.

Management

1. A topical cycloplegic agent (e.g., homatropine 5% twice daily, scopolamine 0.25% four times daily) is administered to enhance patient comfort and to decrease the chance of posterior synechiae.
2. Topical steroid drops are indicated with significant anterior chamber inflammation. These can be tapered slowly over the course of several days or weeks to decrease the probability of a rebound iritis (1). As with any prolonged course of topical steroid medication, intraocular pressures should be followed carefully, especially if the patient is a known steroid responder.

IRIS SPHINCTER TEAR/IRIDODIALYSIS

Diagnosis

1. Damage to the iris sphincter is a common finding after blunt trauma to the anterior chamber.
2. Biomicroscopy discloses irregularities in the iris sphincter that can present clinically as a mydriatic pupil.
3. Traumatic separation of the iris root from the ciliary body (iridodialysis) often occurs in the presence of a hyphema and can be difficult to detect on initial examination (Fig. 16–1).

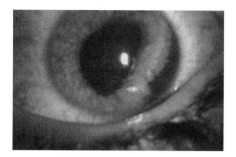

FIG. 16–1. Iridodialysis with small hyphema secondary to blunt trauma from a recoiling bungee cord.

Management

1. Large iridodialyses can cause significant polycoria and monocular diplopia. When patients are symptomatic and have recovered from other damage sustained in the blunt trauma (e.g., hyphema), surgical repair is sometimes indicated.
2. For surgical technique see Chapter 18.

ANGLE RECESSION

Diagnosis

1. Tears between the longitudinal and circular muscles of the ciliary body can often be detected with careful gonioscopy after blunt trauma to the anterior segment (Fig. 16–2).
2. An irregular widening of the ciliary body band is present on gonioscopy.
3. Direct damage to the trabecular meshwork or subsequent endothelialization over the iridocorneal angle may culminate in increased intraocular pressure (2).

Management

1. Patients with angle recession are at risk of developing increased intraocular pressures and need long-term follow-up.
2. The lifetime risk of developing glaucoma is directly correlated with the degree of angle recession. Angle recession of 180 degrees is associated with an approximately 10% lifetime risk of glaucoma (3).
3. Aqueous suppressants such as acetazolamide or methazolamide are often effective in lowering pressure in angle-recession glaucoma.
4. Topical beta-blockers can be used as an alternative treatment modality.
5. Miotics such as pilocarpine are generally contraindicated; instances of a paradoxic increase in intraocular pressures in these patients have been reported.
6. Argon laser trabeculoplasty is usually ineffective because the primary damage is often a traumatized trabecular outflow tract.

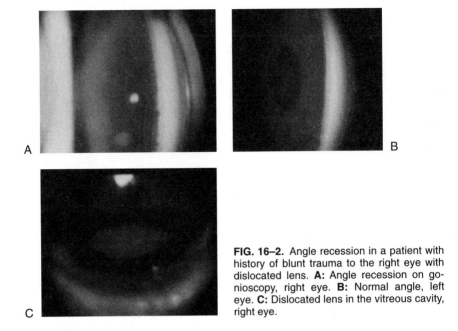

A

B

C

FIG. 16–2. Angle recession in a patient with history of blunt trauma to the right eye with dislocated lens. **A:** Angle recession on gonioscopy, right eye. **B:** Normal angle, left eye. **C:** Dislocated lens in the vitreous cavity, right eye.

7. A filtering procedure for sustained increased intraocular pressure can be performed if nonsurgical interventions do not lower pressure adequately.

CYCLODIALYSIS

Diagnosis

1. Gonioscopy discloses a cleft between the ciliary body and its insertion at the scleral spur; this results in an opening into the suprachoroidal space.
2. Decreased aqueous secretion and increased uveoscleral outflow after cyclodialysis can result in hypotony.

Management

1. Spontaneous closure of the cyclodialysis cleft can occur, resulting in increased aqueous secretion and elevated intraocular pressure.
2. This increased intraocular pressure is often transient due to a gradual improvement of trabecular outflow facility several days after blunt trauma to the anterior segment.
3. Transient pressure elevations can be treated with aqueous suppressants.
4. If intraocular pressures remain high, patients should be treated with standard regimens for chronic open-angle glaucoma.

5. Persistant hypotony can be managed with argon laser photocoagulation to the surface of the ciliary body in the cleft (4) or by sutured closure of the cleft (see Chapter 18). Be prepared for a marked intraocular pressure spike after successful closure.

HYPHEMA

Blunt trauma to the anterior segment can result in disruption of the vessels of the iris and ciliary body culminating in hyphema. Spontaneous hyphema in the absence of blunt trauma should raise the index of suspicion for juvenile xanthogranuloma in children, melanoma or metastatic tumor to the iris in adults, iris neovascularization, or bleeding diatheses.

Diagnosis

Biomicroscopy discloses circulating erythrocytes in the anterior chamber alone (microhyphema) or the presence of layered hemorrhage (hyphema).

Management

1. The primary goals of treatment are to minimize the probability of rebleeding and to prevent prolonged periods of elevated intraocular pressure. Complications after hyphema are more common after rebleeding; these may include corneal bloodstaining, central retinal artery occlusion due to increased intraocular pressure, optic atrophy, and peripheral anterior synechiae. Approximately 75% of patients with hyphema regain visual acuity of better than 20/50 (5). Visual prognosis is significantly worse for patients with rebleeding (6) or who present more than 24 hours after the injury (7). Rebleeds occur in 5% to 33% of untreated eyes with hyphema (7,8), typically 2 to 5 days after the injury when clot retraction and lysis are occurring.
2. Although of no proven benefit in the prevention of rebleeding, hospitalization with moderate restriction of physical activity and close observation is often recommended, especially with patients for whom daily examination for elevated intraocular pressure cannot be ensured.
3. Shielding of the injured eye to prevent accidental trauma, cycloplegia, and examination (including biomicroscopy and applanation tonometry every 6 to 12 hours) to monitor for complications (e.g., rebleeding, elevated intraocular pressure, corneal bloodstaining) have been demonstrated to be of benefit (6,9).
4. Topical steroid preparations can reduce anterior chamber inflammation (instill drops every 2 hours while awake).
5. Aminocaproic acid (Amicar) reduces the incidence of rebleeds in animal studies as well as in prospective clinical trials (10,11). This antifibrinolytic agent can stabilize clot formation at the site of hemorrhage. Dosing at 50 mg/kg every 4 hours (not to exceed 30 g per day) for 5 days is currently recom-

mended (12). Commonly encountered side effects include nausea, vomiting, and postural hypotension and should be explained to the patient. Although no studies in humans have been performed, Amicar has been demonstrated to reduce fetal viability and should not be used in pregnant women (13).

6. Oral prednisone may be considered as an alternative to Amicar in patients observed on an outpatient basis. Prednisone (0.6 mg/kg every day) given to patients with hyphema results in rebleed rates of 7.1%; this is comparable with Amicar (14).

7. Aspirin products are contraindicated in patients with hyphema.

8. If intraocular pressures remain elevated, topical beta-blockers and oral aqueous suppressants (except in patients with sickle cell diseases) are the first line of therapy. If pressures remain elevated and patient has no systemic contraindications (e.g., congestive heart failure, sickle cell disease), oral or intravenous hyperosmotic agents can be used.

9. African American patients with traumatic hyphemas should routinely have a sickle screening test upon presentation. Patients with sickle cell hemoglobinopathy (including sickle trait) are predisposed to developing raised intraocular pressures from sickling of erythrocytes in the trabecular meshwork, resulting in increased resistance to aqueous outflow. The resultant hypoperfusion of the anterior segment leads to acidosis and hypercarbia, causing further sickling. Increased intraocular pressure also can reduce vascular perfusion of the optic nerve or retina. Patients with sickle cell hyphemas can develop optic atrophy after mild increases in intraocular pressure after only 24 hours (15). Systemic aqueous suppressants should be used with extreme caution in these patients due to the risk of acidosis in the anterior chamber, thereby increasing sickling. If an aqueous suppressant is necessary, methazolamide (Neptazane, Lederly) is less likely to induce acidosis than acetazolamide (Diamox, Lederly). Hyperosmotic agents are contraindicated if used more than once a day because they cause hemoconcentration and increased vascular sludging.

10. Elevated intraocular pressures can occur during clot lysis (hemolytic glaucoma) or when the debris of degenerated erythrocytes (ghost cell glaucoma) clogs the trabecular meshwork (16). These phenomena are most common after vitreous hemorrhage with communication to the anterior segment and can occur several weeks after the initial injury. Topical beta-antagonists and aqueous suppressants are useful in the treatment of these glaucomas, which usually resolve spontaneously.

11. Anterior chamber blood should be removed:
   - To prevent optic atrophy:
     Operate before intraocular pressure averages more than 50 mm Hg for 5 days.
     Operate before intraocular pressure averages more than 35 mm Hg for 7 days.
   - To prevent corneal bloodstaining in eyes with a large hyphema:
     Operate before intraocular pressure averages more than 25 mm Hg for 6 days.

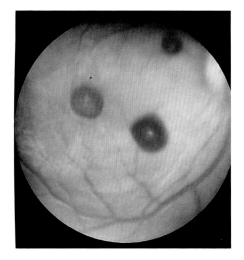

COLOR FIGURE 4–5. Preretinal hemorrhages in shaken baby syndrome.

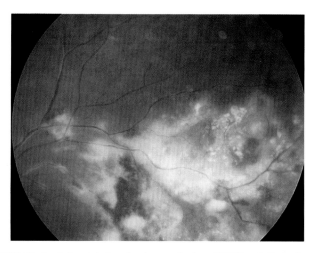

COLOR FIGURE 11–1. Active fulminant cytomegalovirus (CMV) retinitis active CMV retinitis in a patient with AIDS. Note the hemorrhage and full-thickness retinal involvement.

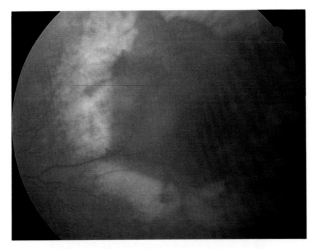

COLOR FIGURE 11–2. Active indolent cytomegalovirus (CMV) retinitis in a patient with AIDS. Absence of hemorrhage distinguishes this form of CMV retinitis from fulminant CMV retinitis. Both forms are treated identically.

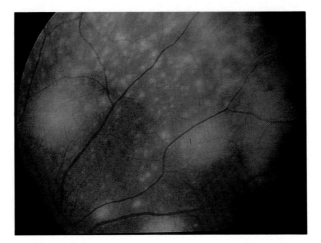

COLOR FIGURE 11–3. Progressive outer retinal necrosis in a patient with AIDS. The deep retinal appearance of the lesions helps to distinguish the process from CMV retinitis, and the absence of prominent vitritis and vasculitis helps to distinguish it from acute retinal necrosis.

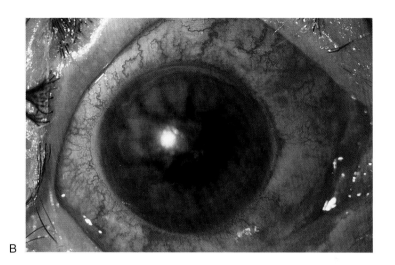

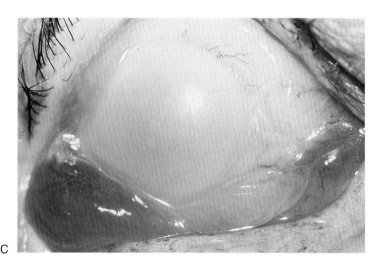

COLOR FIGURE 12–1. Thoft's classification of chemical injury. **B:** Grade II. **C:** Grade IV.

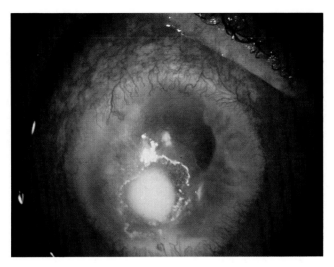

COLOR FIGURE 14–3. A: Bacterial keratitis. Ulcerative keratitis with well-circumscribed corneal infiltrate plus hypopyon due to *S. aureus*.

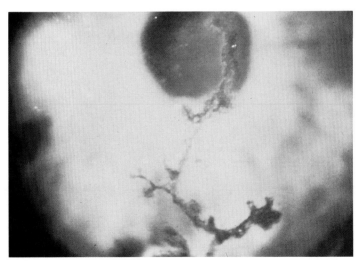

COLOR FIGURE 14–4. B: Herpes simplex keratitis. Rose bengal staining of dendrite.

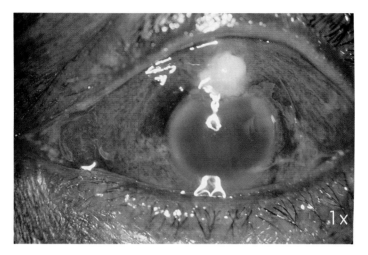

COLOR FIGURE 19–1. Infected conjunctival bleb with endophthalmitis after glaucoma filtering surgery.

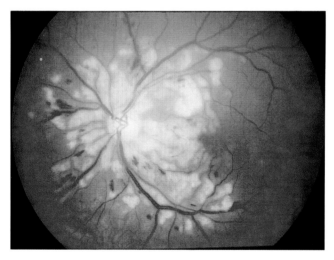

COLOR FIGURE 22–1. Purtscher's retinopathy.

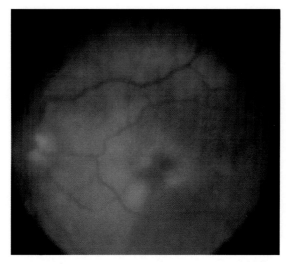

COLOR FIGURE 22–2. A: Commotio retinae (Berlin's edema).

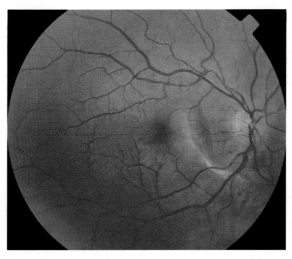

COLOR FIGURE 22–3. A: CNV secondary to choroidal rupture. Choroidal neovascular membrane was identified 3 weeks after the injury.

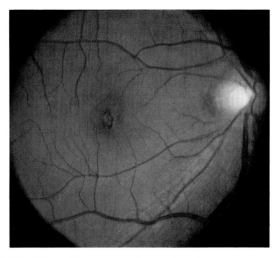

COLOR FIGURE 22–6. Moderate photic maculopathy secondary to sungazing.

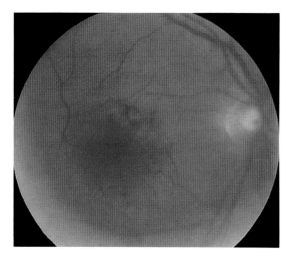

COLOR FIGURE 22–7. Pigmentary changes seen several months after intense light exposure from an operating microscope filament during cataract extraction.

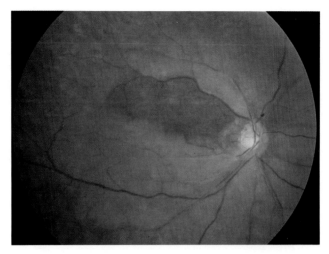

COLOR FIGURE 23–1. A: Central retinal artery occlusions (CRAO) with retained superior macular perfusion by a cilioretinal artery.

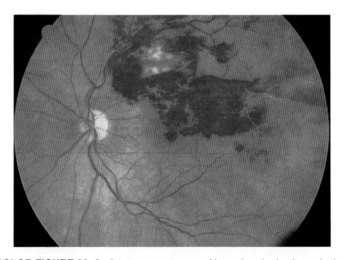

COLOR FIGURE 23–3. Acute superotemporal branch retinal vein occlusion.

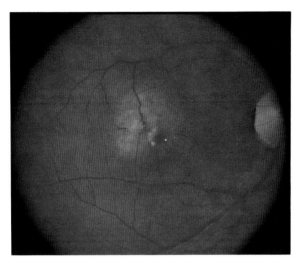

COLOR FIGURE 23–4. A: Subfoveal choroidal neovascularization (CNV) secondary to para-foveal retinal telangiectasis.

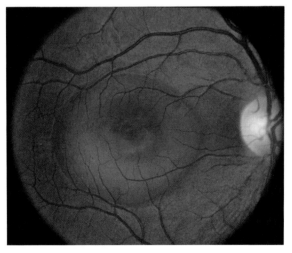

COLOR FIGURE 23–5. A: Central serous chorioretinopathy (CSR). Serous retinal elevation is present in the macular area.

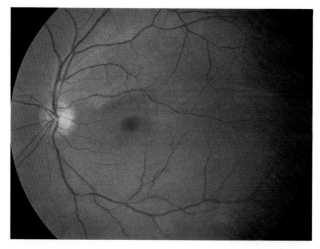

COLOR FIGURE 23–6. A: An inferior rhegmatogenous retinal detachment through the macular area secondary to an inferotemporal dialysis.

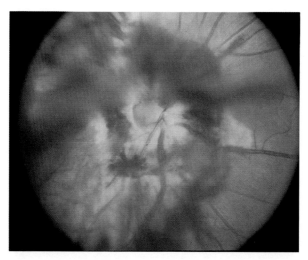

COLOR FIGURE 24–1. Direct traumatic optic neuropathy. This man lost all vision in this eye when an automobile antenna entered his right orbit. There is a depression in the area of the optic disk, and hemorrhage emanates from it. Visual acuity remained at no light perception.

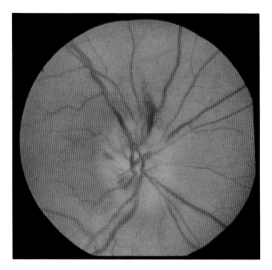

COLOR FIGURE 24–3. Optic disk swelling in optic neuritis. In patients with optic neuritis, disk swelling is seen in approximately 33% and peripapillary hemorrhages in 6%.

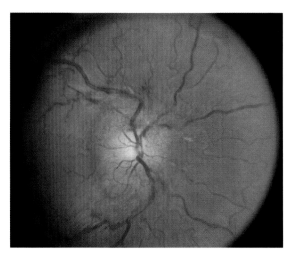

COLOR FIGURE 24–4. Optic disk swelling in papilledema. True papilledema is distinguished from pseudopapilledema by the presence of associated blurring of the peripapillary nerve fiber layer, vascular engorgement, peripapillary hemorrhages, cotton-wool spots, and lack of spontaneous venous pulsations.

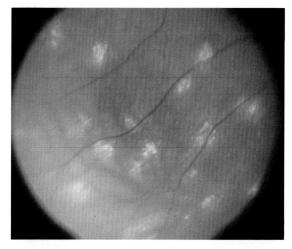

COLOR FIGURE 28–1. Dalen-Fuch's nodules are seen as yellow-white exudates beneath the retinal pigment epithelium.

Operate if there is any indication of early bloodstaining. The earliest sign is yellow granular deposits in the posterior stroma.
- To prevent peripheral anterior synechiae:
Operate before a total hyphema persists for 5 days.
Operate before a diffuse hyphema involving most of the anterior chamber angle persists for 9 days.
- In hyphema patients with sickle cell hemoglobinopathies:
Operate if intraocular pressure averages 25 mm Hg or greater for 24 consecutive hours.
Operate if intraocular pressure has repeated transient elevations more than   30 mm Hg.

Surgical Procedures

Paracentesis

Removal of approximately 0.1 ml from the anterior chamber using aseptic technique can effectively reduce intraocular pressure (see Chapter 23 under Retinal Artery Occlusion), but this may provide only transient relief.

Expression of Clot

1. A 90- to 120-degree limbal shelf incision is created, with clot expression performed by depressing the posterior lip of the wound and drawing a muscle hook across the cornea.
2. The anterior chamber is then gently irrigated. Small clot fragments should not be removed to decrease the risk of secondary hemorrhage.
3. The wound is then closed with interrupted 10-0 nylon suture.

Anterior Chamber Washout

1. Two 2-mm incisions are created at the limbus.
2. The anterior chamber is irrigated with a blunt infusion cannula or bent 23-gauge butterfly needle inserted through one incision. Drainage of anterior chamber debris can be performed by simultaneously depressing the posterior lip of the second incision.
3. A vitreous cutting instrument can be used to evacuate the clot through the opposite incision if irrigation alone is insufficient (Fig. 16–3). An automated irrigation and aspiration unit alone through one incision is an alternative. Caution should be used when introducing instruments into the anterior chamber under poor visualization because there is a high risk of iatrogenic injury to the lens, iris, or corneal endothelium.
4. Limbal wounds should be closed with 10-0 nylon suture if they are not self-sealing to avoid postoperative hypotony with rebleeding.

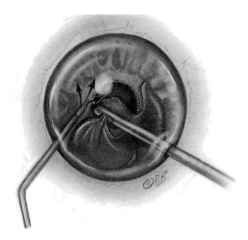

FIG. 16–3. Automated removal of hyphema. Irrigation is provided via a bent 23-gauge butterfly needle while the clot is removed with a vitrectomy instrument.

REFERENCES

1. Rosenbaum JT, Tammaro J, Robertson JE Jr. Uveitis precipitated by non-penetrating ocular trauma. *Am J Ophthalmol* 1991;112:392.
2. Blanton FM. Anterior chamber angle recession and secondary glaucoma: a study of the after effects of traumatic hyphemas. *Arch Ophthalmol* 1964;72:39.
3. Kaufman JH, Tolpin DW. Glaucoma after traumatic angle recession: a ten-year prospective study. *Am J Ophthalmol* 1974;78:648.
4. Alward WLM, Hodapp EA, Parel J-M, Anderson DR. Argon laser endophotocoagulator closure of cyclodialysis clefts. *Am J Ophthalmol* 1988;106:748.
5. Edwards WC, Layden WF. Traumatic hyphema. *Am J Ophthalmol* 1973;75:110..
6. Read J, Goldberg MF. Comparison of medical treatment for traumatic hyphema. *Trans Am Acad Ophthalmol Otolaryngol* 1974;78:799–815.
7. Volpe NJ, Larrison WI, Hersh PS, Kim T, Shingleton BJ. Secondary hemorrhage in traumatic hyphema. *Am J Ophthalmol* 1991;112:507–513.
8. Thomas MA, Parrish RK, Feuer WJ. Re-bleeding after traumatic hyphema. *Arch Ophthalmol* 1986; 104:206.
9. Gilbert HD, Jensen AD. Atropine in the treatment of traumatic hyphema. *Ann Ophthalmol* 1973;5: 1297–1300.
10. McGetrick JJ, Jampol LM, Goldberg MF, et al. Aminocaproic acid decreases secondary hemorrhage after traumatic hyphema. *Arch Ophthalmol* 1983;101:1031–1033.
11. Kutner B, Fourman S, Brein K, et al. Aminocaproic acid reduces the risk of secondary hemorrhage in patients with traumatic hyphema. *Arch Ophthalmol* 1987;105:206.
12. Palmer DJ, Goldberg MF, Frenkel M, et al. A comparison of two dose regimens of epsilon aminocaproic acid in the prevention and management of secondary traumatic hyphemas. *Ophthalmology* 1986;93:102.
13. Dubin WH, Cummings DB, Blake DA, King TM. Effect of epsilon aminocarproic acid, afibrinolytic inhibitor on implantation and fetal viability in the rat. *J Biol Reprod* 1980;23:553–557.
14. Farber MD, Fiscella R, Goldberg MF. Aminocaproic acid versus prednisone for the treatment of traumatic hyphema. A randomized clinical trial. *Ophthalmology* 1991;98:279–286.
15. Goldberg MF. Sickled erythrocytes, hyphema, and secondary glaucoma. I: The diagnosis and treatment of sickled erythrocytes in human hyphemas. *Ophthalmic Surg* 1979;10:17–31.
16. Campbell DG. Ghost cell glaucoma following trauma. *Ophthalmology* 1981;88:115.

Management of Ocular Injuries and Emergencies,
edited by Mathew W. MacCumber.
Lippincott–Raven Publishers, Philadelphia ©1998.

17

Glaucomatous Emergencies

Michael J. Cooney and Harry A. Quigley

*Department of Ophthalmology, Wilmer Eye Institute, The Johns Hopkins University
School of Medicine, Baltimore, Maryland 21287*

Basic Considerations 236
  Examination 237
Primary Angle-Closure Glaucoma 237
  Diagnosis 239 · Management 240 · Procedure: Nd-YAG Laser Peripheral
  Iridectomy 241
Malignant Glaucoma 241
  Diagnosis 241 · Management 242
Inflammatory Uveitis 242
  Diagnosis 243 · Management 244
Posner-Schlossman Syndrome 244
  Diagnosis 245 · Management 245
Ghost Cell Glaucoma 245
  Diagnosis 245 · Management 246
Pseudoexfoliative Glaucoma 246
  Diagnosis 246 · Management 247
Phacolytic Glaucoma (Lens Protein Glaucoma) 247
  Diagnosis 247 · Management 247
Lens Particle Glaucoma 248
  Diagnosis 248 · Management 248
Subluxed or Dislocated Lens and Glaucoma 248
  Diagnosis 249 · Management 250
Neovascular Glaucoma 250
  Diagnosis 250 · Management 252
Congenital Glaucoma 253
  Diagnosis 253 · Management 253
Steroid-Response Glaucoma 253
  Diagnosis 253 · Management 254
Aphakic/Pseudophakic Pupillary Block 254
  Diagnosis 254 · Management 254

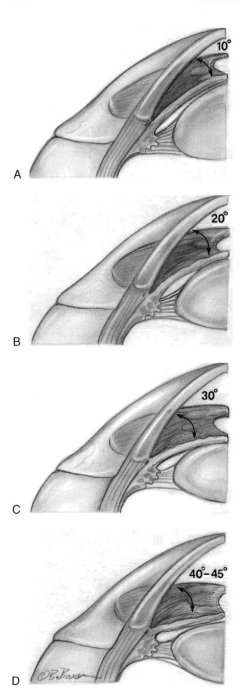

FIG. 17–1. Classification system for grading angle width. **A:** Grade I. **B:** Grade II. **C:** Grade III. **D:** Grade IV.

BASIC CONSIDERATIONS

Aqueous humor is produced in the posterior chamber of the eye and flows through the pupil to the anterior chamber. In the anterior chamber the aqueous passes through the trabecular meshwork to Schlemm's canal and then to the episcleral vessels where it is absorbed into the systemic circulation. Increased intraocular pressure (IOP) results from blockage anywhere along this pathway.

There are numerous ways in which glaucoma can be classified. Primary glaucoma results from an unknown or developmental defect, whereas secondary glaucoma results from an associated or inciting abnormality. Glaucoma can be further classified depending on the status of the anterior chamber angle. In open-angle glaucoma, aqueous has free access to the trabecular meshwork, whereas in closed-angle glaucoma access to the trabecular meshwork is impeded.

In this chapter, we review many of the disorders that can result in glaucomatous emergencies. Although primary open-angle glaucoma is much more common than the other forms of glaucoma, it is typically insidious and asymptomatic. It is not classified as an emergency and therefore is not discussed in this chapter.

Examination

Gonioscopy is the best way to evaluate the peripheral anterior chamber. Determination of the type of glaucoma and the mechanism of aqueous outflow obstruction often relies heavily on information obtained from the physical examination of the angle structures.

The most common gonioscopic lenses in current use are the Goldmann and Zeiss lenses. Each provides a somewhat different view of the angle structures. The Zeiss gonioprism allows for more rapid, convenient examination of the angle recess as well as the dynamic technique of indentation gonioscopy. However, care must be taken to minimize the force with which the Zeiss lens is held against the eye because even light pressure on the lens results in posterior translocation of the peripheral iris and expansion of the iridocorneal angle.

There have been several classification systems for grading of the anterior chamber depth; however, none is completely objective, and interobserver variability is inherent to all. There are various systems of grading the angle width and a general classification is shown in Fig. 17–1.

Intraocular pressure is measured by tonometry. The Goldmann applanation tonometer is the proven standard for variable-force tonometry in patients with normal corneas. In an emergency setting, IOP can be obtained easily with the use of the Tono-Pen (Mentor, Inc., Norwell, MA).

PRIMARY ANGLE-CLOSURE GLAUCOMA

Various types of angle-closure glaucoma have been described, but the appropriate management is based upon the reason for the elevated IOP (1). When an existing cause is not found, the glaucoma is termed "primary angle-closure glau-coma."

Primary angle-closure glaucoma may exist with or without pupillary block. In angle closure caused by pupillary block, the pupillary portion of the iris is in con-tact with the lens, preventing aqueous from flowing through the pupil to the ante-rior chamber (Fig. 17–2*A*). The aqueous builds up behind the iris, pushes it anteri-orly, and shallows the peripheral anterior chamber angle. Static gonioscopy shows no visible angle structures and a convex, forward-bowing iris that is in contact with the anterior wall of the angle (2–4). The central anterior chamber is chroni-cally narrow in susceptible patients and remains the same during an acute attack. Indentation gonioscopy displaces aqueous humor, causing a widening of the angle (3) and a flattening of the mid-peripheral iris (2).

In primary angle-closure glaucoma without pupillary block, the anterior chamber angle is narrowed without iris-lens apposition at the pupil. This is seen in the unusual anatomic variant called plateau iris syndrome, in which angle-closure glaucoma recurs after pupillary dilatation despite a patent iridectomy (Fig. 17–2*B*).

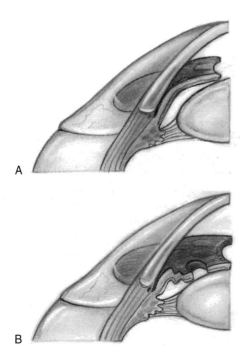

A

B

FIG. 17–2. A: Iris configuration in pupillary block glaucoma. **B:** Iris plateau syndrome. Angle is closed despite iridotomy.

Diagnosis

See Table 17–1.

1. The diagnosis of angle-closure glaucoma is made by history, slit-lamp examination, gonioscopy, and provocative testing.
2. Usually occurs in individuals over 50 years of age, and there may be a history of preceding minor attacks during periods of pupillary dilatation.
3. A sustained attack usually occurs unilaterally with the sudden onset of severe, boring eye pain, headache, and blurred vision. The pain may be so severe as to cause nausea and vomiting and various other gastrointestinal symptoms.
4. The affected eye is typically injected with ciliary flush surrounding the limbus.
5. The cornea may be cloudy secondary to stromal edema, and microcystic bullae in the corneal epithelium create an irregular corneal surface.
6. The anterior chamber is shallow, often with peripheral iris/cornea touch. The anterior chamber often has cell and flare.
7. The pupil may be mid-dilated, fixed, and irregular secondary to iris sphincter ischemia.
8. *Glaukomflecken,* small gray-white anterior lens opacities, occur from previous episodes of increased IOP (1).
9. IOP is high.
10. The fellow eye should always be examined, especially if corneal edema pre-

TABLE 17–1. *Diagnosis of acute angle-closure glaucoma*

History
  Acute onset
Symptoms
  Pain
  Halos
  Visual loss
  Nausea
  Emesis
Clinical signs
  Intraocular pressure (usually high during attack but low after attack in recovery)
  Mid-dilated, unreactive pupil
  Ciliary-conjunctival injection
  Corneal edema
  Engorged iris vessels
  Cells in aqueous (but no keratic precipitates)
  Closed angle gonioscopically (may be open but narrow and "closable" angle after attack)
  Fellow eye—narrow angle judged "closable" by gonioscopy
  Iris atrophy
  Posterior synechiae
  Glaukomflecken of Vogt
  Optic atrophy

Reprinted with permission (30).

vents visualization of the angle structures in the affected eye to confirm that the angle is narrow. Approximately 50% of fellow eyes develop angle closure within 2 years of the attack in the presenting eye (5).

11. Provocative testing may be used if the anterior chamber angle is suspicious but not definite for angle-closure glaucoma. In the mydriatic test, mydriatic drops are instilled and the IOP is measured. An increase in IOP of 8 mm Hg or greater and concomitant angle closure on gonioscopy is diagnostic. Physiologic mydriasis can be induced by placing a patient in a dark room for 60 to 90 minutes. The dark room test can be combined with the prone provocative test by placing the patient in a face-down position in the dark room (6).

Management

The goal of treatment of acute angle-closure glaucoma is to improve the clinical setting for more precise diagnosis and to prevent permanent visual field loss from optic nerve damage or vascular occlusive events (1).

1. The definitive treatment of primary angle-closure glaucoma is to perform a laser iridectomy. Medical therapy should be initiated when laser treatment is delayed by corneal clouding or other considerations.
    • Topical beta-blocker given one time
    • Topical alpha-agonist given one time
    • Topical steroid (prednisolone acetate 1%) every 15 to 30 minutes four times, then hourly
    • Carbonic anhydrase inhibitor (acetazolamide 250 to 500 mg IV or PO
    • Systemic osmotic agent, if above ineffective (50% glycerol solution 1 to 1.5 g/kg in nondiabetics only, oral isosorbide 50 to 100 mg orally, or mannitol 1 to 2 g/kg i.v. over 45 minutes). These agents should be avoided in patients with congestive heart failure (CHF).
    • Miotics (pilocarpine) should always be used (5). Pilocarpine 1% to 2% should not be used more than every 15 minutes three times within the first hour. It must be recognized that because it constricts the ciliary muscle and reduces the anterior chamber depth, it could increase the pupillary block (7). Pilocarpine may be ineffective initially due to iris ischemia.

2. Definitive surgical treatment is performed as soon as possible. In the interim, the patients are followed daily and maintained on the following regimen: topical beta-blocker, alpha-agonist carbonic anhydrase inhibitor, pilocarpine, and prednisolone acetate (8).

3. The definitive surgical management is laser peripheral iridectomy (PI; YAG or argon) to the involved eye. Prophylactic laser PI to the fellow eye is performed in all cases of primary angle-closure glaucoma. If a laser PI is not initially possible, we recommend a trabeculectomy with tight releaseable sutures and an iridectomy.

Procedure: Nd-YAG Laser Peripheral Iridectomy

Contraindications:

1. Uncooperative patient
2. Marked corneal edema
3. Flat anterior chamber

Prelaser preparation:

1. Topical pilocarpine 2% to stretch iris
2. Topical glycerin if corneal edema present
3. Topical apraclonidine 0.1% to reduce postiridectomy IOP elevation

Procedure:

1. Topical anesthesia (e.g., proparacaine hydrochloride 0.5%)
2. Apply iridectomy lens with a coupling agent (e.g., hydroxypropyl methylcellulose)
3. Select thin area of iris (crypt) as far peripheral as possible
4. Power settings needed generally range from 4 to 12 mJ
5. Penetration signaled by slit in stroma and/or pigment epithelium with flow of aqueous humor from the posterior chamber

Complications:

1. Bleeding—usually transient and easily controlled by applying pressure with the contact lens
2. Postoperative IOP spike—control with medications
3. Cataract
4. Endothelial damage
5. Inpatient PI. Make sure PI is in peripheral iris and is full thickness.

MALIGNANT GLAUCOMA

Malignant glaucoma is a secondary form of angle-closure glaucoma. It usually occurs after surgery for angle-closure glaucoma but can occur after cataract surgery or rarely as a spontaneous event. There is disagreement about the mechanism of malignant glaucoma; however, all agree on the management.

Diagnosis

1. Ocular pain and redness occur in a patient who has had previous surgical treatment of angle-closure glaucoma or cataract extraction.
2. The exclusion of pupillary block, choroidal separation, and suprachoroidal hemorrhage.
3. Shallowing of the central anterior chamber depth.

4. Higher than expected IOP.
5. Miotics are ineffective, or worsen the glaucoma, whereas cycloplegics are helpful or curative (1).

Management

The principles of treatment of malignant glaucoma are to relieve the obstruction to aqueous flow and restore normal IOP.

1. Pupillary block is ruled out by performing a PI.
2. If signs of malignant glaucoma are still present after the PI:
   • Cycloplegics (atropine 1% and phenylephrine 2.5% four times daily)
   • Topical beta-blocker 0.5% twice daily
   • Topical alpha-agonist three times daily
   • Xalatan
   • Carbonic anhydrase inhibitors (acetazolamide 500 mg i.v. or 500 mg orally once followed by 250 mg orally four times daily)
   • Osmotic agents, if above ineffective (50% glycerol solution 1 to 1.5 g/kg in non-diabetics only, oral isosorbide 50 to 100 mg orally or mannitol 20% 1 to 2 g/kg i.v. over 45 minutes). These agents should be avoided in patients with a history of CHF.
3. If the block is broken with the above therapy, topical atropine 1% daily is maintained chronically.
4. If the above therapy is ineffective, then the following treatment is considered.
   • If the affected eye is phakic, a pars plana vitrectomy is indicated and usually produces a permanent cure (9).
   • If the affected eye is aphakic or pseudophakic, direct YAG or argon disruption of the anterior hyaloid, either near or through an iridectomy, has been successful (10–13). If this is unsuccessful, a vitrectomy should be considered.

INFLAMMATORY UVEITIS

Uveitis may be complicated by increased IOP (Table 17–2). The IOP depends on the balance between aqueous humor production by an inflamed ciliary body and aqueous outflow through an inflamed trabecular meshwork. During different stages of the inflammatory disease, IOP may be normal, high, or low. Secondary open-angle glaucoma due to obstruction of the trabecular meshwork by inflammatory cells is the most common cause of glaucoma secondary to uveitis (1). Secondary angle-closure glaucoma associated with uveitis has been reported due to peripheral anterior synechiae (PAS), pupillary block from posterior synechiae (iris bombe), neovascular glaucoma, ciliary body swelling (14,15), and anterior rotation of the ciliary body secondary to uveal effusion.

TABLE 17–2. *Inflammatory disorders associated with glaucoma*

I. Anterior uveitis and keratouveitis
  A. Acute anterior uveitis of unknown etiology
  B. Uveitis associated with joint diseases
    1. HLA-B27—associated diseases
      a. Ankylosing spondylitis
      b. Reiter's syndrome
      c. Psoriatic arthritis
    2. Juvenile rheumatoid arthritis
  C. Uveitis associated with infectious diseases
    1. Herpes simplex keratouveitis
    2. Herpes zoster keratouveitis
    3. Congenital rubella
    4. Leprosy
    5. Syphilis
    6. Cytomegalic inclusion retinitis
    7. Toxocariasis
    8. Meningococcal endophthalmitis
    9. Mumps
    10. Nephropathia epidemica
    11. Onchocerciasis
    12. Toxoplasmosis
    13. Coccidiomycosis
  D. Uveitis associated with other disorders
    1. Fuch's heterochromic iridocyclitis
    2. Glaucomatocyclitic crisis
    3. Sarcoidosis
    4. Vogt-Koyanagi-Harada syndrome
    5. Sympathetic ophthalmia
    6. Behçet's disease
    7. Intermediate uveitis (pars planitis)
    8. Lens-induced uveitis
    9. Traumatic uveitis
II. Scleritis and episcleritis
III. Interstitial keratitis
IV. Syndrome of inflammatory precipitates on the trabecular
    meshwork

Reprinted with permission (30).

Diagnosis

The classic signs of the glaucoma may be masked by the uveitis and its complications.

1. History consistent with uveitis (pain, photophobia, blurred vision); symptoms may be minimal.
2. Anterior chamber cell and flare, miotic pupil, PAS, keratic precipitates, conjunctival injection hyperemia, and ciliary flush. Neovascularization of the iris may be present.
3. Elevated IOP.
4. Gonioscopy

- Secondary open-angle glaucoma: may see small gray or yellow trabecular precipitates along trabecular meshwork
- Secondary closed-angle glaucoma: presence of PAS or angle neovascularization

Management

1. Treatment of the underlying uveitis: Anterior uveitis is generally treated with topical steroids combined with mydriatics/cycloplegics. Posterior uveitis is usually treated with periocular or systemic steroids. Infectious uveitis should be treated with the appropriate antibiotics/antivirals and in conjunction with steroids (see Chapter 11).
2. If treatment of the uveitis does not control the IOP, then antiglaucoma medications should be used.
   - Topical beta-blocker, alpha-agonist, and systemic or topical carbonic anhydrase inhibitors (e.g., acetezolamide 250 mg orally four times daily) are effective in reducing aqueous formation.
   - Topical epinephrine 0.5% to 2% twice daily is effective by increasing out flow (16). May worsen cystoid macular edema.
   - Hyperosmotic agents are used when the IOP is acutely elevated (50% glycerol solution 1 to 1.5 g/kg in nondiabetics only, oral isosorbide 50 to 100 mg orally, or mannitol 20% 1 to -2 g/kg i.v. over 45 minutes). These agents should be avoided in patients with a history of CHF.
   - Miotics (e.g., pilocarpine) should be avoided in uveitic glaucoma because they induce ciliary spasm, increase discomfort, and enhance the formation of posterior synechiae and pupillary membranes (1).
3. It is best to avoid surgical treatment until active inflammation subsides. However, surgical treatment is indicated when:
   - IOP is uncontrollable with progressive damage.
   - Pupillary block angle-closure glaucoma occurs.
   Surgical options include:
   - Laser iridectomy: used for secondary pupillary block angle-closure glaucoma
   - Filtration surgery with antifibrosis treatment and seton devices as alternatives should the above management prove unsuccessful.

POSNER-SCHLOSSMAN SYNDROME

Posner-Schlossman syndrome (glaucomatocyclitic crisis) is characterized by recurrent mild cyclitis with minimal symptoms despite marked increased IOP (40 to 60 mm Hg). The attack lasts from a few hours to 2 weeks, and during remission the eye is completely normal (1).

The etiology is unknown. Attention has been focused on the possible role of prostaglandins in the chain of the events leading to glaucomatocyclitic crisis (17).

Diagnosis

1. Usually unilateral, in young to middle-aged patients (18). More common in Asians.
2. The attack lasts from a few hours to 2 weeks.
3. Cyclitis, with a white eye and only trace aqueous cell and flare. A few keratic precipitates on the corneal endothelium and trabecular meshwork usually appear within 2 to 3 days of the onset.
4. There may be corneal epithelial edema and ciliary flush.
5. Elevated IOP in the range of 40 to 60 mm Hg.
6. Open angle on gonioscopy without synechiae.

Management

Treat during an attack to shorten it. Lowering the IOP is recommended in all cases in order to prevent irreversible damage to the optic nerve head (19).

Medical management options are listed as follows:

- Topical beta-blocker twice daily (or extended release form daily)
- Topical alpha-agonist three times daily
- Topical steroids (prednisolone acetate 1% four times daily)
- Carbonic anhydrase inhibitor (e.g., acetazolamide 250 orally four times daily) if IOP is significantly elevated
- Hyperosmotic agents may be necessary acutely (50% glycerol solution 1 to 1.5 g/kg in nondiabetics only, oral isosorbide 50 to 100 mg orally or mannitol 1 to 2 g/kg i.v. over 45 minutes). These agents should be avoided in patients with a history of CHF.
- Indomethacin, an inhibitor of prostoglandin (PGE) synthesis, in a dose of 75 to 100 mg/day, may be effective in lowering IOP (17).
- Strong miotics and mydriatics should be avoided because they tend to aggravate the symptoms (20,21).

GHOST CELL GLAUCOMA

The mechanism of ghost cell glaucoma involves a morphologic change in erythrocytes. In order for ghost cell glaucoma to occur, two things must happen: there must be a vitreous hemorrhage, and there must be a defect in the hyaloid face. The red blood cells in the vitreous degenerate over 1 to 3 weeks, resulting in a change in shape of these cells and an increase in rigidity. The degenerate cells pass through breaks in the hyaloid face into the anterior chamber and mechanically obstruct the trabecular meshwork.

Diagnosis

1. History of a vitreous hemorrhage and a defect in the hyaloid face, typically in the setting of surgery or trauma.

2. Small, tapioca-colored cells floating in the anterior chamber with little associated inflammation.
3. Gonioscopy may show cellular precipitates on the trabecular meshwork or a tan hypopyon.

Management

Medical management options are listed as follows:
- Topical beta-blockers twice daily.
- Topical alpha-agonist three times daily.
- Carbonic anhydrase inhibitors (e.g., acetazolamide 250 orally four times daily).
- Unremitting elevations of pressure may require surgical intervention. Anterior chamber paracentesis or lavage may be effective in lowering IOP for 6 to 24 hours. A vitrectomy is often necessary (1).

PSEUDOEXFOLIATIVE GLAUCOMA

The pseudoexfoliation syndrome is clinically distinguished by the deposition of a fibrillogranular material throughout the anterior segment. The syndrome is seen frequently in the Scandinavian population but has been identified in almost every population studied. It is often unilateral initially, and its prevalence increases with age.

The pseudoexfoliative material is composed of a filamentous proteoglycosaminoglycan that forms fibrils when it aggregates (22).

Diagnosis

1. Usually asymptomatic.
2. Corneal endothelial pigment deposition in a diffuse pattern or in that of a Krukenberg spindle.
3. Transillumination iris defects and pigment deposition on anterior iris surface. The transillumination iris defects are in the peripupillary and sphincter regions of the iris.
4. Pseudoexfoliative material is often found on the pupillary border.
5. Gonioscopic examination shows an open angle with irregular pigment deposition on the trabecular meshwork, usually inferiorly, and along Schwalbe's line (refered to as Sampaolesi's line).
6. Deposition of pseudoexfoliative material on the anterior lens capsule. Three distinct zones are typically found: a central translucent zone, a peripheral granular zone, and a clear zone separating the two (1).

Management

1. Medical management:
   - Topical beta-blocker twice daily (or extended release form daily)

- Topical alpha-agonist three times daily
- Topical pilocarpine, epinephrine, and/or Xalatan™
- Carbonic anhydrase inhibitors if IOP uncontrolled by topical therapy

2. If medical therapy fails, argon laser trabeculoplasty should be considered.
3. Trabeculectomy should be considered when the above treatment modalities fail to control IOP and/or glaucomatous changes.

PHACOLYTIC GLAUCOMA (LENS PROTEIN GLAUCOMA)

Phacolytic glaucoma is a secondary open-angle glaucoma (Table 17–3). It is thought to result from high molecular weight lens proteins that leak through an intact lens capsule. These proteins are taken up by macrophages in the anterior chamber, which in turn may obstruct the trabecular meshwork.

Diagnosis

1. A history of unilateral visual loss, ocular pain, tearing, and photophobia.
2. An injected red eye is typical. The IOP is markedly elevated.
3. There is intense flare in the anterior chamber with little cellular activity. Iridescent particles representing calcium oxalate and peices of white material may be seen floating in the anterior chamber (23).
4. A hypermature or mature cataract is usually present.
5. Gonioscopy shows an open angle.

Management

1. The definitive treatment of phacolytic glaucoma is the removal of the entire lens. This is usually performed within 1 to 2 days after attempts to lower the IOP and reduce the inflammation. It is imperative to remove all of the lens material. Trabeculectomy is usually not necessary at the time of the cataract surgery.
2. Medical management:
   - Topical beta-blocker twice daily (or extended release form daily)
   - Topical alpha-agonist three times daily
   - Carbonic anhydrase inhibitors (e.g., systemic acetazolomide 250 mg orally four times daily) or topical dorzolamide 2% three times daily
   - Topical steroids (prednisolone acetate 1% every hour)

LENS PARTICLE GLAUCOMA

Lens particle glaucoma is a secondary open-angle glaucoma that occurs days to years after planned or unplanned extracapsular cataract surgery or trauma (Table 17–3). Lens particles are released into the anterior chamber and obstruct the trabecular meshwork. The inflammatory reaction is typically greater than that seen in phacolytic glaucoma.

TABLE 17–3. *Lens-induced glaucomas*

Entity	Angle status	Mechanism of glaucoma
Phacolytic glaucoma	Open	Outflow obstruction by lens protein and macrophages
Lens particle glaucoma	Open	Outflow obstruction by lens particles, possibly inflammatory cells
Glaucoma associated with phacoanaphylactic uveitis	Open or closed	Outflow obstruction due to inflammation; pupillary block
Phacomorphic glaucoma	Closed	Pupillary block; rarely direct compression of angle by intumescent lens
Glaucoma secondary to ectopia lentis	Closed	Pupillary block

Reprinted with permission (30).

Diagnosis

1. History of cataract surgery or ocular trauma.
2. Unilateral blurred vision, ocular pain, and injection. Marked elevation of IOP.
3. Anterior chamber cell and flare associated with pieces of lens cortical material.
4. Gonioscopy shows an open angle.

Management

1. Medical management:
   - Topical beta-blocker twice daily (or extended release form daily)
   - Topical alpha-agonist three times daily
   - Carbonic anhydrase inhibitors (e.g., systemic acetazolonide 250 mg orally four times daily or topical dorzolamide 2% three times daily)
   - Topical steroids (prednisolone acetate 1% every hour)
2. If medical therapy fails to control IOP, surgical removal of residual cortical and nuclear material with thorough irrigation are often needed.

SUBLUXED OR DISLOCATED LENS AND GLAUCOMA

Subluxation of the lens occurs from a partial disruption of the zonular fibers. The lens is decentered but remains partially in the pupillary aperture. Dislocation of the lens occurs with complete disruption of the zonular fibers. The lens is displaced out of the pupillary aperture. Trauma results in subluxation if more than 25% of the zonular fibers are ruptured (8). Other causes of lens subluxation/dislocation include high myopia, Marfan's syndrome, homocystinuria, Weill-Marchesani syndrome, acquired syphilis, and others (Table 17–4).

Anterior dislocation of the lens into the pupillary space or into the anterior chamber causes pupillary block glaucoma (1). Lenses that dislocate posteriorly may remain in the vitreous without complications or may rarely lead to phacolytic glaucoma (24).

TABLE 17–4. *Conditions associated with ectopia lentis*

Systemic disorders

Marfan's syndrome	Ehlers-Danlos syndrome
Marfan-like syndrome	Refsum's syndrome
Familial pseudomarfanism	Kniest syndrome and
Stickler's syndrome	variants
Vitreoretinopathy-	Klippel-Feil syndrome
encephalocele	Wildervanck's syndrome
syndrome	Alport's syndrome
Homocystinuria	Focal dermal hypoplasia
Weill-Marchesani	syndrome
syndrome	Sprengel's deformity
Hyperlysinemia	Polydactyly
Sulfite oxidase	Cross-Khodadoust
deficiency	syndrome
Syphilis	Primordial dwarfism
Sturge-Weber syndrome	Klinefelter's syndrome
Crouzon's syndrome	Lenz microphthalmia
Oxycephaly	syndrome
Pfandler's syndrome	Rieger's syndrome
Scleroderma	Mandibulofacial dysostosis

Ocular disorders

Trauma (including surgical)	Exfoliation syndrome
Familial simple ectopia	Cornea plana
lentis	Blepharoptosis-high myopia
Ectopia lentis et pupillae	syndrome
Congenital glaucoma/	Persistent hyperplastic
buphthalmos	primary vitreous
Megalocornea	Intraocular pentastomid
Mature or hypermature	larva
cataract	Intraocular tumor
Aniridia	Chronic uveitis

Reprinted with permission (30).

Diagnosis

1. There may be a history of trauma.
2. Monocular diplopia, decreased visual acuity, marked astigmatism, acquired high myopia, displaced or decentered lens, iridodonesis (quivering of the iris), phakodonesis (quivering of the lens), and asymmetry of the anterior chamber may be present.
3. History/physical findings consistent with the above mentioned syndromes should be sought.

Management

1. This form of pupillary block glaucoma may be treated with a cycloplegic agent. If the lens returns to the posterior chamber, a miotic is used to prevent further anterior dislocation of the lens.

2. Two peripheral iridectomies must be performed to prevent future episodes of pupillary block glaucoma.
3. In patients without a PI, miotics must be used cautiously because they may worsen the pupillary block by loosening the zonules and allowing further anterior displacement of the lens (inverse glaucoma) (25).
4. A lensectomy may be required.

NEOVASCULAR GLAUCOMA

Neovascularization of the anterior and posterior segments of the eye is thought to result from widespread retinal ischemia, which induces the release of vasoproliferative factors (26). Diseases that have been implicated in this process include retinal anterio-venous obstructive disease, diabetic retinopathy, carotid artery obstructive disease, rhegmatogenous retinal detachment, and others (Table 17–5).

Neovascularization of the iris can begin at the pupillary zone, iris periphery, or angle. Proliferating connective tissue composed of myofibroblasts (27) accompany the new vessels, forming a fibrovascular membrane. This membrane adheres to the cornea and the iris in the angle resulting in peripheral anterior synechiae. If the synechiae progress, secondary angle-closure glaucoma can occur.

Diagnosis

1. The patient may be asymptomatic or complain of a painful, red eye associated with decreased vision.
2. High-magnification slit-lamp examination shows new iris vessels at the pupillary margin. The fine vessels extend tortuously toward the iris periphery. If the vessels cover enough of the iris, the iris will have a red tinge (rubeosis iridis).
3. PAS and ectropion uveae may be present.
4. Gonioscopy may show new vessels in the angle.
5. There may be a spontaneous hyphema.
6. Fluorescein angiography can detect new iris vessels at least 1 month before they are visible with the slit lamp.

Management

1. Panretinal photocoagulation is used to induce the regression of iris vessels (28) and may be used when the retina cannot be visualized.
2. The IOP can be controlled with the following:
   - Topical beta-blockers twice daily (or extended release form daily)
   - Topical alpha-agonist three times daily
   - Systemic or topical carbonic anhydrase inhibitors (e.g., systemic acetazolomide 250 mg orally four times daily) or topical dorzolamide 2% three times daily)
   - Topical Xalatan™

TABLE 17–5. *Neovascular angle-closure glaucomas secondary to retinal diseases*

Ocular vascular disease	Other ocular disorders	Ocular neoplasms	Extraocular vascular disease
Retinal venous obstruction	Rhegmatogenous retinal detachment	Retinoblastomas	Carotid artery obstruction
Central/hemispheric/branch	Uveitis	Choroidal melanoma	Carotid-cavernous fistula
Diabetic retinopathy	Endophthalmitis	Metastatic carcinoma	Carotid artery ligation
Central retinal artery obstruction	Vitreous wick syndrome	Reticulum cell sarcoma (intraocular lymphoma)	Giant cell arteritis
Combined retinal artery/vein obstruction			Takayasu's disease (pulseless disease)
Coats' disease			
Eales' disease			
Sickle cell retinopathy			
Sturge-Weber, choroidal hemangioma			
Angiomatosis retinae (Von Hippel's disease)			
Radiation retinopathy			
Syphilitic vasculitis			
Familial exudative vitreoretinopathy of Criswick and Schepens			
Pars planitis			

Reprinted with permission (30).

- Miotics should be avoided because they increase the permeability of the blood-aqueous barrier (1)
3. If the IOP remains elevated, despite the regression of blood vessels, a trabeculectomy with antifibrosis agents should be considered. Other alternatives include shunt tube procedures and cycloablation.

CONGENITAL GLAUCOMA

Congenital glaucoma can be subdivided into primary congenital glaucoma and secondary/complicated congenital glaucoma (Table 17–6).

Primary congenital glaucoma results from an abnormality in the trabecular meshwork, trabeculodysgenesis. It is not associated with any other ocular or systemic disorders.

Secondary/complicated congenital glaucoma can result from anterior segment abnormalities (Axenfeld's anomaly, Rieger's anomaly, Peters' anomaly, etc.), Lowe's syndrome (oculocerebrorenal syndrome), rubella, phakomatoses, and others.

Diagnosis

1. Presenting symptoms are commonly epiphora, blepharospasm, and photophobia.
2. Enlarged globe (buphthalmus), corneal clouding, corneal diameter greater than

---

TABLE 17–6. *Shaffer-Weiss classification of congenital glaucoma patients*

A. Primary congenital glaucoma
   1. Late-developing primary congenital glaucoma
B. Glaucoma associated with congenital anomalies
   1. Aniridia
   2. Sturge-Weber syndrome
   3. Neurofibromatosis
   4. Marfan syndrome
   5. Pierre Robin syndrome
   6. Homocystinuria
   7. Goniodysgenesis (Axenfeld's anomaly and syndrome, Rieger's anomaly and syndrome, Peters' anomaly)
   8. Lowe syndrome
   9. Microcornea
  10. Microspherophakia
  11. Rubella
  12. Chromosomal abnormalities
  13. Rubinstein-Taybi (broad thumb) syndrome
  14. Persistent hyperplastic primary vitreous
C. Secondary glaucoma in infants
   1. Retinopathy of prematurity
   2. Tumors
     a. Retinoblastoma
     b. Juvenile xanthogranuloma
   3. Inflammation
   4. Trauma

Reprinted with permission (30).

12 mm, IOP greater than 20 mm Hg, linear horizontal or vertical tears in Descemet's membrane (Haab's striae), myopic astigmatism, and optic nerve cupping. Detailed examination and accurate measurement of IOP often requires sedation with ketamine.

Management

1. Definitive management is surgical.
   - Goniotomy or trabeculotomy.
   - If the above fail to control IOP, alternatives include filtration surgery with mitomycin C, setons, and cycloablative therapy.
2. Medical therapy is temporary and consists of:
   - Topical beta-blocker twice daily (or extended release form daily)
   - Topical alpha-agonist three times daily
   - Topical carbonic anhydrase inhibitor (dorzolamide 2% three times daily)

STEROID-RESPONSE GLAUCOMA

Corticosteroids have been shown to elevate the IOP when taken systemically or applied topically (29). It is thought that steroids increase the resistance to aqueous outflow.

Diagnosis

1. Increased IOP in a patient using systemic or topical steroids that decreases on discontinuation of the steroid.
2. Signs of glaucomatous damage.

Management

1. Discontinue the steroid or decrease its frequency.
2. Reduce the concentration or dosage of the steroid.
3. Change to a less potent steroid or a topical steroid that has less intraocular penetration.
4. Start topical and systemic glaucoma therapy if necessary.

APHAKIC/PSEUDOPHAKIC PUPILLARY BLOCK

Pupillary block can occur after cataract surgery when the pupil and any iridectomies are occluded by vitreous, lens remnants, or an intraocular lens. In the presence of an intraocular lens this is termed "pseudophakic pupillary block," and in the absence of a lens this is termed "aphakic pupillary block." Iris-bombe is usually present in cases of aphakic pupillary block. In pseudophakia the pupillary edge may be held posteriorly by the artificial lens, keeping the anterior chamber deep.

Diagnosis

Increased IOP, history of lens removal or lens implant, variable depth of anterior chamber.

Management

1. If the cornea is clear and the eye is not significantly inflamed, a laser PI is performed.
2. If a PI cannot be performed immediately, then a cycloplegic/mydriatic agent (mydriacyl 1%) is used with a sympathomimetic (phenylephrine 2.5%).
3. Topical beta-blockers, carbonic anhydrase inhibitors, and hyperosmotic agents are used to further control IOP (see management of primary angle closure glaucoma above).
4. Topical steroids are used to decrease inflammation.
5. The definitive treatment is a peripheral iridectomy even if medical therapy relieves the pupillary block. Usually several large iridectomies are required.

REFERENCES

1. Higginbotham EJ, Lee D. *Management of Difficult Glaucoma.* Boston: Blackwell Scientific; 1994.
2. Campbell DG. A comparison of diagnostic techniques in angle-closure glaucoma. *Am J Ophthalmol* 1979;88:197–204.
3. Forbes M. Gonioscopy with corneal indentation. *Arch Ophthalmol* 1962;6:488–492.
4. Gorin G. *Clinical Glaucoma.* New York: Marcel Dekker; 1977:179–196.
5. Catalano RA. *Ocular Emergencies.* Philadelphia: WB Saunders; 1992.
6. Harris LS, Galin MA. Prone provocative testing for narrow angle glaucoma. *Arch Ophthalmol* 1972;87:493–496.
7. Poinoosawmy D, Nagasubramanian S, Brown NAP. Effect of pilocarpine on visual acuity and on the dimensions of the cornea and anterior chamber. *Br J Ophthalmol* 1976;60:676–679.
8. Cullom RD, Chang B. The Wills Eye Manual. *Office and Emergency Room Diagnosis and Treatment of Eye Disease.* Philadelphia: JB Lippincott; 1994.
9. Weiss H, Shin DH, Kollarits CR. Vitrectomy for malignant (ciliary block) glaucomas. *Int Ophthalmol Clin* 1981;21:113–119.
10. Epstein DL, Steinert RF, Puliafito CA. Neodymium-YAG laser therapy to the anterior hyaloid in aphakic malignant (ciliovitreal block) glaucoma. *Am J Ophthalmol* 1984;98:137–143.
11. Shrader CE, Belcher III CD, Thomas JV, Simmons RJ, Murphy EB. Pupillary and iridovitreal block in pseudophakic eyes. *Ophthalmology* 1984;91:831–837.
12. Wand M, Haight B. Pseudophakic malignant glaucoma. *Glaucoma* 1986;8:28–29.
13. Cinotti DG, Reiter DJ, Maltzman BA, et al. Neodymium:YAG laser therapy for pseudophakic pupillary block. *J Cataract Refrac Surg* 1986;12:174–179.
14. Ritch R. Pathophysiology of glaucoma in uveitis. *Trans Ophthalmol Soc UK* 1981;101:321–324.
15. Phelps CD. Angle-closure glaucoma secondary to ciliary body swelling. *Arch Ophthalmol* 1974;92:287–290.
16. Schenker HI, Yablonski ME, Podos SM, Linder L. Fluorophotometric study of epinephrine and timolol in human subjects. *Arch Ophthalmol* 1981;99:1212–1216.
17. Masuda K, Izawa Y, Mishima S. Prostaglandins and glaucomatocyclitic crisis. *Jpn J Ophthalmol* 1975;19:368–375.
18. Kass MA, Becker B, Kolker AE. Glaucomatocyclitic crises and primary open angle glaucoma. *Am J Ophthalmol* 1973;75:668–673.
19. Ritch R, Shields MB, Krupin T, eds. *The Glaucomas.* St. Louis: CV Mosby; 1989:1187–1223.

20. Posner A, Schlossman A. Further observations on the syndrome of glaucomatocyclitic crises. *Trans Am Acad Ophthalmol Otolaryngol* 1953;57:531–536.
21. Theodore FH. Observations on glaucomatocyclitic crises. *Br J Ophthalmol* 1952;36:207–210.
22. Davanger M. Studies on the pseudo-exfoliation material: a review. *Graefes Arch Klin Exp Ophthalmol* 1978;208:65–68.
23. Bartholomew RS, Rebello PF. Calcium oxalate crystals in the aqueous. *Am J Ophthalmol* 1979;88: 1026–1028.
24. Chandler PA. Choice of treatment in dislocation of the lens. *Arch Ophthalmol* 1964;71:765–786.
25. Sallmann L. Glaucoma juvenile inversum. *Z Augenheilkd* 1930;72:46–63.
26. Brown G, Margaral L, Schachat A, Shah H. Neovascular glaucoma: etiologic considerations. *Ophthalmology* 1984;91:315–320.
27. John T, Sassani JW, Eagle RC. The myofibroblastic component of rubeosis iridis. *Ophthalmology* 1983;90:721–728.
28. Flanagan DW, Blach RK. Place of panretinal photocoagulation and trabeculectomy in the management of neovascular glaucoma. *Br J Ophthalmol* 1983;67:526–528.
29. Becker B, Mills DW. Corticosteroids and intraocular pressure. *Arch Ophthalmol* 1963;70:500–507.
30. Tasman W, Jaeger EA, eds. *Duane's Clinical Ophthalmology*. Vol. 3. Philadelphia: JB Lippincott; 1995.
31. Ritch R. Glaucoma secondary to lens intumescence and dislocation. In: Ritch R, Shields MB, eds. The Secondary Glaucomas. St. Louis: CV Mosby; 1982:134.

Management of Ocular Injuries and Emergencies,
edited by Mathew W. MacCumber.
Lippincott–Raven Publishers, Philadelphia © 1998.

18

Management of the Injured Lens: Anterior Segment Reconstruction

Dante J. Pieramici, Mathew W. MacCumber, Dimitri T. Azar, and Walter J. Stark

Department of Ophthalmology and Visual Science, Vitreoretinal Section, Yale University School of Medicine, New Haven, Connecticut 06520-8061; Department of Ophthalmology, Wilmer Eye Institute, The Johns Hopkins University School of Medicine, Baltimore, Maryland 21287; Retina Service, Department of Ophthalmology, Rush Medical College, Chicago, Illinois 60612; Department of Ophthalmology, Massachusetts Eye and Ear Infirmary, Harvard Medical School, Boston, Massachusetts 02114

Basic Considerations   257
Contusion and Lacerating Lens Injuries   258
   Diagnosis   258 · Associated Complications   259 · Management   261
Traumatic Iris Defects and Cyclodialysis Clefts   269
   Radial Iris Defects   269 · Iridodialysis and Cyclodialysis Clefts   272

BASIC CONSIDERATIONS

The crystalline lens is susceptible to injury from a wide range of mechanical and physical forces. The result of these forces is often loss of lens transparency and alteration of accommodative power. Lenticular trauma can also subsequently result in severe, permanent damage to other intraocular structures. Lens trauma may result from a variety of mechanisms including:

1. Contusion injuries. The compression and expansion changes of the globe induced by blunt force can induce zonular and capsular tears with lens displacement and subluxation. Contusion may result in direct pathologic changes in lens transparency and cataract formation.
2. Open globe injuries. Lens injury usually results from direct contact from a penetrating object. Secondary changes also may occur as a result of retained intraocular foreign bodies.
3. Other physical forces. Electrical, thermal, ultraviolet, and microwave energy can induce permanent changes in lenticular structure and transparency.
4. Pharmacologic agents. Several medications are known to cause lenticular

deposits and opacification. Steroid treatment is an important part of the management of ocular injuries, but long-term use may result in cataracts.

This chapter is limited to the discussion of the management and complications of blunt and penetrating lenticular injuries. Repair of iris defects and cyclodialysis clefts also are presented as they pertain to anterior segment reconstruction.

CONTUSION AND LACERATING LENS INJURIES

Lens injury is a frequent complication of open and closed globe injuries and carries a significantly worse prognosis to similar injuries without lens involvement (1). In blunt injuries, "coup" and "contrecoup" forces may result in cataract, capsular rupture, subluxation, and dislocation. These traumatic changes may be stationary or progressive, and complications of blunt lens injury such as severe inflammation or glaucoma may permanently affect vision.

Lacerating ocular trauma may result in similar lenticular injuries with a greater preponderance of capsular rupture, cataract formation, and intraocular inflammation. When retained intraocular foreign bodies are present, more specific lens changes may occur. Foreign bodies composed of iron or steel may induce siderosis with ferrous pigmentation, resulting in a rust colored cataract. With copper or bronze foreign bodies a sunflower cataract of the anterior capsule may develop, which is a particularly impressive manifestation of chalcosis.

Diagnosis

A high index of suspicion must be maintained in all cases of mechanical ocular injury, particularly when the cornea and anterior segment are involved. Initial examination should include slit-lamp analysis and dilated ophthalmoscopy, but in cases of an open globe, overaggressive attempts to examine a patient may be counterproductive. In such cases, more detailed examination can be achieved in the operating room. In closed and open wounds that have been primarily closed, more detailed examination should include assessment of lens clarity, position, stability, and integrity.

Clarity

The location of cataractous change (i.e., anterior subcapsular, nuclear, cortical, posterior subcapsular, as well as location in reference to the lens center) should be noted.

Visual acuity, potential acuity testing, glare testing, and entopic phenomenon will help document and quantitate visual disability associated with the cataract. Examination of the lens should be performed before and after pupillary dilation including retroillumination. Fibrotic capsulolenticular membranes can mimic lenticular opacities and must be considered in the differential diagnosis of traumatic cataracts. Some of these fibrous membranes resolve with steroid treatment. Examination of the fellow eye helps determine whether the cataract may have predated the trauma.

In contusion injury, a trauma-specific lens change known as a Vossius ring may form. It is a result of forceful impact of the iris against the anterior lens surface with the deposition of a circle of pigment on the anterior lens capsule. It has no visual significance and often resolves with time.

Position and Stability

Determine whether zonular dehiscence has occurred. This is a critical part of the lens examination because it has significant impact on the surgical management. Clinical evidence of zonular dehiscence and lens instability is summarized in Table 18–1.

Capsular Integrity

Identifying the presence of posterior capsular rupture is important not only in planning the surgical approach, but knowledge of capsular rupture will help determine whether severe post-traumatic inflammation is likely lens induced.

In the presence of lens opacification, anterior capsular rupture may occasionally be difficult to ascertain. If the lens has opacified or the ocular media are not clear, posterior capsular rupture may be undetectable. In such cases, fluid immersion B-scan ultrasound can be helpful in identifying occult capsular rupture.

Associated Complications

For further details on medical management, see also Chapter 17.

Lens Particle Glaucoma

Liberation of lens particles and debris after disruption of the lens capsule can lead to intraocular pressure increase, often soon after capsular violation. White fluffed lens cortical material is seen in the anterior chamber in proportion to the intraocular pressure increase. The proposed mechanism of pressure increase is blockage of the trabecular meshwork with the particulate material (2). Management includes aqueous suppressants and steroids. When the pressure cannot be controlled medically, irrigation and aspiration of the material should be undertaken. Use of a vitrectomy cutting and aspiration device may be required to remove adherent material.

TABLE 18–1. *Signs of zonular dehiscence*

Subluxation (decentration of the lens)
Phacodonesis ("wobble" of the lens with eye movement)
Iridodonesis ("wobble" of the iris with eye movement)
Asymmetric anterior chamber depths
Vitreous herniation
Change in angle depth
Eccentric pupil

Phacolytic Glaucoma

Phacolytic glaucoma is associated with hypermature, mature, or dislocated cataracts and may occur long after the traumatic episode. The patient presents with an acute onset of monocular pain and redness. Examination may disclose conjunctival hyperemia, anterior chamber inflammation with chunks of white material in the aqueous, and similar deposits on the corneal endothelium and lens capsule. It is postulated that soluble lens proteins are released from the mature lens stimulating a macrophage reaction. The trabecular meshwork is subsequently blocked by macrophages laden with lens material (3). The pressure is initially brought under control with hyperosmotics, carbonic anhydrase inhibitors, topical beta-blockers, and steroids. Definitive treatment requires cataract removal and thorough irrigation of all lens material.

Lens-Induced Angle Closure

The traumatized lens may induce pupillary block if dislocated into the pupillary space or anterior chamber (4). It also may result from herniation of vitreous into the pupillary space. If the lens is not completely dislocated but has loose zonules, it may be permitted to move anteriorly, initiating pupillary block. Miosis should be avoided in this situation because contraction of the ciliary muscle will further relax the zonules and worsen the pupillary block. In such cases cycloplegia and aqueous suppressants may break the attack until more definitive treatment is performed, including laser iridotomy or lens removal.

If the lens dislocates into the anterior chamber, attempts are made to reposition it. With the patient in the supine position, the iris is dilated, allowing the lens to settle posterior to the pupillary space. A miotic is then used chronically to keep the lens behind the iris.

Lens-Induced Uveitis (Phacoanaphylactic Uveitis, Phacoantigenic Uveitis)

An immune-mediated granulomatous inflammatory reaction may be initiated by lens proteins liberated from the ruptured capsule (5). The onset is days to weeks after the traumatic episode. The patient presents with a red painful eye, keratic precipitates, and intense anterior chamber inflammation centered around retained lens particles. Occasionally glaucoma may occur with blockage of the trabecular meshwork and synechiae formation. Initial management includes control of the inflammation with frequent topical steroids and management of increased intraocular pressure as required. Definitive treatment requires removal of the remaining lens material.

Dislocated Lens-Associated Ocular Injuries

Trauma is the most frequent cause of lens dislocation. As noted above, anterior dislocations can lead to relative pupillary block and glaucoma. Additionally, a lens in the anterior chamber can lead to mechanical abrasion and stripping of the corneal endothelium, with resultant corneal edema, and should be repositioned or removed in all cases. Dislocation of the crystalline lens or pseudophakos into the posterior chamber is often well tolerated. However, retinal injury can result from severe posterior inflammation and its complications. Alternatively, a mobile lens or pseudophakos may cause contusion injury to the retina, resulting in retinal hemorrhage, edema, retinal breaks, choroidal effusion, and retinal detachment.

Management

Traumatic Cataract with Minimal or No Zonular Dehiscence and/or Capsular Rupture

Even without evidence of weakened zonules or capsular rupture the surgeon should still be prepared for such complications when managing traumatic cataracts. Primary cataract extraction is indicated if there is obvious capsular rupture with extruded flocculent lens material or when there is posterior segment injury or intraocular foreign body and the cataract prohibits proper management of these problems. Primary surgical removal generally should be avoided otherwise because all traumatic cataracts are not inevitably progressive and many may remain localized and asymptomatic. In addition, inflammation and fibrous changes anterior to the lens may mimic a cataract and will resolve with aggressive steroid treatment alone.

Deferring surgery will allow for reduction in intraocular inflammation and hemorrhage and permit more accurate intraocular lens (IOL) measurements. The exact timing of surgery is not critical in these cases because the secondary complications listed above are unlikely. Indications for deferred surgery include visual compromise attributable to lens opacity that is symptomatic to the patient or an inability to examine the posterior pole as a result of the cataract.

The anterior (limbal) approach is the method of choice either by planned extracapsular cataract extraction or phacoemulsification with or without IOL implantation. In children or young adults it may be removed by aspiration with minimal or no ultrasound.

Procedure: Bimanual Technique for Lenticular Aspiration, Limbal Approach

1. Two limbal paracenteses are prepared 135 to 180 degrees apart (6,7).
2. An infusion cannula (bent 23-gauge butterfly needle) is placed through one site (Fig. 18–1A).
3. An microvitreoretinal (MVR) blade or the infusion needle is used to perform a stab anterior capsulotomy.
4. An automated cutting-aspiration handpiece (vitreous cutter) is inserted and used to cut and aspirate lens cortex and nucleus (Fig. 18–1A).

Flexible iris retractors (Grieshaber) placed through the limbal paracenteses may be useful in adequately dilating a pupil for complete lens cortex removal (Fig. 18–1B).

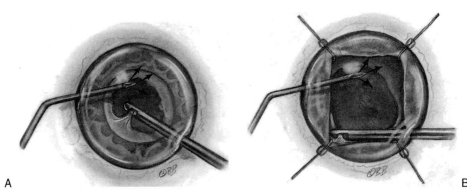

FIG. 18–1. A: Bimanual technique for lenticular aspiration, limbal approach. The bent 23-gauge butterfly needle is seen left and vitreous cutter right. **B:** Four flexible iris retractors are used for adequate pupillary dilation.

Alternatively, an instrument with an irrigating sleeve can be used through a small (3.5 mm) corneoscleral groove. Full-function instruments (i.e., the original Peyman vitreophage or a standard phaco handpiece) combine cutting, aspiration, and infusion in one instrument and can eliminate the use of the separate infusion site in the above technique. In children the nucleus may be soft enough to remove with aspiration alone and thus can be performed with an irrigating-aspirating handpiece.

If significant lens instability or capsular rupture is encountered intraoperatively, alternative methods may be considered (see below).

Intraocular Lens Implantation

There have been many limited retrospective reports of successful use of IOL implantation either primarily or secondarily in adults and children following trauma (8–12). No prospective study has addressed timing of IOL implantation in traumatic cataracts. Primary implantation is difficult due to significant postoperative inflammation and limitations of fellow eye measurements for the IOL power. Potential advantages of primary cataract extraction and IOL implantation include earlier visual rehabilitation, early removal of potentially toxic lens material, and elimination of the need for secondary lens implantation surgery. In children, the implantation of an IOL may be the only realistic approach to limiting the development of amblyopia. Posterior chamber IOL (PCIOL) implantation may be completed by:

- Capsular bag fixation, if zonular disruption is mild (4 clock hours or less), iris fixation, McCannel technique (see below)
- Sulcus fixation, Malbran/Stark technique (see below)
- Combination capsular bag and suture fixated

Anterior chamber IOLs (ACIOLs), particularly closed loop models, have higher complication rates and should be avoided in the traumatized eye (13–16), although newer ACIOLs may prove safe and effective. Alternatively, vision can be rehabilitated with contact lens or epikeratophakia (17,18). Aphakic spectacles are not tolerated because of anisometropia.

Traumatically Subluxed or Dislocated Cataractous Lens

When the traumatized lens loses adequate zonular and capsular support, it may subluxate or totally dislocate. Removal of these cataracts is a challenge, and the surgeon's goals are to minimize iatrogenic damage while removing the unstable lens, to manage prolapsing vitreous, and to secure an IOL.

Indications for removal include capsular rupture with resultant glaucoma or ocular inflammation, visual compromise, retinal contusion injury, and corneal endothelial damage. However, in a patient with a subluxed or even dislocated mobile lens with capsular integrity one can consider leaving the lens alone and rehabilitating vision with spectacles or a contact lens.

Anterior Techniques

These methods include anterior or limbal approaches to remove an unstable lens and prevent the lens from falling into the posterior segment during the removal.

Procedure: Intracapsular Technique

1. Two 27-gauge 1.5-inch needles are secured together at their base (19).
2. The needles are then inserted 4 mm posterior to the limbus behind the lens to prevent posterior migration (Fig. 18–2A). If the lens is floating freely in the vit-

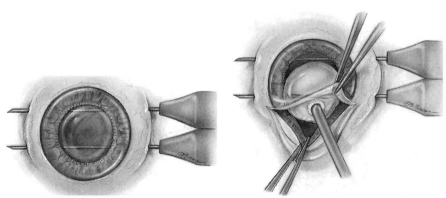

A   B

FIG. 18–2. A: Intracapsular technique. Two 27-gauge needles support the dislocated lens. **B:** The cryoextractor is applied to the anterior and superior mid-periphery of the lens for cryoextraction.

reous cavity, the patient can be turned prone and the lens trapped just posterior to the pupil.

3. A corneoscleral incision is prepared, and the lens is then delivered with the cryoprobe or lens loop (Fig. 18–2*B*). Care must be taken not to incarcerate vitreous in the cryoprobe. Any vitreous attached to the lens must be cut free with scissors to reduce the chance of traction on the retina.

4. The zonules are usually disrupted but may require lysis by irrigating alpha-chymotrypsin in a concentration of 1:5,000 to 1:10,000. It is injected into the posterior segment through a peripheral iridectomy.

5. If the anterior hyaloid has been violated, air should be placed in the anterior chamber to indicate the presence of vitreous to the wound. Vitreous should be removed by weck-cell or automated vitrectomy.

Extracapsular Techniques (Planned and Phacoemulsification)

With significant lens instability, planned extracapsular extraction carries a significant risk of posterior migration of the lens during delivery and should be avoided. However, such cases often can be completed successfully with careful and gentle phacoemusification:

• Viscoelastic can be used to tamponade prolapsing vitreous and protect potentially compromised corneal endothelium.
• Extensive hydrodissection or viscodissection should be used.
• Minimize zonular stress, particularly with nuclear rotation.
• Careful anterior vitrectomy should be performed.
• Air can be injected into the anterior chamber to assure that no vitreous is present at the wound.

Posterior Techniques

These are preferred when there is significant posterior capsular rupture, subluxation, or dislocation. Intracapsular and extracapsular cataract extraction are associated with more complications in these patients due to excessive vitreous loss, retinal detachment, and glaucoma.

Procedure: Pars Plana Lensectomy

The surgical goal is to remove the entire lens, prolapsed vitreous, and in some cases to insert an IOL (20,21).

1. Conjunctival peritomy is prepared nasally and temporally with scissors.

2. Creation of three sclerotomies with an MVR blade, one each in the inferotemporal, superotemporal, and superonasal quadrants, each 90 to 180 degrees apart. In adults the sclerotomies are created in the pars plana 3.0 mm posterior

to the limbus. In children under 3 years of age, the sclerotomies are created more anteriorly because the pars plana is not fully developed.

3. A 4- or 6-mm infusion cannula is sutured in place into the inferotemporal sclerotomy. The infusion is not turned on until the cannula port is visualized in the vitreous cavity.

4. A surgical blade is introduced through one of the sclerotomies and passed through the equator of the nucleus to judge central hardness.

5. A bent 23-gauge butterfly needle is inserted into the lens as a secondary infusion until the pars plana infusion cannula can be visualized (Fig. 18–3A). This also serves to anchor and hydrodissect the lens.

6. In children or young adults, the lens can be removed with the cutting/aspiration probe. In older individuals with harder lenses, the lens nucleus requires ultrasonic fragmentation before irrigation and aspiration of the cortex and posterior capsule (Fig. 18–3A).

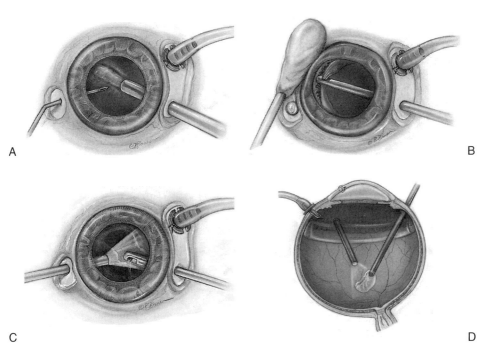

A

B

C

D

FIG. 18–3. A: Pars plana lensectomy. The bent 23-gauge butterfly needle is seen left and the infusion line and ultrasonic fragmentation instrument right. **B:** Depression with cotton tip applicator. **C:** Pars plana vitrectomy. **D:** Pars plana retrieval of posteriorly dislocated lens fragments with ultrasonic fragmentation.

7. Depression with a cotton-tipped applicator can aid in removal of peripheral lens material (Fig. 18–3*B*). Flexible iris retractors (Grieshaber) placed through limbal paracenteses may be useful in adequately dilating a pupil for complete lens cortex removal.

8. Consideration should be given to performing a vitrectomy. Vitrectomy should be performed for removal of anterior prolapsed vitreous, significant vitreous opacity (usually blood), and retrieval of dropped lens fragments (Fig. 18–3*C*). Posterior lens fragments are divided and aspirated with the ultrasonic fragmentation handpiece or vitreous cutter after the surrounding vitreous has been removed. Fragmentation is only performed in the anterior vitreous cavity after the lens fragment has been safely elevated off of the retina (Fig. 18–3*D*). Only surgeons experienced in vitreoretinal techniques should attempt posterior vitrectomy; if performed, consideration should be given to removal of an attached posterior hyaloid in older individuals (over age 40) because this may decrease the risk of future spontaneous posterior vitreous detachment with rapid development of retinal detachment or epiretinal membrane formation.

9. A posterior or anterior chamber lens may be placed (see below).

10. The sclerotomies are then closed with 7-0 Vicryl sutures followed by conjunctiva closure with 6-0 collagen sutures.

Pars Plana Recovery of a Posteriorly Dislocated Lens

A posteriorly dislocated lens need not always be removed. In the absence of related ocular complications, a patient may be managed with a contact lens and regular ophthalmologic examinations (every 3 to 6 months). Indications for removal include:

• Posterior uveitis presumed secondary to lens proteins
• Phacolytic glaucoma
• Retinal contusion injuries secondary to the dislocated lens
• Lens obstructing vision or the ability to examine the retina

Surgical technique is similar to step 8 under Pars Plana Lensectomy. If nuclear or large cortical fragment are present in the vitreous cavity, referral should be made to a vitreoretinal specialist within 24 to 36 hours.

Placement of an Intraocular Lens in Eyes without Capsular Support

Anterior chamber IOLs, particularly closed-loop models, increase corneal epithelial loss and may compromise the angle structures in an eye already predisposed to glaucoma. In addition, these lenses require iris support, which may not be present in the traumatized eye.

Without proper capsular support (greater than 7 clock hours with haptics in the areas of greatest support), a PCIOL placed either in the sulcus or bag may decenter or dislocate into the vitreous cavity.

Alternatives for support of PCIOL are listed as follows:

- Sulcus fixation alone may be appropriate if there are greater than 7 clock hours of intact capsule; the haptics are positioned in the areas of greatest support.
- Iris fixation can be used if only partial capsular support is present. The haptics are placed in sulcus and the PCIOL is fixated by suturing one or both haptics to the iris.
- Scleral fixation can be used if partial or no capsular support is present. With partial capsular support, only a superior "safety suture" may be necessary to prevent PCIOL dislocation. With minimal or no capsular support, both a superior and inferior suture must be placed.

Procedure: Iris Fixation of Posterior Chamber Intraocular Lens

This procedure is similar to the technique illustrated below for closure of radial iris defects (22,23).

1. Sodium hyaluronate is injected into the anterior chamber.
2. The lens is placed in the remaining capsular bag or sulcus.
3. Two Sinskey hooks are used to rotate the optic centrally and then elevate it to induce pupillary capture.
4. A miotic is then injected to maintain optic capture.
5. The course of the haptics should be mentally outlined under the iris.
6. A single armed 10-0 prolene suture on a CIF-4 or CTC-6 needle is placed through the peripheral cornea, underneath the haptic and out through the peripheral cornea.
7. The needle is cut off and both suture ends are grasped through a paracentesis tract with a Bonn or Sinskey hook.
8. The suture ends are tied and trimmed, and the iris is pushed back into position.
9. The lens is then pushed into place behind the pupil with the Sinskey hook.

Procedure: Scleral Fixation of Posterior Chamber Intraocular Lens

This procedure is an alternative for eyes with extensive capsular or zonular dehiscence (24,25).

1. Conjunctival peritomy is prepared superiorly and inferiorly.
2. A rectangular or triangular partial-thickness scleral flap is fashioned inferiorly 180 degrees away from the location of the superior corneoscleral incision.
3. A 7-mm superior corneoscleral groove incision is created, and a limited anterior vitrectomy is performed.
4. Viscoelastic is injected into the anterior chamber over the iris to push any vitreous posteriorly and protect the corneal endothelium.
5. Select posterior chamber intraocular lens (PCIOL) with 6.5 to 7 mm optic and polypropylene C-loop haptics. The ends of the haptics are beaded with dispos-

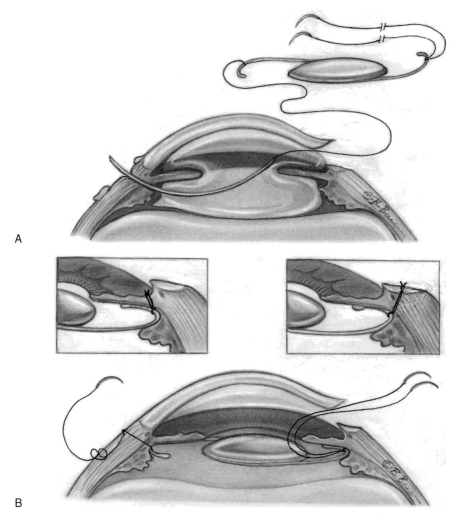

FIG. 18–4. A: Insertion of a PCIOL. The vitreous is forced posteriorly with sodium hyaluronate. A CIF-4 needle with a prolene suture tied to the inferior IOL loop is passed through a corneoscleral incision superiorly, through the pupil, behind the iris inferiorly, and out through the ciliary sulcus. **B:** Fixation of the PCIOL in the ciliary sulcus. The IOL is fixated inferiorly using a scleral suture and superiorly using an iris suture (inset, top left) or a scleral suture (inset, top right).

able cautery. Alternatively, a one-piece all polymethylmethacrylate (PMMA) PCIOL with or without haptic suture islets may be used.

6. A double-armed 10-0 prolene suture on a CIF-4 needle is cut in half and the free end is tied to the inferior haptic (Fig. 18–4A).

7. A double armed 10-0 prolene suture on a BV-100-4 needle is secured to the superior haptic.

8. The needle attached to the inferior haptic is passed out through the inferior ciliary sulcus approximately 0.5 to 1.0 mm posterior to the limbus within the previously prepared scleral flap (Fig. 18–4*A*).

9. The IOL haptics are placed within the ciliary sulcus while the inferior suture is gently pulled with tying forceps.

10. The superior suture is tied to the peripheral iris or passed through the pupil under the iris and through the sclera, exiting 0.5 to 1 mm posterior to the limbus within the corneoscleral incision (Fig. 18–4*B*). The two ends are tied together with the knot buried in the incision.

11. The inferior needle is then regrasped and an adjacent superficial scleral bite is taken and the suture tied to itself under the flap.

12. The corneal scleral incision and scleral flaps are closed with interrupted 10-0 nylon and the conjunctiva closed with 6-0 collagen suture.

TRAUMATIC IRIS DEFECTS AND CYCLODIALYSIS CLEFTS

Closed and open injuries to the globe often include a radial iris defect or iridodialysis (see Chapter 16). Sectoral iridectomies are sometimes created at the time of ocular surgery to aid in cataract extraction. Once corneal lacerations and traumatic cataracts are managed, the ophthalmic surgeon may choose to close iris defects to restore more normal anatomy during the same or subsequent ocular surgeries.

A cyclodialysis cleft can be a vision-threatening injury due to resulting hypotony. If the cleft fails to respond to laser treatment (see Chapter 16), it can be closed surgically. Surgical repair of a cyclodialysis cleft is similar to repair of an iridodialysis, so they are both presented here.

Radial Iris Defects

If the iridodialysis is superior, it can be closed through the corneoscleral wound at the time of cataract extraction. Otherwise, a modified McCannel technique can be used (22).

Procedure: Repair of a Radial Iris Defect

1. A 10-0 prolene suture on a CIF-4 needle is passed through the peripheral cornea, through both sides of the iris defect, and out through the peripheral cornea on the opposite side (Fig. 18–5*A*).

2. A limbal paracentesis is prepared with a Ziegler knife adjacent to the iris defect. Sodium hyaluronate may be injected over the iris defect to maintain the anterior chamber (Fig. 18–5*B*).

3. A Bonn iris or Sinskey hook is passed into the anterior chamber through the paracentesis and used to externalize the suture on either side of the iris defect (Fig. 18–5*C*).

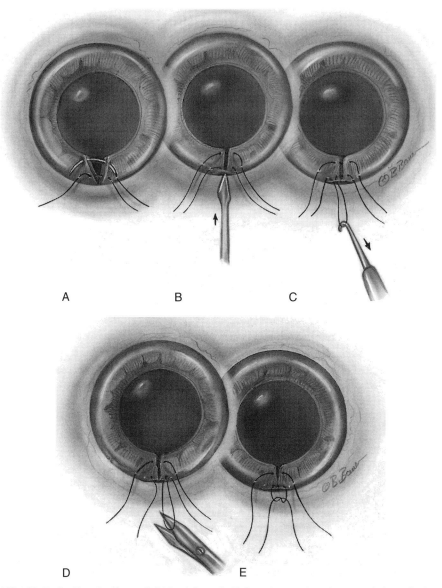

FIG. 18–5. A: Repair of a radial iris defect. A 10-0 prolene suture is passed through the cornea and iris defect. **B:** Limbal paracentesis is prepared. **C:** A Bonn iris hook is used to externalize the suture. **D:** The prolene loops are cut and ends removed. **E:** The knot is tied and the iris redeposited.

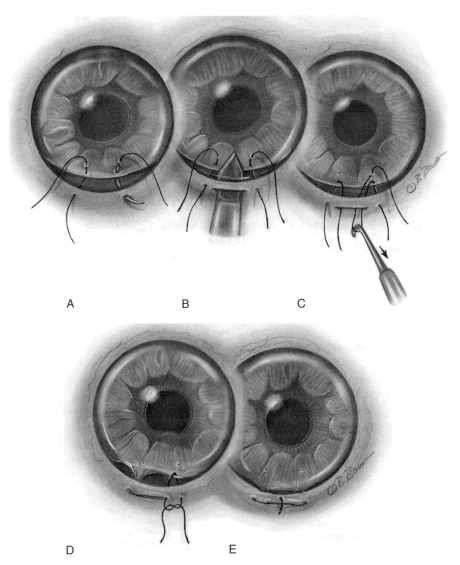

FIG. 18–6. A: Repair of an iridodialysis. A 10-0 prolene suture on a BV-100 needle is passed through the cornea, the iris, across the iridodialysis and out through sclera about 1 mm posterior to the limbus. **B:** A self-sealing corneoscleral tunnel is prepared. **C:** A Bonn iris hook is used to externalize the prolene suture and the loop is cut. The end passing through the cornea is removed. **D:** The ends of the suture are tied and the knot buried into the wound. **E:** If necessary, the corneoscleral tunnel is closed with 10-0 nylon suture.

4. The prolene loops are cut and the ends passing through the cornea are removed (Fig. 18–5D).
5. The suture is tied, the ends trimmed short, and the knot and iris deposited into their final position (Fig. 18–5E).
6. The above sequence can be repeated so both the peripheral and central iris wound is reapproximated.

Iridodialysis and Cyclodialysis Clefts

Procedure: Repair of an Iridodialysis

1. A fornix-based conjunctival flap is prepared at the limbus with scissors in the area of the iridodialysis.
2. Cautery is used for hemostasis.
3. A 10-0 prolene suture on a BV-100 needle is passed through the peripheral cornea, through the iris, across the iridodialysis, and out through the sclera about 1 mm posterior to the limbus. Alternatively, the suture may be passed through the sclera first and out through peripheral cornea. If the iridodialysis is large, a second suture can be placed (Fig. 18–6A).
4. A small self-sealing corneoscleral tunnel (less than 3.5 mm in width) is prepared using a crescent blade and keratome adjacent to (between) the prolene sutures (Fig. 18–6B).
5. Sodium hyaluronate is injected to maintain the anterior chamber.
6. A Bonn iris or Sinskey hook is passed through the corneoscleral tunnel and used to externalize the prolene suture. The loop is cut and the end passing through the cornea is removed (Fig. 18–6C).
7. The ends of the suture are tied, approximating the iridodialysis. The knot is rotated into the corneoscleral wound (Fig. 18–6D).
8. The sodium hyaluronate is removed with an irrigation-aspiration apparatus. If necessary, the corneoscleral tunnel is closed with 10-0 nylon suture and the knot buried (Fig. 18–6E).
9. The conjunctiva is closed with cautery or collagen suture.

Procedure: Repair of a Cyclodialysis Cleft

The procedure is identical to the above procedure for repair of an iridodialysis with the exception that the prolene suture is passed through the avulsed iris root instead of across the iridodialysis cleft.

REFERENCES

1. deJuan E, Sternberg P, Michels RG. Penetrating ocular injuries. *Ophthalmology* 1983;90:1318–1322.
2. Epstein DL, Jedziniak JA, Grant WM. Obstruction of aqueous outflow by lens particles and by heavy-molecular-weight soluble lens proteins. *Invest Ophthalmol Vis Sci* 1978;17:272.

3. Flocks M, Littwin CS, Zimmerman LE. Phacolytic glaucoma. A clinicopathologic study of one hundred thirty eight cases of glaucoma associated with hypermature cataract. *Arch Ophthalmol* 1955;54:37.
4. Chandler PA. Choice of treatment in dislocation of the lens. *Arch Ophthalmol* 1964;71:765.
5. Apple DJ, Mamalis N, Steinmetz RL, et al. Phacoanaphylactic endophthalmitis associated with extracapsular cataract extraction and posterior chamber intraocular lens. *Arch Ophthalmol* 1984;102:1528–1532.
6. Irvine JA, Smith RE. Lens injuries. In Shingleton et al, eds: *Eye Trauma*. St. Louis: CV Mosby; 1991.
7. Ryan SJ, Von Noorden GK. Further observations on the aspiration technique in cataract surgery. *Am J Ophthalmol* 1971;71:626–630.
8. Koenig SB, Ruttum MS, Lewandowski MF, Schultz RO. Pseudophakia for traumatic cataracts in children. *Ophthalmology* 1993;100:1218–1224.
9. Hemo Y, Ben ED. Traumatic cataracts in young children. Correction of aphakia by intraocular lens implantation. *Ophthalmic Paediatr Genet* 1989;15:196–200.
10. Gupta AK, Grover AK, Gurha N. Traumatic cataract surgery with intraocular lens implantation in children. *J Pediatr Ophthalmol Strabismus* 1992;29:73–78.
11. Bleckman H, Hanuschik W, Vogt R. Implantation of posterior chamber lenses in eyes with phakodonesis and lens subluxation. *J Cataract Refract Surg* 1990;16:485–489.
12. Muga R, Maul E, The management of lens damage in perforating corneal lacerations. *Br J Ophthalmol* 1978;62:784–787.
13. Drews RC. Intermittent touch syndrome. *Arch Ophthalmol* 1982;100:1440–1441.
14. Stark WJ, Worthen DM, Holladay JT, et al. The FDA report on intraocular lenses. *Ophthalmology* 1982;90:311–317.
15. McDonnell PJ, Green WR, Maumenee AE, Iliff WJ. Pathology of intraocular lenses in 33 eyes examined postmortem. *Ophthalmology* 1983;90:386–403.
16. Apple DJ, Olson RJ. Closed-loop anterior chamber lenses. *Arch Ophthalmol* 1987;105:52–57.
17. Smiddy WE, Hamburg TR, Kratcher GP, et al. Contact lenses for visual rehabilitation after corneal laceration repair. *Ophthalmology* 1989;96:293–298.
18. Morgan KS, Stephenson G. Epikeratophakia in children with corneal lacerations. *J Pediatr Ophthalmol Strabismus* 1985;22:105–108.
19. Calhoun FP, Hagler WS. Experience with the Jose' Barraquer method of extracting a dislocated lens. *Am J Ophthalmol* 1960;50:701–715.
20. Peyman GA, Schulman JA. *Intravitreal Surgery*. Norwalk, CT: Appleton & Lange; 1994.
21. Michels RG, Shacklett DE. Vitrectomy technique for removal of retained lens material. *Arch Ophthalmol* 1977;103:1767–1773.
22. McCannel MA. A retrievable suture idea for anterior uveal problems. *Opthalmic Surg* 1976;7:98–103.
23. Panton RW, Sulewski ME, Parker JS, et al. Surgical management of subluxed posterior-chamber intraocular lenses. *Arch Ophthalmol* 1993;111:919–926.
24. Malbran ES, Malbran E Jr, Negri I. Lens guide for transport and fixation in secondary IOL implantation after intracapsular extraction. *Int Ophthalmol* 1986;9:151–160.
25. Stark WJ, Gottsch JD, Goodman DF, et al. Posterior chamber intraocular lens implantation in the absence of capsular support. *Arch Ophthalmol* 1989;107:1078–1083.

Management of Ocular Injuries and Emergencies,
edited by Mathew W. MacCumber.
Lippincott–Raven Publishers, Philadelphia ©1998.

19

Endophthalmitis

Shannath L. Merbs, Lisa S. Abrams, and Peter A. Campochiaro

*Department of Ophthalmology, Wilmer Eye Institute, The Johns Hopkins University School
of Medicine, Baltimore, Maryland 21287*

Basic Considerations 275
  Types of Endophthalmitis 275 · Epidemiology 276 · Organisms 276
  Diagnosis 277 · Treatment 280

BASIC CONSIDERATIONS

Endophthalmitis is infection within the eye. Although technically endophthalmitis could be used to describe intraocular infection with any type of pathogen, by convention it is generally reserved for bacterial or fungal infection. Exogenous endophthalmitis indicates direct inoculation of the eye either from surgery, penetrating trauma, or perforation from external infection such as a corneal ulcer. Endogenous endophthalmitis indicates spread of infection to the eye from a site elsewhere in the body. Severe damage to vital intraocular structures from infection is best avoided by a high degree of clinical suspicion and rapid diagnosis and treatment.

Types of Endophthalmitis

Traumatic endophthalmitis is somewhat uncommon but can be particularly devastating because organisms with high pathogenicity are often involved.

Postoperative endophthalmitis accounts for the majority of cases and can be divided into early (within 6 weeks of surgery) and late.

Endogenous endophthalmitis results from spread of infection to the eye through the posterior circulation, particularly with fungus, but also may occur directly from surrounding periorbital tissues. Patients are often immunosuppressed, debilitated, or have a history of parenteral feeding or intravenous drug use.

Epidemiology

Traumatic

Posttraumatic endophthalmitis makes up between 3% and 44% of all cases of endophthalmitis, with most sources citing a rate of 20% to 30% (1–6). The incidence of endophthalmitis after penetrating trauma ranges from 2.8% to 7.4% and is highest when a retained intraocular foreign body is present or when the injury occurs in a rural setting (4.7% to 13%) (1,2,7–11). In a lacerating injury, disruption of the crystalline lens increases the relative risk of developing endophthalmitis (8).

Postoperative

Postoperative endophthalmitis is the most common form of endophthalmitis, accounting for more than half of all cases (Fig. 19–1) (2–5). The reported incidence of early postoperative endophthalmitis reported in the most recent literature ranges from 0.1% to 0.6% (2,12–14). The rates after cataract and filtering surgery are similar, and the rates after secondary intraocular lens implantation and cataract surgery with anterior vitrectomy are higher (12,13).

Endogenous

Endogenous endophthalmitis, the least common form, represents 6% to 14% of all cases of endophthalmitis (2,5,6). The incidence of endogenous endophthalmitis is only about five in 10,000 hospitalized patients but is more prevalent in severely ill patients and intravenous drug users (15–17). *Candida albicans* may have a particular predisposition for spread to the eye (18).

Organisms

Bacteria are responsible for the majority of cases of endophthalmitis. Coagulase-negative *Staphylococcus,* the most common organism causing endophthalmitis, is also the most common organism to colonize the conjunctiva. DNA studies in *Staphylococcus epidermidis* endophthalmitis suggest that the most common source of infection is the patient's own flora (19). In many instances, organisms can be grown in enriched media from anterior chamber fluid removed during cataract surgery (20). Taken together, these data suggest that during cataract surgery a constant seeding of the anterior chamber with bacteria from the patient's own flora occurs. In the majority of cases, this small innoculum is handled by host defenses. However, in a small percentage of eyes and for reasons that are not well understood, infection occurs.

Sometimes bacteria of low pathogenicity, such as *Propionibacterium acnes* or some strains of coagulase-negative *Staphylococcus,* enter the eye and cause chronic low-grade inflammation (21). The bacteria may become sequestered, often around the intraocular lens and posterior capsule, and become quiescent. Later, they may begin to proliferate and cause severe infection, either spontaneously due to a decrease in host defenses, or when freed by YAG capsulotomy.

Traumatic endophthalmitis is usually associated with organisms of high pathogenicity. A high incidence of *Bacillus* species, a particularly virulent organism, is found in traumatic endophthalmitis (11). Table 19–1 lists the relative frequency of various organisms isolated from cases of traumatic and postoperative endophthalmitis.

Over half of the cases of endogenous endophthalmitis are caused by fungi, predominantly *Candida* species (17,22). The majority of bacterial endogenous endophthalmitis cases are caused by Gram-positive organisms, predominantly *Staphylococcus* and *Streptococcus* species (16). About one third of bacterial cases are caused by Gram-negative bacteria, predominantly *Escherichia coli* (16).

Diagnosis

Symptoms

Symptoms include blurred vision (90% to 100%), redness (75% to 85%), pain (75%), decreased vision (90%, 5/200 or worse; 25% light perception).

Signs

Signs include conjunctival hyperemia (100%); anterior chamber cell and flare (100%); vitreous cell and opacities (90% to 100%); hypopyon (85%); lid edema (30%); chemosis, corneal edema, anterior chamber reaction (common); reduced red reflex (70%); afferent pupillary defect (15%); and corneal ring infiltrate (5%) (Fig. 19–1).

Onset

Traumatic: acute, with pain and inflammation exceeding that expected from the trauma itself. It can be difficult to differentiate symptoms of endophthalmitis from those caused by the trauma.

TABLE 19–1. *Organisms isolated from endophthalmitis cases (1,2,4–9,11,12,18–19,22–30)*

	Staphylococcal	Streptococcol	Gram-negative	Bacillus	Polymicrobial	Fungal
Traumatic	20–50%	5–31%	4–29%	15–46%	3–31%	13–17%
Postoperative						
Acute	44–47%	20–38%	7–15%	3%	8–16%	3%
Late-onset	7–17%	17–57%	30%			

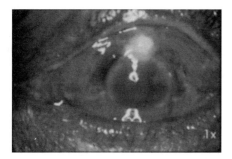

FIG. 19–1. Infected conjunctival bleb with endophthalmitis after glaucoma filtering surgery. *For a color representation of this figure, please see the color insert facing p. 256.*

Postoperative: median of 6 days after surgery with the vast majority within 6 weeks of surgery. When due to a bacteria of low pathogenicity or fungus, it can present later than 6 weeks.

Endogenous: dependent on the organism, ranging from fulminant to insidious with only floaters and mildly decreased vision.

Imaging Studies

When endophthalmitis is suspected, an ultrasound can aid in diagnosis of vitreous inflammation by showing vitreous opacities, choroidal thickening, or choroidal detachment, especially in cases when the view of the posterior pole is poor. Ultrasound also can be useful in following the response of the endophthalmitis to treatment (see Chapter 5).

Computed tomography (CT) is indicated in cases of trauma when a foreign body is suspected (see Chapter 21). Additionally, when spread from an adjacent orbital or periorbital site appears to be the source of the infection, CT scan is necessary to identify possible sinus disease, which would require surgical intervention (see Chapter 10).

Differential Diagnosis

Traumatic: inflammation secondary to the trauma itself, inflammatory reaction to an intraocular foreign body, phacoanaphylaxis if the lens capsule has been violated. The diagnosis of endophthalmitis in the setting of trauma can be difficult due to the disruption of ocular contents secondary to the injury itself. Often, however, signs of endophthalmitis are not present at the time of presentation, prompting prophylactic use of intravitreal antibiotics in the presence of an intraocular foreign body (see Prophylaxis for Penetrating Trauma, below).

Postoperative: postoperative inflammation, phacoanaphylaxis from retained lens material, foreign material retained in the eye, incarceration of intraocular tissues in the operative wound. Late-onset infection with indolent organisms may present as chronic low-grade inflammation that is steroid responsive. In these cases, a white plaque(s) may be present on the posterior capsule or intraocular lens.

Endogenous: retinochoroidal infection, noninfectious posterior uveitis, neoplastic condition.

Culture Sites and Methods

When the diagnosis of endophthalmitis of any type is suspected, or an open globe injury with an intraocular foreign body has occurred, intraocular cultures and cultures of the foreign body should be performed. Both vitreous and aqueous humor should be cultured because occasionally organisms are isolated from one and not the other (6,23–25). The techniques for obtaining cultures are the same for all types of endophthalmitis and may be performed under local retrobulbar anesthesia with or without monitored intravenous sedation. As demonstrated in the Endophthalmitis Vitrectomy Study, for cases of postoperative endophthalmitis, vitrectomy may not be necessary when the presenting visual acuity is hand motions or better but should be performed if visual acuity is light perception (25):

Surface: open wounds, conjunctival discharge or filtering blebs cultured with a cotton-tip applicator.

Systemic: cultures of blood, urine, cerebrospinal fluid if indicated, and other extraocular sites if an endogenous etiology is suspected.

Anterior chamber tap:
1. Surface is prepared with half-strength povidone-iodine 10% (Betadine, Purdue Frederick Co.).
2. A sterile lid speculum is placed.
3. A 27-gauge needle on a tuberculin syringe is used to make a paracentesis tract, removing approximately 0.1 ml of aqueous fluid.

Vitreous tap (attempt only in an eye with liquefied vitreous):
1. Surface is prepared with half-strength Betadine.
2. A sterile lid speculum is placed.
3. A 22- to 25-gauge needle on a tuberculin syringe is used to remove 0.1 ml of vitreous fluid, entering 3 mm posterior to the limbus in the pseudophakic or aphakic (the diameter of the hub of a tuberculin syringe is approximately 3 mm). The needle should be directed toward the center of the globe to avoid the lens in phakic eyes; entry should be less than 1 cm.

Vitreous biopsy:
1. Surface is prepared with half-strength Betadine.
2. A sterile lid speculum is placed.
3. A fornix-based conjunctival flap is prepared with scissors if a standard 20-gauge vitreous cutter is used. This step is not necessary for a 23-gauge or smaller vitreous cutter.
4. A sclerotomy is made either 4.0 mm (in phakic eyes) or 3.0 mm (in pseudophakic eyes) posterior to the limbus with a stiletto knife.

5. The unprimed mechanical vitreous cutter is used to obtain at least 0.5 cc of vitreous gel, which is aspirated into an attached syringe.
6. If a 20-gauge vitreous cutter is used, then the sclerotomy and conjunctiva should be closed with absorbable sutures (e.g., 7-0 polyglactin 910 [Vicryl, Ethicon]).
7. Antibiotics are injected using a 30-gauge needle inserted through the pars plana and visualized behind the lens. Two separate injections are made because the antibiotics cannot be mixed.

Material obtained should be immediately inoculated on culture plates. Cultures should be prepared on blood and chocolate agar and thioglycolate broth and incubated at 37°C, and on blood and Saboraud agar incubated at 25°C. A portion of each sample should be used for immediate Gram, Giemsa, and periodic acid-Schiff stains. Methenamine silver stain (Gomori method) also should be used if fungi are suspected. If culture materials are not available, specimens can be inoculated into blood culture bottles.

Treatment

See Appendix B for instructions on the preparation of antibiotics.

Prophylaxis for Penetrating Trauma

In the management of penetrating trauma, the use of prophylactic antibiotics is generally recommended, with intravitreal antibiotics recommended in the setting of an intraocular foreign body or an injury associated with dirt or vegetable matter, and considered whenever the posterior segment of the eye is involved in the wound. (1,3,21,24,26–29). Because the offending organisms are varied and can be quite virulent, broad-spectrum coverage is indicated. Our regimen for prophylaxis in the management of penetrating trauma is as follows:

Intravenous ceftazidime 1 g every 8 hours
Intravenous vancomycin 1 g intravenously every 12 hours
Topical ciprofloxacin 0.3% every 4 hours
Topical prednisilone acetate 1% every 2 hours
Topical atropine 1% every 12 hours
Oral ciprofloxacin 500 mg twice daily for 1 week after discharge.

The blood-retinal barrier blocks significant penetration of antibiotics into the vitreous. Therefore, in cases in which traumatic endophthalmitis is suspected or the nature of the injury is at high risk for contamination of the globe (including the presence of an intraocular foreign body), intravitreal antibiotics are used. For cases of traumatic endophthalmitis or high-risk injury, we add the following to the above regimen once cultures have been obtained:

Intravitreal ceftazidime 2 mg/0.1 ml
Intravitreal vancomycin 1 mg/0.1 ml
Intravitreal clindamycin 0.5 mg/0.1 ml (if injury is high risk or Bacillus species)
Subconjunctival cefazolin 100 mg
Subconjunctival dexamethasone 12 to 24 mg

Acute and Delayed Postoperative and Endogenous Bacterial Endophthalmitis

When the diagnosis of endophthalmitis is suspected, appropriate cultures are obtained and our regimen for initial treatment of any endophthalmitis is initiated:

Intravitreal ceftazidime 2 mg/0.1 ml
Intravitreal vancomycin 1 mg/0.1 ml
Subconjunctival ceftazidime 100 mg
Subconjunctival vancomycin 25 mg
Subconjunctival dexamethasone 12 to 24 mg
Topical ciprofloxacin 0.3% every 4 hours
Topical fortified cefazolin 50 mg/ml every 1 to 4 hours (or topical fortified vancomycin 50 mg/ml) alternating with ciprofloxacin
Topical prednisilone acetate 1% every 2 hours
Topical atropine 1% every 12 hours

We routinely start systemic steroids, prednisone 1 mg/kg orally every day, 24 hours after appropriate treatment has been initiated provided stains are negative for fungus.

Some ophthalmologists also advocate the use of intravitreal steroids, but we do not routinely use them. A possible beneficial effect of intravitreal steroids is currently being studied in a randomized controlled trial.

The use of intravenous ceftazidime and amikacin in the treatment of acute postoperative endophthalmitis has been shown to have no effect on visual outcome (25). For endogenous bacterial endophthalmitis, the choice of intravenous antibiotics should be made in consultation with the patient's internist with consideration to the likely primary source of the infection.

Endogenous Fungal or Delayed-Onset Postoperative Fungal Endophthalmitis

Only in cases of culture-proven or Gram stain– or Giemsa stain–proven fungal endophthalmitis do we use intravitreal and intravenous antifungals:

Intravitreal amphotericin-B 0.005 mg/0.1 ml (5 μg/0.1 ml)
Systemic fluconazole 100 mg orally twice daily for 2 to 4 weeks or amphotericin-B 0.25 to 1.0 mg/kg/day intravenously in divided doses (consult with internist)
Topical atropine 1% every 12 hours
Topical amphotericin-B 1.5 mg/ml

Vitrectomy is recommended in cases of significant vitreous involvement (30).

Follow-up Treatment

If appropriately treated, patients usually have a dramatic improvement in their pain by the first postoperative day. The antibiotics are changed as indicated by the results of cultures and sensitivities. The clinical course should be closely monitored.

Intravitreal antibiotics maintain therapeutic levels for 24 to 48 hours after injection. Therefore, if there is no clinical response within 48 to 72 hours, or the clinical examination shows signs of deterioration, repeat cultures should be obtained and/or a vitrectomy should be performed if not done previously. Selection of antibiotics should be guided by sensitivities.

Systemic antibiotics, if given, are usually continued for at least 7 days. Intraocular pressure, which may be elevated acutely, should be monitored and treated medically as indicated. Inflammatory signs may persist for weeks, and retinal detachment may be a late complication.

REFERENCES

1. Brinton GS, Topping TM, Hyndiuk RA, Aaberg TM, Reeser FH, Abrams GW. Posttraumatic endophthalmitis. *Arch Ophthalmol* 1984;102:547.
2. Fisch A, Salvanet A, Prazuck T, et al. Epidemiology of infective endophthalmitis in France. *Lancet* 1991;338:1373.
3. Joosse MV, Van Tilburg CJG, Mertens DAE, et al. Endophthalmitis: incidence, therapy, and visual outcome in the period 1983–1992 in the Rotterdam Eye Hospital. *Doc Ophthalmol* 1992;82:115.
4. Nobe JR, Gomez DS, Liggett P, Smith RE, Robin JB. Post-traumatic and postoperative endopthalmitis: a comparison of visual outcomes. *Br J Ophthalmol* 1987;71:614.
5. Kent DG. Endophthalmitis in Auckland 1983–1991. *Aust N Z J Ophthalmol* 1993;21:227.
6. Puliafito CA, Baker AS, Haaf J, Foster CS. Infectious endophthalmitis: review of 36 cases. *Ophthalmology* 1982;89:921.
7. Barr CC. Prognostic factors in corneoscleral lacerations. *Arch Ophthalmol* 1983;101;919.
8. Thompson WS, Rubsamen PE, Flynn HW, Schiffman J, Cousins SW. Endophthalmitis after penetrating trauma: risk factors and visual acuity outcomes. *Ophthalmology* 1995;102:1696.
9. Williams DF, Mieler WF, Abrams GW, Lewis H. Results and prognostic factors in penetrating ocular injuries with retained intraocular foreign bodies. *Ophthalmology* 1988;95:911.
10. Behrens-Baumann W, Pratetorius G. Intraocular foreign bodies: 297 consecutive cases. *Ophthalmologica* 1989;198:84.
11. Thompson JT, Parver LM, Enger CL, Mieler WF, Liggett PE. Infectious endophthalmitis after penetrating injuries with retained intraocular foreign bodies. *Ophthalmology* 1993;100:1468.
12. Javitt JC, Vitale S, Caner JK, et al. National outcomes of cataract extraction: endophthalmitis following inpatient surgery. *Arch Ophthalmol* 1991;109:1085.
13. Kattan HM, Flynn HW Jr, Pflugfelder SC, Robertson C, Forster RK. Nosocomial endophthalmitis survey: current incidence of infection after intraocular surgery. *Ophthalmology* 1991;98:227.
14. Katz LJ, Cantor LB, Spaeth GL. Complications of surgery in glaucoma. *Ophthalmology* 1985;92:959.
15. Okada AA, D Amico DJ. Endogenous endophthalmitis. In: Albert DM, Jakobiec FA, eds. *Principles and Practice of Ophthalmology*. Philadelphia: WB Saunders; 1994:3120.
16. Okada AA, Johnson RP, Liles WC, D'Amico DJ, Baker AS. Endogenous bacterial endopthalmitis. *Ophthalmology* 1994;101:832–838.
17. Peyman GA, Raichand M., Bennett TO. Management of endophthalmitis with pars plana vitrectomy. *Br J Ophthalmol* 1980;64:472.
18. Parke DW II, Jones DB, Gentry LO. Endogenous endopthalmitis among patients with candidemia. *Ophthalmology* 1982;89:789.
19. Speaker MG, Milch FA, Shah MK, Eisner W, Kreiswirth BN. The role of external bacterial flora in the pathogenesis of acute postoperative endophthalmitis. *Ophthalmology* 1991;98:639–649.

20. Sherwood DR, Rich WJ, Jacob S, Hart RJ, Fairchild YL. Bacterial contamination of intraocular and extraocular fluids during extracapsular cataract extraction. *Eye* 1989;3:308–312.
21. Zambrano W, Flynn HW, Pflugfelder SC. Management options for Propionibacterium acnes endophthalmitis. *Ophthalmology* 1989;96:110.
22. Wilson FM. Causes and prevention of endophthalmitis. *Int Ophthalmol Clin* 1987;27:67.
23. Affeldt JC, Flynn HW, Forster RK, Mandelbaum S, Clarkson JG, Jarus GD. Microbial endophthalmitis resulting from ocular trauma. *Ophthalmology* 1987;94:407.
24. Bohigian GM, Olk RJ. Factors associated with a poor visual result in endophthalmitis. *Am J Ophthalmol* 1986;101:332.
25. Endophthalmitis Vitrectomy Study Group. Results of endophthalmitis vitrectomy study: a randomized trial of immediate vitrectomy and of intravenous antibiotics for the treatment of postoperative bacterial endophthalmitis. *Arch Ophthalmol* 1995;113:1479.
26. Mieler WF, Glazer LC, Bennett SR, Han DP. Favourable outcome of traumatic endophthalmitis with associated retinal breaks or detachment. *Can J Ophthalmol* 1002;27:348.
27. Parrish CM, O Day DM. Traumatic endophthalmitis. *Int Ophthalmol Clin* 1987;27:112.
28. Peyman GA, Daun M. Prophylaxis of endophthalmitis. *Ophthalmic Surg* 1994;25:671.
29. Seal DV, Kirkness CM. Criteria for intravitreal antibiotics during surgical removal of intraocular foreign bodies. *Eye* 1992;6:465.
30. Forster RK, Abbott RL, Gelender H. Management of infectious endopthalmitis. *Ophthalmology* 1980;87:313.

Management of Ocular Injuries and Emergencies,
edited by Mathew W. MacCumber.
Lippincott–Raven Publishers, Philadelphia ©1998.

20

Acute Management of Posterior Segment Injuries and Emergencies

Sharon Fekrat, Mathew W. MacCumber, and Eugene de Juan, Jr.

Department of Ophthalmology, Wilmer Eye Institute, The Johns Hopkins University School of Medicine, Baltimore, Maryland 21287 and Retina Service, Department of Ophthalmology, Rush Medical College, Chicago, Illinois 60612

Basic Considerations 285
Vitreous 286
  Vitreous Hemorrhage 286 · Avulsion of the Vitreous Base 290
Choroid 290
  Chorioretinitis Sclopeteria 290 · Choroidal Detachment 291
Retina 294
  Retinal Dialysis 294 · Retinal Breaks without Retinal Detachment 295
  Rhegmatogenous Retinal Detachment 299 · Retinal Incarceration 305

BASIC CONSIDERATIONS

Blunt ocular trauma can result in various posterior segment manifestations that may or may not require surgical intervention. These include a dislocated lens, vitreous hemorrhage, vitreous base avulsion, retinal dialysis, retinal break(s) with or without retinal detachment, chorioretinitis sclopeteria, serous or hemorrhagic choroidal detachment, and occult or obvious partial- or full-thickness scleral rupture.

Open globe injury may result in findings ranging from a partial-thickness scleral laceration over the pars plana without other ocular manifestations to a full-thickness scleral laceration with a vitreous hemorrhage and retinal detachment to an almost unrecognizable and irreparable globe that may require primary enucleation. Each of these situations requires adept surgical judgment and a variety of adaptable surgical skills.

Retinal tear, retinal dialysis, and retinal detachment may or may not present with a history of blunt trauma. In either case, management is similar.

It is important to evaluate and manage all clinical scenarios on an individual case-by-case basis. More than one surgical technique described in this chapter may be needed depending on the clinical features of the individual case (e.g., retinal detachment with vitreous hemorrhage; an intraocular foreign body with a corneal entry site requiring primary corneal closure, possible temporary keratoprosthesis with keratoplasty, lensectomy, and foreign body removal), and management will depend on the judgment and surgical skills of the attending surgeon. Combinations of the surgical techniques described in this chapter as well as elsewhere in this text may be useful in approaching these challenging clinical scenarios to achieve the best possible outcome. Only ophthalmologists with adequate experience should perform vitreoretinal techniques discussed in this chapter, and only fully trained vitreoretinal surgeons should attempt intraocular procedures within the posterior segment.

VITREOUS

Vitreous Hemorrhage

A traumatic vitreous hemorrhage after either blunt or penetrating ocular trauma may result from a retinal break, injury to the uveal tract (iris, ciliary body, choroid), injury to the retinal blood vessels, and/or scleral laceration/rupture. Causes of spontaneous vitreous hemorrhage include proliferative retinopathies (most commonly diabetic), retinal vein occlusion, posterior vitreous detachment with avulsed or torn retinal blood vessel, or breakthrough hemorrhage from choroidal neovascularization.

Diagnosis

1. Ask the patient about history of blunt or penetrating ocular trauma, diabetes mellitus, or sickle cell disease.
2. Red blood cells are present in the vitreous cavity on examination.
3. The presence of a retinal break, retinal detachment, intraocular foreign body, and/or scleral rupture must be excluded. When the hemorrhage obscures adequate retinal examination by indirect ophthalmoscopy, ultrasonography is necessary (see Chapter 5).
4. The best visualization of retinal detail usually is obtained from the initial fundus examination because the hemorrhage is often limited immediately after the injury.

Management

The management of a vitreous hemorrhage varies depending on the etiology. A vitreous hemorrhage due to retinal vascular disease, such as proliferative diabetic retinopathy or retinal vein occlusion, may require scatter laser photocoagulation or pars plana vitrectomy (see Chapter 23). The management of a vitreous hemorrhage due to a retinal break, whether traumatic or not, is described below.

Medical

1. Observation of a vitreous hemorrhage may be warranted when the hemorrhage is the sole ocular injury. No associated retinal break, detachment, intraocular foreign body, or scleral penetration should coexist.
2. When a vitreous hemorrhage does not permit adequate retinal examination, associated intraocular pathology should be excluded with serial ultrasonography.
3. A limited period of bedrest with elevation of the head for 24 hours after presentation may allow gravitational settling of the hemorrhage to permit indirect ophthalmoscopy. If visualization of the fundus is incomplete, ultrasonography should be performed.
4. If the retina is initially attached by ophthalmoscopy or ultrasonography, an isolated hemorrhage may be observed without surgical intervention initially at weekly and then longer intervals for a 3- to 6-month period to permit spontaneous resolution of the hemorrhage. Clinical scenarios that may prompt earlier surgical removal of an isolated hemorrhage include status of the fellow eye, occupation, patient age, and, in some instances, patient anxiety. If the patient is less than 8 years of age, a vitrectomy should be considered after no more than 3 to 4 weeks after injury to decrease the risk of developing deprivation amblyopia (1).
5. Should the retina detach during follow-up, a pars plana vitrectomy with retinal reattachment should then be performed.

Surgical

If an intraocular foreign body or retinal detachment is initially present, or if a retinal detachment develops during follow-up, a prompt pars plana vitrectomy is usually indicated (see Chapter 6).

Pars Plana Vitrectomy

1. If scleral buckle placement is not necessary, the sclera is exposed nasally and temporally by incising overlying conjunctiva. A standard three-port technique is recommended beginning with the inferotemporal port. The eye is entered 3 mm posterior to the limbus in aphakic eyes, 3.5 mm in pseudophakic eyes, and 4 mm in phakic eyes using a microvitreoretinal (MVR) blade, taking care not to touch the lens. The infusion cannula is then inserted into the inferotemporal port with the infusion off and is sutured into place using 4-0 white silk. The tip of the infusion cannula should now be visualized in the eye, free of any overlying tissue, before turning the infusion on (Fig. 20–1). Two additional ports are made superonasally and superotemporally (Fig. 20–2) in a similar fashion. The vitrector handpiece and light pipe are inserted into the eye through these two ports. An irrigating or sew-on contact lens is used for visualization of the posterior segment.

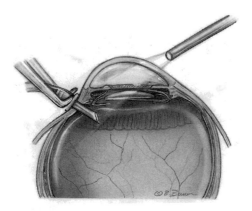

FIG. 20–1. Pars plana vitrectomy. The infusion cannula tip should be seen in the eye, free of overlying tissue, before turning the infusion on.

2. With the infusion on, a core vitrectomy is performed. Avoid hitting the lens with the instruments during insertion and intraocular manipulation. In many eyes, a posterior vitreous detachment (PVD) may be present and may facilitate removal of the posterior hyaloid. If a PVD is not present, one may now be created with careful suction with the vitreous cutter near the edge of the optic disc. If this is unsuccessful, the posterior hyaloid may be engaged with a soft-tipped extrusion cannula (2). More specifically, the vitreous cutter is removed and replaced with a cannula with a flexible silicone tip. The cannula is connected to the aspiration system of the vitrectomy machine with the aspiration set at 100 to 150 mm Hg. The infusion bottle is positioned about 50 cm above the level of the patient's head. The cannula tip is placed 1 mm anterior to the retinal surface and just adjacent to the disc. Aspiration is slowly applied while gently elevating the cannula. If a layer of posterior cortical vitreous is present, the cannula will bend posteriorly. The posterior hyaloid is then elevated with the cannula to further detach it to the equator. In some eyes, additional manipulation is necessary at the disk to complete the posterior hyaloid detachment.

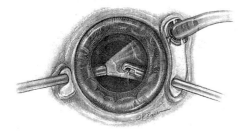

FIG. 20–2. Pars plana vitrectomy. Two additional ports are made superotemporally and superonasally.

3. After the PVD has been created, the vitreous cutter is reinserted. The detached posterior hyaloid face is then incised and any subhyaloid blood may be aspirated from the preretinal space. This blood rarely clots. A blunt cannula connected to the vitrectomy system for automated extrusion or to a fluted handle for passive extrusion may be used to aspirate the preretinal blood. Any remaining vitreous, including the posterior hyaloid, is removed with the vitrector. The soft-tipped cannula is then reinserted, placed 1 mm above the retinal surface, and moved side to side while applying suction. If all of the posterior hyaloid has been removed, the cannula tip will not bend.

4. If the posterior hyaloid is still adherent to the retina in certain areas, it may be resected from adjacent vitreous to release localized vitreoretinal traction. Vitreous traction should be relieved from retinal breaks if possible. If traction persists, a local scleral buckle may be placed. In eyes with history of trauma, sites of persistent vitreoretinal traction should be evaluated for the coexistence of an occult scleral rupture that may be present. The retinal periphery should be examined after completion of the vitrectomy to identify any preexisting or iatrogenic retinal breaks or dialyses.

5. If a retinal detachment is present, its extent must be assessed ophthalmoscopically. Consideration can be given to placement of a scleral buckle at this point (see step 6 below). Make sure the anesthesiologist has stopped nitrous oxide inhalation at least 15 minutes before flattening the retina with fluid air exchange. It is useful to mark retinal breaks with intraocular cautery so they can be identified easily. If the retinal break is anterior, then a posterior drainage site is prepared (ideally superior and nasal to the optic disk). The retina is flattened with fluid-air exchange while subretinal fluid is drained through the retinal break or drainage site with a soft-tipped extrusion cannula. Retinal photocoagulation and/or cryotherapy is applied to all retinal breaks and lastly the drainage site.

6. Residual traction or inferior retinal breaks often require support with a scleral buckle. The details of scleral buckle selection and placement are discussed in the section on retinal detachment later in this chapter. However, in general, a 360-degree conjunctival peritomy is performed and all four rectus muscles are isolated with 2-0 black silk on a Gass muscle hook after adequate preparation and sterile draping of the surgical field. All retinal breaks are isolated and treated with cryotherapy. The scleral buckle, commonly a 41- or 240-band to support the vitreous base with additional circumferential or radial elements to support other breaks, is passed under all four muscles to support the retinal break(s) after proper suture placement.

7. The air is exchanged for long-acting intraocular tamponade (typically 14% C_3F_8 or 20% SF_6) if necessary.

8. Sclerotomy sites are closed with 7-0 Vicryl suture. The conjunctiva is closed with 6-0 plain collagen suture. Subconjunctival antibiotic and steroid are usually injected and the eye dressed with a patch and shield.

Avulsion of the Vitreous Base

Blunt trauma may transmit force to the vitreous body, leading to acute severe vitreoretinal traction. Rapid displacement of the vitreous may lead to avulsion of the vitreous base with or without an associated retinal break.

Diagnosis

1. After excluding the possibility of scleral rupture, careful indirect ophthalmoscopy with scleral depression should be performed on all patients to exclude the presence of a vitreous base avulsion.
2. The presence of a retinal dialysis or other associated retinal break also must be excluded at the time of presentation.

Management

Medical

Observation is warranted if a retinal break or dialysis is not present.

Surgical

1. If a retinal break or dialysis is present, surgical treatment for these entities may proceed as discussed later in this chapter.
2. If other associated ocular pathology exists such as a vitreous hemorrhage, management should be dictated by the concurrent pathology.

CHOROID

Chorioretinitis Sclopeteria

Chorioretinitis sclopeteria results from a direct contusion injury to the eye, often from a high-speed missile brushing against the eye wall, that produces a chorioretinal but not scleral rupture. The direct injury due to the missile's path leads to pressure necrosis. Indirect injury due to transmission of shock waves from the impact site usually occurs in the posterior pole and results in disruption of photoreceptors known as Berlin's edema (see Chapter 22).

Diagnosis

1. Large areas of irregular, jagged retinal holes may be observed in the affected area.
2. Marked vitreous, intraretinal, and subretinal hemorrhage may obscure the view. Ultrasonography is then necessary to exclude an underlying retinal detachment.

3. As the hemorrhage resolves, the characteristic retinal pigment epithelium (RPE) proliferation and subretinal scar formation become evident.
4. The retinal breaks rarely result in detachment in these eyes because inflammation at the edges of necrotic retina produces a firm chorioretinal adhesion. If a detachment does occur, it is usually from another site. Thus, retinal breaks outside the area of sclopeteria may be the cause of a retinal detachment and their presence should be excluded.
5. Chorioretinitis sclopeteria should not be confused with choroidal rupture (see Chapter 22).

Management

Medical

1. Observation is indicated in most cases.
2. Should a retinal detachment develop during follow-up, it is usually from another site.

Surgical

1. A pars plana vitrectomy may be necessary if an associated vitreous hemorrhage does not resolve.
2. Prophylactic retinopexy with cryotherapy or laser photocoagulation to the area of sclopeteria is not necessary. A retinal break outside the affected area should be treated with retinopexy.
3. A retinal detachment or other associated ocular pathology should be treated.

Choroidal Detachment

There are two types of choroidal detachment: serous and hemorrhagic. Although both types may result from blunt trauma to a nonruptured globe, they are usually associated with blunt rupture or penetrating injury of the eye, particularly scleral lacerations or even after perforation of a corneal ulcer (3).

Nontraumatic choroidal detachments may occur intraoperatively as well as postoperatively in hypotonous eyes. After traumatic or surgical rupture of a globe, the pressure differential produces a sudden decrease in the extraluminal pressure surrounding the choroidal vessels. The choroidal vessels then dilate. A long or short posterior ciliary arterial vessel may rupture, for example, leading to a hemorrhagic choroidal detachment. Choroidal detachments also occur secondary to intraocular inflammation (e.g., uveitis or endophthalmitis) and after pan-retinal photocoagulation or scleral buckling procedure.

One must confirm that a choroidal melanoma is not coincidentally present in an eye with a hemorrhagic choroidal detachment despite the history of blunt trauma without rupture. One may be mistaken for the other (4).

Diagnosis

1. Both serous and hemorrhagic detachments may present as smooth, bullous, orange elevations of the retina and choroid that may extend 360 degrees around the periphery in a lobular configuration. The ora serrata may be visualized without scleral depression.
2. Findings in a nonruptured globe with a serous detachment include a low intraocular pressure (usually less than 6 mm Hg), a shallow anterior chamber, mild cell and flare, and normal transillumination.
3. Findings in a nonruptured globe with a hemorrhagic detachment include a high intraocular pressure, a shallow anterior chamber, mild cell and flare, and no transillumination. The patient usually complains of pain.
4. Hemorrhagic detachments also may occur suddenly during an intraocular surgical procedure, most commonly cataract extraction, trabeculectomy, or penetrating keratoplasty. Initially there will be increased positive pressure with shallowing of the anterior chamber followed by loss of the red reflex and expulsion of intraocular contents if the wound is not immediately closed.
5. Ultrasonography may distinguish between a choroidal hemorrhage and a choroidal melanoma in the nonruptured globe and between a serous and hemorrhagic choroidal detachment (see Chapter 5).

Management

The management of a nontraumatic choroidal detachment is the same as that of traumatic choroidal detachment.

Medical

1. Most choroidal detachments, even those associated with an overlying retinal detachment, may be observed initially. Indications for medical management include a choroidal detachment limited to one or two quadrants, normal intraocular pressure, no pain, no retina-iris contact, no vitreous hemorrhage, and no retinal detachment (Table 20–1).
2. Atropine 1% four times daily and prednisolone acetate 1% four times daily. In some cases when risk of infection is low, and the choroidal detachment is hem-

TABLE 20–1. *Indications for medical management of a choroidal detachment*

Choroidal detachment limited to one or two quadrants
Normal intraocular pressure
No pain
No retina–iris contact
No vitreous hemorrhage
No retinal detachment

orrhagic, oral prednisone (1 mg/kg with rapid taper over 1 week) may be given to prevent secondary scarring and adhesion formation.

3. Serous detachments are usually managed conservatively; however, surgical drainage may be needed for a flat or progressively shallow anterior chamber, especially with associated intraocular inflammation.
4. "Kissing" choroidal detachments, whether serous or hemorrhagic, require drainage within 7 to 10 days. Drainage is more successful if the choroidal hemorrhage is liquefied on ultrasonography. If not kissing, they may be followed ultrasonographically until they decrease in height or the hemorrhage liquefies.
5. Hemorrhagic detachments are often associated with corneal or scleral lacerations. In these eyes, the laceration is primarily repaired (see Chapter 15). The hemorrhagic detachment is treated medically until the eye undergoes a secondary reparative procedure.

Surgical

1. Indications for surgical management of a hemorrhagic or serous choroidal detachment in an intact globe include an intraocular pressure greater than 30 mm Hg despite maximum medical management, a flat anterior chamber, pain, retinal apposition, and/or retina-iris apposition (5) (Table 20–2). In an intact globe with a hemorrhagic detachment, the presence of a choroidal melanoma should be excluded by ultrasonography before surgical intervention.
2. To drain a choroidal detachment in an intact globe, a 23- or 25-gauge needle or anterior chamber infusion cannula is inserted through the limbus into the anterior chamber. In aphakic or pseudophakic eyes with a posterior capsulotomy, fluid is infused into the anterior chamber to maintain intraocular volume and to facilitate drainage through the sclerotomy site. Air also may be used by pumping it into the eye at a continuous pressure of 25 mm Hg to push the blood posteriorly out of the drainage site. Sodium hyaluronate or penfluorocarbon liquid may be used as an alternative to facilitate drainage by replacing intraocular volume and displacing the choroidal hemorrhage (7). A cyclodialysis spatula placed through the sclerotomy against the inner aspect of the sclera may aid in lysing a clot to speed drainage (Fig. 20–3B).
3. Before drainage of a choroidal detachment in a ruptured globe, the globe must be primarily repaired. The following procedures may be performed within 7 to

TABLE 20–2. *Indications for surgical management of a hemorrhagic or serous choroidal detachment in an intact globe*

Intraocular pressure >30 mm Hg despite maximum medical management
Flat anterior chamber
Pain
Retinal apposition
Retina–iris apposition

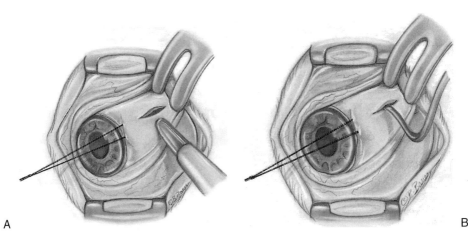

A

B

FIG. 20–3. A: Drainage of suprachoroidal hemorrhage. A suture passed near the limbus provides traction to rotate the globe and improve exposure. Infusion of fluid into the anterior chamber is not shown. **B:** A cyclodialysis spatula can be inserted against the inner aspect of the sclera to break up the clot and improve drainage.

10 days after primary repair unless earlier intervention is indicated. A pars plana vitrectomy (as described earlier in this chapter) should be performed before drainage of the choroidal detachment so that traction from vitreous incarcerated into the wound will not cause an iatrogenic retinal break during drainage (6). Placement of the infusion cannula through the pars plana may be difficult due to the bullous choroidal detachment and resultant forward rotation of the pars plana; thus, it is not recommended because of the high likelihood of causing retinal damage during instrument insertion. Instead, balanced saline solution may be infused into the anterior chamber through an anterior chamber infusion cannula inserted at the corneoscleral limbus. The vitrectomy instrument also may be inserted at the limbus in an aphakic eye. Note that the lens in these traumatized eyes is likely cataractous or dislocated (see Chapter 18) or has been extruded from the eye at the time of the injury, producing aphakia. Once vitreous traction is released, then saline or air infusion may proceed to facilitate drainage of the choroidal blood. An anterior radial sclerotomy site(s) is then created over the affected area using a rounded blade at least 3 mm posterior to the limbus and measuring about 3 to 4 mm in length (Fig. 20–3A). If any preexisting retinal apposition has been alleviated and the anterior chamber depth maintained, further drainage is usually not necessary.

RETINA

Retinal Dialysis

A retinal dialysis, larger than one oral bay, is the most common retinal break due to blunt trauma (8) and may be present in up to 85% of traumatic retinal detachments (9). The most common locations are the superonasal and inferotemporal quadrants because most blunt trauma strikes the globe inferotemporally (10,11).

Diagnosis

1. Using indirect ophthalmoscopy with scleral indentation, disinsertion of the retina from the ora is found for one or more clock hours (Fig. 20–4).
2. Myopic eyes are typically susceptible to a dialysis in the superonasal quadrant.
3. If an associated vitreous hemorrhage prevents adequate retinal examination, ultrasonography is necessary.
4. Because the vitreous in young trauma patients is a solid gel without areas of liquefaction, a retinal detachment caused by a traumatic dialysis usually advances slowly, especially in the inferior half of the eye, and may go undiagnosed.

Management

Surgical

1. If no other concurrent ocular injuries requiring surgical intervention are present, laser photocoagulation or external cryopexy (Fig. 20–4) to the dialysis is indicated.
2. With associated retinal detachment, support with a circumferential scleral buckle or pneumatic retinopexy is necessary.

Retinal Breaks without Retinal Detachment

Transmission of blunt force to the vitreous gel results in sudden vitreoretinal traction. Acute displacement of the vitreous may tear the retina and cause a variety of retinal breaks, including a retinal dialysis with or without avulsion of the vitreous base; a horseshoe-shaped retinal tear at the posterior margin of the vitreous base, at a meridional fold or cystic retinal tuft, and/or at the equator; an operculated retinal tear; or a macular hole, among others (8,12).

Spontaneous symptomatic retinal breaks are often associated with posterior vitreous detachment and usually require treatment (see also Chapter 23 under Posterior Vitreous Detachment).

Diagnosis

1. Pigment may be present in the anterior vitreous cavity (Shafer's sign).
2. A retinal break(s) (horseshoe tear, operculated hole, dialysis, etc.) may be identified on examination. Scleral indentation during indirect ophthalmoscopy is essential.
3. After blunt trauma, small, radial, slit-shaped tears in the paravascular retina between the equator and posterior pole may occur at sites of strong perivascular vitreoretinal adhesion due to sudden separation of the vitreous from retina (13). A vitreous hemorrhage may occur concurrently.

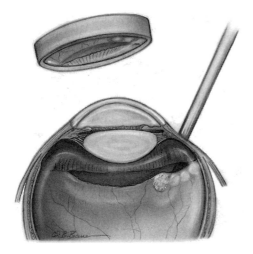

FIG. 20–4. Retinal dialysis. Using indirect ophthalmoscopy with scleral indentation, disinsertion of the retina from the ora may be found for one or more clock hours. External cryotherapy is applied to the dialysis, as shown.

Management

The management of a nontraumatic retinal break without an associated retinal detachment is the same as that for a traumatic break.

The treatment goal is to create an adhesion between the retina and RPE to seal the edge of the break and prevent fluid entry into the subretinal space. One of three approaches may accomplish this: diathermy, cryotherapy, or laser photocoagulation. Diathermy is rarely used. The two remaining modalities demonstrate similar retinal adhesion 14 days after treatment (14); however, differences in adhesion are present immediately posttreatment. Laser photocoagulation increases retinal adhesion within 24 hours posttreatment (15), whereas cryopexy decreases retinal adhesion for 1 week after application. Laser photocoagulation is more convenient to administer provided the media are clear and causes less blood-ocular barrier breakdown (16) but can be difficult to place anteriorly.

Surgical

Laser Photocoagulation.

Laser retinopexy may be delivered using a slit lamp, an indirect ophthalmoscope, an endoprobe (17), or trans-sclerally (18,19). The desired end point ophthalmoscopically is similar with each system: two to three rows of adjacent burns around the retinal break resulting in retinal whitening (Fig. 20–5). The retina must be attached or shallowly detached for effective application. The anterior border of the break also should be treated appropriately.

Always be sure that the appropriate laser filters are in position and operational before starting treatment.

Slit-lamp laser delivery system.

1. Topical anesthesia is usually adequate. Retrobulbar anesthesia may be necessary in some patients.
2. A Goldmann or pan-funduscopic contact lens may be used.
3. Argon green is recommended; however, krypton red or yellow dye may be required to penetrate vitreous hemorrhage or lenticular opacity.
4. The following parameters are used for the argon green laser: 0.1-second duration, 300 spot size, and variable power settings.
5. Adjusting the eye position or tilting the lens may improve the view of the break being treated.

Laser indirect ophthalmoscope delivery system.

1. Topical anesthesia, subconjunctival infiltration of 2% lidocaine in the affected area, or a retrobulbar anesthetic may be necessary. Retrobulbar anesthesia causes akinesia that may interfere with adequate treatment of anterior breaks.
2. The use of an indirect ophthalmoscope may facilitate treatment of selected peripheral retinal breaks.
3. Simultaneous scleral indentation may be necessary, may stabilize the globe for treatment, and may appose the RPE and retina in the presence of subretinal fluid to allow the uptake of laser energy.
4. Argon green is recommended; however, krypton also may be used. The following parameters are suggested: variable power settings, and 0.1- to 0.3-second duration.
5. A 20- or 28-diopter hand-held lens may be used.

Intraocular laser photocoagulation with endoprobe.

1. This is performed intraoperatively during intraocular posterior segment surgery to reattach the retina.
2. Argon green is recommended. The parameters are a 0.5-second duration with variable power settings starting at 300 mW. The spot size and retinal burn intensity may be varied by changing the distance between the tip of the endoprobe and the retinal surface. The closer the probe tip to the retinal surface, the larger the spot size and the more intense the retinal burn.

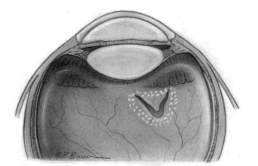

FIG. 20–5. The ophthalmoscopic end point after laser photocoagulation to a retinal break is two to three rows around it of contiguous burns that result in retinal whitening.

Transscleral diode laser delivery system.

1. The trans-scleral diode laser may be used in eyes as an alternative to the indirect ophthalmoscope and where slit-lamp delivery is not possible due to opaque media or to anterior location of a retinal break, when intraocular posterior segment surgery is not planned, and where cryopexy is not feasible due to the presence of a scleral buckling element in the affected area. The diode laser may penetrate solid silicone scleral buckles (18,19). The use of the diode laser is becoming more common.

2. Subconjunctival infiltration of 2% lidocaine in the area to be treated is usually sufficient.

3. The probe may be placed directly on the conjunctiva or scleral surface over the affected area for delivery.

4. The recommended settings are 1.0- to 2.0-second duration at variable power settings starting at 500 mW and increasing to achieve the ophthalmoscopically visible end point of retinal whitening. The spot size is not variable.

Cryotherapy.

1. Cryotherapy applications generate temperatures as low as −89°C due to expansion of high-pressure nitrous oxide at the probe tip (2.5 mm in diameter). An insulating sleeve localizes the freezing effect to the probe tip.

2. Topical anesthetic and subconjunctival 2% lidocaine are necessary. Retrobulbar anesthesia causes akinesia that may interfere with adequate treatment of anterior breaks.

3. A lid speculum provides good exposure. A conjunctival peritomy is not necessary.

4. The indentation of the probe is seen ophthalmoscopically and is aligned with the break. The end point of each application is retinal whitening without ice crystal formation. To avoid posterior freezes, the probe tip should be accurately positioned for precise indentation so that the indentation seen ophthalmoscopically is from the probe tip and not the shaft (Fig. 20–6A).

5. The first freeze should be done at the most anterior part of the lesion to evaluate the location and intensity of treatment.

6. All retinal breaks should be surrounded by 1 to 2 mm of contiguous treatment (Fig. 20–6B), although treatment should not overlap to avoid the effects of refreezing. Small retinal breaks and atrophic retinal holes may be completely treated with a single application centered on the break. Larger retinal breaks require several applications to all margins of the break. For flap retinal tears, treatment is performed contiguously around the tear and then extended to the ora anteriorly. Do not treat bare RPE within the break.

7. Treatment of overlying retina is preferable to only treating underlying RPE because a stronger adhesion is obtained (20). If bullous retinal elevation prevents treatment of the retina, the RPE alone may be treated or the treatment postponed until the subretinal fluid can be evacuated.

8. After each application, the tip of the cryoprobe should adequately thaw before removing it from the surface of the eye to prevent pulling adjacent tissue.

9. Cryotherapy may result in the dispersion of RPE cells that may lead to prolifer-

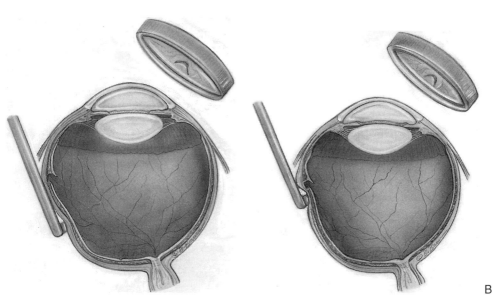

B

FIG. 20–6. A: Improper placement of cryotherapy. To avoid posterior freezes, the probe tip should be accurately positioned for precise indentation so that the indentation seen ophthalmoscopically is from the probe tip and not the shaft. **B:** Proper placement of cryotherapy. For flap retinal tears, treatment is performed contiguously around the tear and then extended anteriorly to the ora. Avoid treating bare RPE in the bed of the break.

ative vitreoretinopathy (21,22) and thus should not be used beyond that required.

Rhegmatogenous Retinal Detachment

Spontaneous rhegmatogenous retinal detachment (RRD) is the result of a retinal break under traction. The retinal break in spontaneous RRD is most commonly an anterior horseshoe tear secondary to posterior vitreous detachment.

An acute RRD due to blunt trauma is not common because most patients with eye trauma are young and have a solid vitreous gel. This gel internally tamponades the retina, preventing the development of an RRD despite the presence of a retinal break. By carefully examining the retina soon after the injury and treating any retinal break(s), the formation of an RRD may be avoided in many eyes. The initiating event in the development of an acute RRD after blunt trauma is the formation of a retinal break(s) (more often a retinal dialysis) due to the anteroposterior compression of the globe, lateral expansion of the equatorial area, and sudden vitreoretinal traction. Traumatic syneresis of the vitreous gel over the break may occur either immediately or many months later. The liquefied vitreous may then dissect under the retinal break and produce an RRD. Note that an RRD also may occur many months after the trauma due to the development of a posterior vitreous detachment or proliferative vitreoretinopathy. Retinal breaks also may occur from direct contusion to the eye and subsequent tissue necrosis (chorioretinitis sclopeteria), although these breaks rarely result in a RRD.

Diagnosis

1. A history of photopsias, floaters, visual field loss, and/or a decrease in central visual acuity in most cases.
2. Pigmented cells in the anterior vitreous (Shafer's sign), particularly pigment clumps, are present in the majority of eyes.
3. A vitreous hemorrhage may prevent adequate ophthalmoscopy, thus requiring ultrasonography.
4. A Weiss ring suggests that a posterior vitreous detachment is present.
5. A lower intraocular pressure in the affected eye may be present.
6. A varying degree of retinal elevation is present with one or more retinal break(s). In one series, retinal breaks were limited to the ora serrata in 59% of 158 eyes with retinal detachment caused by ocular contusion (8) and were posterior to the ora in 23%. About 9% of the breaks were posterior to the equator.
7. The detached retina has a corrugated appearance and moves with eye movement. The clear subretinal fluid does not shift with changes in body position.

Management

The management of a nontraumatic retinal detachment is similar to that for traumatic detachments.

Most traumatic retinal detachments may be reattached with conventional scleral buckling techniques. An encircling element is recommended in all eyes due to the potential for retinal damage 180 degrees from the impact site. The retinal break(s) must be adequately supported on the encircling element. The method of retinopexy used and the decision to drain subretinal fluid are determined using the same principles as for nontraumatic detachments (23,24).

Retinal detachment due to a superior retinal break less than one clock hour in size can also be managed with pneumatic retinopexy (23). The pathogenesis of the detachment, the clinical setting, and the experience of the vitreoretinal surgeon should dictate which modality is used. The encircling scleral buckle procedure has the highest overall success rate, so it is presented here.

Timing of surgical intervention varies depending on whether the macula is attached or detached on presentation (see Chapter 6).

Surgical

Indications for scleral buckle placement include the presence of a macula-on or macula-off RRD or the prevention of retinal detachment in an eye at high risk for detachment (e.g., after posterior penetrating trauma).

An RRD less commonly results from a retinal dialysis, a giant retinal tear (see Fig. 23-6), or a macular hole. Treatment of a giant retinal tear–associated retinal detachment is beyond the scope of this text. A retinal detachment caused by a traumatic macular hole is uncommon and may be more commonly seen in highly myopic eyes. It is best treated with a pars plana vitrectomy and internal subretinal fluid drainage through the macular hole while air is simultaneously infused into the vitreous cavity (24) followed by an air-gas (14% C_3F_8) exchange. Laser photocoagulation to the macular hole is controversial and is not generally advocated.

Procedure: Encircling Scleral Buckle (25).
1. General anesthesia with endotracheal intubation or local (retrobulbar, peribulbar, sub-Tenon's) anesthesia with a 1:1 mixture of 4% lidocaine and 0.75% bupivicaine with 150 units of hyaluronidase per 10 cc plus supplemental intravenous analgesia may be used.
2. A 360-degree conjunctival peritomy is made with radial relaxing incisions superonasally and inferotemporally. Closed, blunt scissors are placed in the space between Tenon's capsule and sclera in each quadrant between the rectus muscles to lyse the episcleral fascial connections between the sclera and Tenon's. A fenestrated muscle hook (26) with 2-0 black silk suture is used to isolate each muscle insertion by placing the hook tangential to the sclera and sliding it posterior to the muscle insertion in a circumferential direction. The hook engages the insertion when brought anteriorly. Avoid the oblique muscles and vortex veins during this manuever. The hook is removed, the stay suture remains, and the ends knotted.
3. The next step is to localize the retinal break(s) using indirect ophthalmoscopy and the end of a cotton-tipped applicator or an O'Connor localizer (27). Before localization, the surface of the sclera is inspected in each quadrant for scleral thinning, staphyloma, occult rupture, or vortex veins. The area of the retinal break is then marked with a sterile marking pen. Both the anterior and posterior extent of the break is localized when larger flap tears, nonradial tears, or dialyses are present. Note that a highly elevated break may appear more posterior than its true location.
4. Treatment of the retinal break(s) is usually performed intraoperatively with cryotherapy (see above) before placing the encircling explant. However, if desired, the encircling element may be placed first and subretinal fluid drained to facilitate close apposition of the retina and RPE, followed by indirect laser treatment of the retinal break(s) for chorioretinal adhesion.
5. After identification, localization, and treatment of all retinal breaks, an encircling explant is chosen. Explants are made of either solid silicone rubber or silicone sponges and come in various sizes and shapes (Fig. 20–7). Three basic shapes of solid silicone rubber are available: straight, symmetric tire, and asymmetric tire. Asymmetric tires provide increased buckle height posteriorly. All three allow placement of an encircling band.
6. Once an explant is chosen (e.g., a 41-, 42-, or 240-band with or without a supplemental 286 or 287 tire), proper placement of the element requires effective

suturing technique. A spatulated needle with a 5-0 nonabsorbable suture such as nylon may be used while firmly fixating the globe with a toothed forcep. Magnification with loupes is helpful. The spatulated needle should be firmly grasped by the needle holder about two thirds of the distance from its tip where the needle is flat to allow good control of the needle (Fig. 20–8A). The anterior one fourth of the needle is oriented tangentially to the sclera, and the sclera is depressed with the needle to elevate fibers in front of the needle's cutting edge. The needle is then passed at partial-thickness depth through the sclera parallel to its surface. The needle tip must be visualized at all times. The suture is passed through the sclera at one-half to three-fourths depth over a distance of 3 to 5 mm, usually in a horizontal mattress fashion (Fig. 20–8B and C). Complete the passage of the needle along the arc of the needle to avoid perforation of the hub of the needle through the globe (Fig. 20–8D). The sutures are usually positioned 1 to 2 mm farther apart than the width of scleral contact for a given explant. The spacing of the mattress sutures from the element and amount of tightening are the principal means of increasing the indentation. Placement of the mattress suture in the same meridian as the retinal break provides additional height beneath the break. The chosen explant and band are then passed under each of the four rectus muscles and through each preplaced suture. Note that the precise localization and placement of the element with respect to the retinal break(s) is more important to the successful reattachment than the actual element used. Radial elements may be required to provide additional support to breaks that are under excessive traction or extend posteriorly.

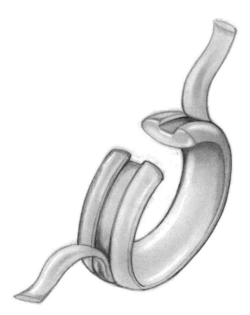

FIG. 20–7. Explants are made of either solid silicone rubber or silicone sponges and come in various sizes and shapes.

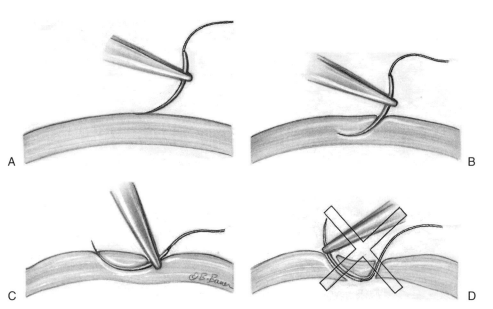

A　　　　B

C　　　　D

FIG. 20–8. A,B: Suture placement to secure explant. The spatulated needle should be firmly grasped by the needle holder about two thirds of the distance from its tip where the needle is flat to allow good control. **C,D:** Complete the passage of the needle along the arc of the needle to avoid perforation of the hub of the needle through the globe.

A Watzke sleeve is placed through both ends of the band (usually super-onasally). The sutures are then tied to themselves and the buckle height adjusted by indirect ophthalmoscopic examination and suture adjustment.

7. To flatten the retina onto the buckling element, the drainage of subretinal fluid may be necessary. Drainage decreases intraocular volume and allows an increase in buckle height, without developing elevated intraocular pressure. The retina may then be apposed to the RPE on the elevated buckle. Indications for subretinal fluid drainage vary (Table 20–3). An external drainage site is chosen after scleral sutures and buckle have been placed to ensure that the amount or location of fluid remains unchanged during globe manipulation. Drainage may be performed in the bed of the scleral buckling element in a location with adequate fluid to allow safe entry into the subretinal space, usually just superior or inferior to either horizontal meridian, avoiding vortex veins. Avoid drainage through areas previously treated with cryotherapy or near retinal break(s) to prevent entry of vitreous into the subretinal space and out of the drainage site. Before entering the subretinal space, a 4-mm radial sclerotomy perpendicular to the sclera is prepared under magnification with a rounded blade down to choroid. A 5-0 nylon mattress suture is placed through the scleral edges of the sclerotomy to close the sclerotomy when drainage is finished. Diathermy to the scleral margins of the sclerotomy shrink the adjacent sclera to improve ex-

TABLE 20–3. *Indications for subretinal fluid drainage during scleral buckling retinal reattachment surgery*

Decrease intraocular volume for high scleral buckle indentation
No identifiable retinal break
Accurate localization in highly bullous detachments
Inferior retinal break(s)
Reoperation
Highly myopic or aphakic eyes
Poor RPE function
Glaucoma

posure. If major choroidal vessels are noted, select another drainage site. The choroid may be diathermized to decrease bleeding on entry. A 30-gauge needle may be used to enter the subretinal space and puncture the choroid, either tangentially or perpendicularly. The needle is removed and the entry site inspected. To prevent retinal incarceration during drainage, a normal and constant intraocular pressure should be maintained. If a hemorrhage occurs during drainage, maintain pressure on the eye to allow blood to leave through the sclerotomy site until a clot forms, instead of blood filling the subretinal space and threatening the macula. Indentation of the globe at the ora in the meridian of the drainage opening elevates the retina over the site and pushes fluid toward the opening. When pigment appears in the fluid, the drainage may almost be complete. If drainage stops prematurely, the sclera near the sclerotomy can be manipulated with forceps. When drainage ceases, the preplaced sclerotomy suture is tied. Check for residual fluid with indirect ophthalmoscopy. If no further fluid needs drainage, the buckle sutures are tightened, secured with temporary ties, and the retina is again examined. If the breaks are well-supported on the encircling element, the sutures may be tied. The suture knot should be rotated posteriorly.

8. A commonly encountered problem when placing an encircling scleral buckle is fishmouthing of retinal breaks (Fig. 20–9). Ways to correct this include decreasing the buckle height to relieve the radial folding of the retina, moving the encircling band more posterior, adding a radial element posterior to the encircling element, and/or injecting an intravitreal gas bubble (e.g., C_3F_8) with proper postoperative patient positioning. Avoid multiple small gas bubbles during injection to prevent subretinal gas and retinal redetachment.

9. The band is tightened and indirect ophthalmoscopy is performed to assess perfusion of the central retinal artery and buckle height. If the the central retinal artery is not perfused, the band must be loosened or fluid removed from the anterior chamber via a 30-gauge needle on a tuberculin (TB) syringe passed through the limbus.

10. The 2-0 silk sutures are removed and the conjunctiva (and Tenon's capsule) is closed with 6-0 plain collagen suture. Usually, subconjunctival antibiotic

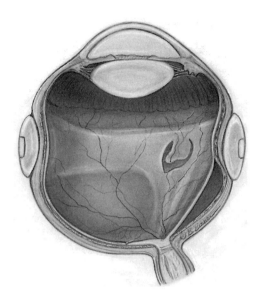

FIG. 20–9. A commonly encountered problem when placing an encircling scleral buckle is fishmouthing of retinal breaks.

with or without steroid is administered and the eye dressed with patch and shield.

Retinal Incarceration

Focal retinal incarceration may occur during the drainage of subretinal fluid or as a result of a blunt or penetrating injury with scleral rupture and may remain incarcerated despite attempts at repositing it during primary closure. Several mechanisms may result in incarceration of retina into the wound as a result of a scleral rupture:

1. At the time of injury, both vitreous and retina near the wound may be extruded.
2. Retina distant to the wound that is adherent to vitreous may be pulled into the wound as vitreous is extruded.
3. The fibrosis that occurs during the healing of the rupture site, whether it sealed without surgical intervention or was too posterior for surgical apposition, may progressively pull the retina toward the wound.
4. The retina remained incarcerated in the wound despite primary repair of the scleral rupture and simultaneous attempts at repositing it.

Diagnosis

1. A prior history of blunt or penetrating trauma in the affected eye is present with or without a history of primary surgical repair.

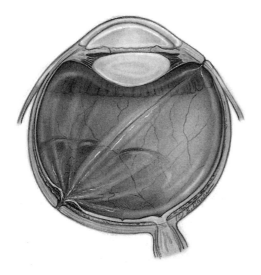

FIG. 20–10. Note how the retina may have a star-fold configuration at the point of incarceration into a scleral laceration or rupture.

2. On examination, a vitreous hemorrhage may be present. The retina has a star-fold configuration at the point of incarceration (Fig. 20–10). Surrounding retina is usually detached with fixed folds radiating toward the central wound.

3. The scleral wound size, the amount of incarcerated retina, and the extent and chronicity of fibrous proliferation at the incarceration site determine the amount of retinal shortening and contraction present.

Management

Surgical

1. If anterior and localized, support with a scleral buckling element may be all that is necessary.

2. If retinal detachment is present or the incarceration site posterior, then repair is complex. Surgical approach would require pars plana vitrectomy with mechanical removal of the retina from the incarceration site or localized retinectomy.

REFERENCES

1. Ferrone PJ, de Juan Jr E. Vitreous hemorrhage infants. *Arch Ophthalmol* 1994;112:1185.
2. Kelly NE, Wendel RT. Vitreous surgery for idiopathic macular holes: results of a pilot study. *Arch Ophthalmol* 1991;109:654.
3. Reynolds M, Haimovici R, Flynn H, DiBernardo C, Byrne S, Feuer W. Suprachoroidal hemorrhage: clinical features and results of secondary surgical management. *Ophthalmology* 1993;100:460.
4. Morgan C, Gragoudas E. Limited choroidal hemorrhage mistaken for a choroidal melanoma. *Ophthalmology* 1987;94:41.
5. Abrams GW, Thomas M, Williams G, Burton T. Management of postoperative suprachoroidal hemorrhage with continuous-infusion air pump. *Arch Ophthalmol* 1986;104:1455.

6. Welch J, Spaeth G, Benson W. Massive suprachoroidal hemorrhage: follow-up and outcome of 30 cases. *Ophthalmology* 1988;95:1202.
7. Baldwin L, Smith T, Hollins J, Pearson P. The use of viscoelastic substances in the drainage of post-operative suprachoroidal hemorrhage. *Ophthalmic Surg* 1989;20:504.
8. Cox MS, Schepens CL, Freeman HM. Retinal detachment due to ocular penetration: I. Clinical characteristics and surgical results. *Arch Ophthalmol* 1966;76:678.
9. Sternberg P Jr. Trauma: principles and techniques of treatment. In: Ryan SJ, ed. *Retina.* 2nd ed. St. Louis: CV Mosby; 1994:2351.
10. Ross WH. Traumatic retinal dialysis. *Arch Ophthalmol* 1981;99:1374.
11. Zion VM, Burton TC. Retinal dialysis. *Arch Ophthalmol* 1980;98:1971.
12. Weidenthal DT, Schepens CL. Peripheral fundus changes associated with ocular contusion. *Am J Ophthalmol* 1966;62:465.
13. Cooling RJ. Traumatic retinal detachment mechanisms and management. *Trans Ophthalmol Soc UK* 1986;105:575.
14. Kita M, Negi A, Kawano S, Honda Y. Photothermal, cryogenic and diathermic effects on retinal adhesive force in vivo. *Retina* 1991;11:441.
15. Folk JC, Sneed ST, Folberg R, Coonan P, Pulido JS. Early retinal adhesion from laser photocoagulation. *Opthhalmology* 1989;96:1523.
16. Jaccoma EH, Conway BP, Campochiaro PA. Cryotherapy causes extensive breakdown of the blood-retinal barrier: a comparison with argon laser photocoagulation. *Arch Ophthalmol* 1985;103: 1728.
17. Smiddy WE, Chong LP. Retinopexy. In: Wright KE, ed. *Retinal Surgery and Ocular Trauma: Color Atlas of Ophthalmic Surgery.* Philadelphia: JB Lippincott; 1995:25.
18. Jennings T, Fuller T, Vukovich JA, et al. Transscleral retinal photocoagulation with 810 nm semiconductor diode laser. *Ophthalmic Surg* 1990;21:492.
19. Peyman GA, Naguib K, Gaasterland DE. Transscleral application of semi-conductor diode laseer. *Lasers Surg Med* 1990;10:569.
20. Laqua H, Machemer R. Repair and adhesion mechanisms of the cryotherapy lesion in experimental retinal detachment. *Am J Opthalmol* 1976;81:833.
21. Campochiaro PA, Kaden IH, Vidaurri-Leal J, Glaser B. Cryotherapy enhances intravitreal dispersion of viable retinal pigment epithelial cells. *Arch Ophthalmol* 1985;103:434.
22. Singh AK, Michels RG, Glaser BM. Scleral indentation following cryotherapy and repeat cryotherapy enhance release of viable retinal pigment epithelial cells. *Retina* 1986;6:176.
23. Michels RG, Wilkinson CP, Rice TA. *Retinal Detachment.* St. Louis: CV Mosby; 1990.
24. Harris MJ, deBustros S, Michels RG. Treatment of retinal detachments due to macular holes. *Retina* 1984;4:144.
25. Williams GA, Aaberg TM Sr. Techniques of scleral buckling. In: Ryan SJ, ed. *Retina.* 2nd ed. St. Louis: CV Mosby; 1994:1979.
26. Gass JDM. Fenestrated muscle hook for retinal detachment surgery. *Arch Ophthalmol* 1967;77: 676.
27. O'Connor PR. Scleral depression: marker for retinal detachment surgery. *Am J Ophthalmol* 1971; 72:1013.

Management of Ocular Injuries and Emergencies,
edited by Mathew W. MacCumber.
Lippincott–Raven Publishers, Philadelphia © 1998.

21

Management of Intraocular Foreign Bodies

Michael U. Humayun, Arturo Santos, and Eugene de Juan, Jr.

5615 April Journey, Columbia, Maryland 21044; Department of Health Science, University of Guadalajara, Guadalajara, Jalisco 45042, Mexico; and Department of Ophthalmology, Wilmer Eye Institute, The Johns Hopkins University School of Medicine, Baltimore, Maryland 21287

Basic Considerations 309
   Anterior Segment Intraocular Foreign Bodies 310 · Posterior Segment Intraocular Foreign Bodies 310 · Composition and Size 310 · Initial Management 310
Anterior Segment Intraocular Foreign Bodies 311
   Corneal Foreign Bodies 311 · Anterior Chamber, Angle, and Iris Foreign Bodies 312 · Lenticular Foreign Bodies 313
Posterior Segment Intraocular Foreign Bodies 314
   Intravitreal Foreign Bodies 314 · Retinal Foreign Bodies 316

BASIC CONSIDERATIONS

Most injuries resulting in intraocular foreign bodies occur from striking metal on metal (1–3). The majority are magnetic (4–6). BBs and gunshot pellets also commonly cause injury, resulting in the poorest outcome (7–9). It is important to determine the size, composition, and location of the foreign body, including examination of structures that it has violated. These injuries can be grouped into anterior segment or posterior segment intraocular foreign bodies.

Visual results after removal of intraocular foreign bodies are generally favorable. Some investigators have shown that up to 63% of patients recover vision of 20/40 and only 14% had visual acuity less than 5/200 (4). Poor visual outcome may be seen in patients with associated macular injury, complicated retinal detachment, or optic nerve injury.

Anterior Segment Intraocular Foreign Bodies

Intraocular foreign bodies may become imbedded deep in the cornea, anterior chamber, angle, iris, or lens. Introduction of microbial organisms and inflammation may occur (5).

Posterior Segment Intraocular Foreign Bodies

Such foreign bodies usually have a greater force and momentum than do anterior segment intraocular foreign bodies. They may be present in the vitreous, retina, choroid, and/or sclera. Injury occurs both through initial penetration and secondary complications including vitreous hemorrhage, retinal detachment, and possible endophthalmitis, usually from bacilli or staphylococci (5).

Composition and Size

Certain foreign bodies may be well tolerated, such as silver, platinum, gold, stone, glass, rubber, plastic, and cilia (1,10,11). However, magnetic foreign bodies such as iron may result in an intense inflammatory reaction and possible siderosis (12). Steel, which contains iron, also can result in a severe inflammatory reaction. Nonmagnetic foreign bodies such as pure copper commonly cause a severe inflammatory reaction and chalcosis in alloys with 80% copper or less (10). Vegetable matter also can cause an intense inflammatory reaction and endophthalmitis (13). Some magnetic substances such as nickel and nonmagnetic substances such as aluminum, mercury, and zinc may produce milder inflammatory reactions.

As for size, the larger the foreign body, the greater the physical damage associated with it. Also, the size of the intraocular foreign body will influence the surgical approach by which it is removed.

Initial Management

When examining patients with a history of trauma involving a possible projectile, one must obtain a detailed account of the exact events that led to the trauma, especially as some of these cases have medicolegal ramifications. Attention to whether ocular protection was used should be noted. Every effort should be made in order to identify the type of intraocular foreign body and whether it is magnetic. Have family members or friends bring a portion of the material that has resulted in the injury. Visual acuity, a complete anterior segment, and dilated fundus examination are essential. A good visual acuity may be misleading because a small foreign body may result only in a mild decrease in vision. In some cases a cataract, vitreous hemorrhage, or inflammation may prevent adequate ophthalmoscopic examination. Even if the media are clear, yet there is a suspicion of an intraocular foreign body, a computerized tomography (CT) or a B-scan ultrasound should be performed to localize the foreign body, as long as one is cognizant of applying minimal pressure on the open globe (see Chapter 5) (14,15) Magnetic resonance imaging (MRI) is contraindicated because most foreign bodies are metallic and magnetic.

Because the incidence of endophthalmitis is high in cases presenting with intraocular foreign bodies, we administer intravenous ceftazidime 1 g every 8 hours and clindamycin 600 mg every 8 hours as soon as an intraocular foreign body is suspected. Clindamycin serves as excellent coverage against *Bacillus* species, which may result in severe posttraumatic infection.

After the initial evaluation, a shield is placed over the involved eye, and the remainder of the examination is conducted in the operating room.

A discussion of detailed management of intraocular foreign bodies depending on location and composition is presented below.

ANTERIOR SEGMENT INTRAOCULAR FOREIGN BODIES

These foreign bodies have traversed with a lesser momentum and force than posterior segment foreign bodies. A history is helpful in determining the possible location and mechanism of injury. For example, an explosive injury results in multiple foreign bodies for which one must conduct a careful search.

Corneal Foreign Bodies

A foreign body may involve only the cornea (see also Chapters 13 and 15).

Diagnosis

1. There may be unilateral or bilateral injuries. Visual acuity can vary depending on the extent of injury and whether the visual axis is involved.
2. Clinical findings of the depth of the intracorneal foreign body, with or without Seidel positivity, corneal edema, a possible irregular pupil, decreased intraocular pressure, and increased anterior chamber inflammation should be noted.
3. The composition of the foreign body should be identified. In cases of chalcosis, tiny granules of copper deposited near Descemet's membrane in the deep stroma may occur (10).

Management

1. Complete examination to ensure that there is no further ocular involvement must be conducted. If necessary, a CT or B-scan ultrasound should be performed. If the injury has perforated the cornea, tetanus prophylaxis should be administered as needed along with intravenous ceftazidime 1 g every 8 hours and clindamycin 600 mg every 8 hours, or oral Ciprofloxacin.
2. Superficial foreign bodies may be removed with a 25-gauge needle at a slit lamp after administering topical proparacaine. Removal of the rust ring with an ophthalmic rust ring drill should be performed. Occasionally time to allow the

rust to migrate to the surface may help in removal of deeper presenting rings. Antibiotic ointment, cycloplegic, and a pressure patch for 24 hours (not with vegetable matter injuries) should be used. Daily follow-up until the epithelium is healed is recommended.

3. Smaller and deeper inert foreign bodies, such as glass and plastic, do not require removal, especially if damage to tissues may occur during removal.

4. Foreign bodies involving full-thickness cornea with or without Seidel positivity should be removed in the operating room.

5. All vegetable matter foreign bodies should be removed emergently to reduce the risk of infection.

Anterior Chamber, Angle, and Iris Foreign Bodies

Diagnosis

1. Intraocular foreign bodies with enough force will lodge in the anterior chamber, angle, or iris.

2. A corneal penetration site, irregular pupil, decreased intraocular pressure, hyphema, anterior chamber inflammation, and transillumination defects may be noted.

3. Peripheral corneal edema in areas of anterior chamber angle foreign bodies may be present. Chalcosis may result in a greenish color to the iris (10).

4. Siderosis causes a brownish colored iris, resulting in heterochromia (10).

5. CT should be performed.

6. Gonioscopy with a Goldmann lens to minimize pressure on the eye may localize the anterior chamber foreign body.

Management

1. Tetanus prophylaxis should be administered as needed (see Table 4–2).

2. All vegetable matter foreign bodies and copper should be removed emergently in the operating room.

3. Iron, steel, mercury, nickel, aluminum, and zinc should be removed within 24 hours (5).

4. Glass, plastic, and cilia are often well tolerated, and if not damaging other structures should not be removed (1,10,11).

5. When removal is anticipated, we prefer general anesthesia, unless the artery wound is small (< 2mm). Careful prep and lid speculum placement is used, taking care not to put pressure on the open globe.

6. Complete localization of the entry site is important.

7. Balanced salt solution, viscoelastic, or air is used to maintain anterior chamber depth and to protect the corneal endothelium. All viable uveal tissue is reposited. Consider closure of a corneal wound with 10-0 nylon suture before removal of the foreign body to stabilize the anterior chamber (see Chapter 15).

8. A foreign body lodged in the anterior chamber can be removed via forceps

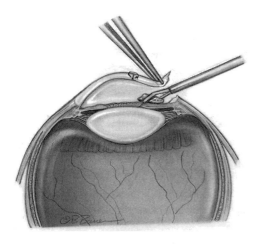

FIG. 21–1. Anterior segment foreign body is removed with intraocular forceps through a corneoscleral shelved incision. The anterior chamber is maintained with viscoelastic and the corneal wound repaired with 10-0 nylon suture.

through the wound or a limbal corneoscleral shelved incision (Fig. 21–1). If it is magnetic, an intraocular or external magnet can be used.

9. Anterior chamber angle foreign bodies are removed via a limbal incision in the area of the foreign body. Intraoperative gonioscopy may be necessary to localize the foreign body. Nonmagnetic foreign bodies are removed with forceps, and magnetic ones are removed using the intraocular or external magnet.

10. Adherent iris foreign bodies can be dislodged using viscoelastic or a needle. Once liberated, the forceps for nonmagnetic and intraocular or external magnet for magnetic foreign bodies may be used.

11. We use interrupted 9-0 nylon suture to close scleral and 10-0 nylon suture for corneal wounds (see Chapter 15). Tissue adhesives with bandage contact lenses may be used in corneal trauma cases where the small size of the wound or inadequacy of wound closure with nylon due to missing or disrupted tissue may make this a better option. Intravenous ceftazidime 1 g every 8 hours, clindamycin 600 mg every 8 hours (alternatively, ciprafloxacin 750 mg orally twice a day), topical ciprofloxacin every 2 hours, prednisolone acetate 1% four times daily, and atropine 1% twice daily are administered postoperatively.

Lenticular Foreign Bodies

In certain trauma cases, the foreign body can penetrate the lens.

Diagnosis

1. A corneal or scleral penetration site, hyphema, irregular pupil, anterior chamber inflammation, decreased intraocular pressure and cataractous lens may be noted.

2. CT is used to localize single or multiple foreign bodies.
3. In cases of siderosis, brownish spots secondary to iron deposits in lens epithelial cells may be noted (10).
4. A greenish-brownish sunflower cataract can be associated with chalcosis (10).

Management

1. Tetanus prophylaxis is given if necessary (see Table 4–2).
2. We recommend general anesthesia, a careful preoperative prep, and lid speculum placement, when removal is planned.
3. The penetration site and extent of injury are identified.
4. If the foreign body is superficially embedded within the lens, either forceps in nonmagnetic cases or an intraocular or external magnet in magnetic cases may be used to remove the foreign body.
5. A careful phacoemulsification is performed if significant cataract is present. If zonular or posterior capsule disruption with vitreous presentation is noted, a pars plana approach may be used (see Chapter 18).
6. A deeply embedded intralenticular foreign body can be removed via an extracapsular technique removing the lens and foreign body. If posterior capsule violation with vitreous presentation is noted, a pars plana approach should be used. Alternatively, the foreign body may be left in the lens if it is inert.
7. Primary placement of a posterior chamber intraocular lens can be considered but is not routinely performed (16). A secondary intraocular lens or contact lens can be used.
8. Postoperative intravenous ceftazidime 1 g every 8 hours, clindamycin 600 mg every 8 hours, topical ciprofloxacin every 2 hours, prednisolone acetate 1% four times daily, and atropine 1% twice daily are administered postoperatively.

POSTERIOR SEGMENT INTRAOCULAR FOREIGN BODIES

Missile injury may result in foreign bodies penetrating into the posterior segment.

Intravitreal Foreign Bodies

With sufficient force, an intraocular foreign body may reach the vitreous cavity, retina, or choroid.

Diagnosis

1. A corneal or scleral laceration site, anterior segment trauma, lenticular violation and vitreous in the anterior chamber (AC), vitreous hemorrhage, and retinal detachment are signs that the posterior segment may be a harbinger of an intraocular foreign body.

2. CT or B-scan ultrasound is recommended to localize the foreign body and to identify whether a retinal detachment is present when visualization is poor.

Management

1. Tetanus prophylaxis is advised when necessary (see Table 4–2).
2. All vegetable matter and copper are removed immediately via vitrectomy and forceps through an enlarged sclerotomy site or, if very large, through a limbal site. It is helpful to remove the posterior hyaloid when possible.
3. Aluminum, zinc, iron, steel, nickel and mercury should be removed within 24 hours (5). If magnetic, a vitrectomy and initial adherence to an intraocular magnet (17,18) and then transferral to forceps (19) are recommended (Fig. 21–2). If nonmagnetic, vitrectomy and forceps removal is performed. The foreign body may be moved through an enlarged sclerotomy site or if very large then through a corneoscleral incision.
4. Cilia, glass, gold, silver, and platinum are relative inert and can be left provided no inflammation, infection, or disruption of anatomy is noted (1,10,11). The benefits are weighed against risks in each individual case scenario.
5. A prophylactic scleral buckle is recommended in cases of severe injury, especially where there is an anterior scleral wound with vitreous loss (see Chapter 20) (20).
6. Intravitreal vancomycin (1 mg/0.1 cc), ceftazidime (2 mg/0.1 cc), and clindamycin (1 mg/0.1 cc) can be administered in cases when contamination is suspected. Intravenous ceftazidime 1 g every 8 hours and clindamycin every 8 hours are recommended if intravitreal antibiotics are not used. Topical

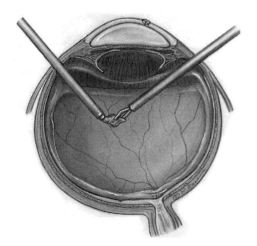

FIG. 21–2. Intravitreal foreign body is stabilized with intraocular magnet and transferred to intraocular foreign body forceps. The forceps sclerotomy site (right in drawing) was previously enlarged for foreign body removal.

ciprofloxacin every 2 hours, prednisolone acetate 1% four times daily, and atropine 1% twice daily are administered postoperatively. Careful postoperative
follow-up for the development of endophthalmitis is advised.

Retinal Foreign Bodies

An intraocular foreign body with enough momentum may incarcerate itself
within the retina at times, resulting in a retinal detachment (21,22). When the foreign body is a BB or a pellet, it is associated with a poor prognosis (24).

Diagnosis

1. An anterior segment entry site, hyphema, lenticular trauma, vitreous prolapse,
   vitreous hemorrhage, and at times a retinal detachment may be noted.
2. A CT is preferred for identification and localization of the foreign body (See
   Chapter 5). A B-scan may be performed in the operating room following wound
   closure.
3. Retinal pigmentary degeneration may be seen in cases of siderosis. Eyes with
   retained iron containing intraocular foreign bodies may eventually develop a
   flat electroretinogram (ERG) (12).
4. Highly refractile particles within the retina may be seen in cases of chalcosis
   (25).

Management

1. Tetanus prophylaxis is recommended when necessary.
2. All vegetable matter and copper should be removed immediately. Aluminum,
   zinc, iron, steel, nickel, lead, and mercury are removed within 24 hours (5).
3. Gold, silver, cilia, glass, plastic, and platinum may be left as to not cause any
   further anatomic disruption in cases where the eye is quiet (1,10,11).
4. Magnetic intraocular foreign bodies which are small and well-visualized may
   be removed via the external electromagnet (25,26). Removal at an anterior site
   may be performed. Also, a scleral incision with preplaced sutures can be made
   over the location of the foreign body. In these cases, diathermy is applied to the
   choroid. The electromagnet is placed over the sclera directly adjacent to the foreign body and is activated. The incision site may need to be enlarged to accommodate removal of the foreign body. The scleral incision site is then sutured
   close. Hemorrhage, retinal, and vitreous incarceration are possible complications. Caution is exercised in the use of the external electromagnet because little
   control over removal of the foreign body can result in greater iatrogenic trauma.
   Thus, we favor the intraocular approach.
5. Larger and poorly visualized magnetic retinal foreign bodies should be managed
   with pars plana vitrectomy, initial intraocular magnet adherence, and subsequent
   transferral to forceps for removal. Nonmagnetic foreign bodies are removed via

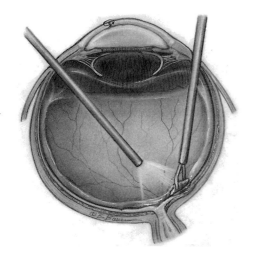

FIG. 21–3. Retinal foreign body grasped with intraocular forceps. The forceps sclerotomy site (right in drawing) was previously enlarged for foreign body removal.

vitrectomy and forceps (Fig. 21–3). Well-incarcerated or subretinal intraocular foreign bodies can be removed either through the initial retinal penetration site or through a retinotomy site (27). Endolaser if posterior, or cryotherapy if anterior, around the retinal break or retinotomy site can be performed. Diathermy surrounding the retinotomy or retinal penetration site before removal of the intraocular foreign body or elevating the bottle may minimize the risk of bleeding.

6. Patients with large intraocular foreign bodies should undergo vitrectomy with removal of the posterior hyaloid. Intraocular magnet and forceps are used for adequate control when removing magnetic foreign bodies. Forceps alone are used for removing nonmagnetic foreign bodies. The large foreign body can be removed either through enlarging the sclerotomy wound or through a limbal incision. Usually, the lens is damaged in these cases and a primary lensectomy is performed. Placement of an IOL is not recommended initially (16), especially when there is injury to the vitreous base. However, in certain cases an IOL may be placed initially. Capsular support in these cases is poor and a sutured posterior chamber intraocular lens may be necessary.

7. Retinal breaks are commonly associated with trauma caused by intraocular foreign bodies (see Chapter 20). Anterior breaks are treated by cryotherapy and are commonly supported by scleral buckles. We recommend a broad encircling scleral buckle to support the vitreous base in such cases. Posterior tears are treated with endolaser and gas tamponade.

8. Intravitreal vancomycin (1 mg/0.1 cc), ceftazidime (2 mg/0.1 cc), and clindamycin (1 mg/0.1 cc) may be administered in cases when contamination is suspected. Intravenous ceftazidime 1 g every 8 hours and clindamycin 600 mg every 8 hours are recommended when intravitreal antibiotics are not used. Topical ciprofloxacin every 2 hours, prednisolone acetate 1% four times daily, and

atropine 1% twice daily are administered postoperatively. Careful daily follow-up is advised for evaluation of the development of endophthalmitis.

REFERENCES

1. Barry DR. Effects of retained intraocular foreign bodies. *Int Ophthalmol Clin* 1968;8:153.
2. Lai YK, Moussa M. Perforating eye injuries due to intraocular foreign bodies. *Med J Malaysia* 1992;47:212.
3. Percival SPB. A decade of intraocular foreign bodies. *Br J Ophthalmol* 1972;56:454.
4. Williams DF, Mieler WF, Abrams GW, Lewis H. Results and prognostic factors in penetrating ocular injuries with retained intraocular foreign bodies. *Ophthalmology* 1988;95:911.
5. Thompson JT, Parver LM, Enger CL, et al. Infectious endophthalmitis after penetrating injury with retained intraocular foreign bodies. *Ophthalmology* 1993;100:1468.
6. Behrens-Bauman W, Praetorius G. Intraocular foreign bodies: 297 consecutive cases. *Ophthalmologica* 1989;198:84.
7. de Juan E Jr, Sternberg P Jr, Michels RG. Penetrating ocular injuries. Types of injuries and visual results. *Ophthalmology* 1983;90:1318.
8. Pieramici DJ, MacCumber MW, Humayun MU, et al. Open globe injury: update on types of injuries and visual results. *Ophthalmology* 1996;103:1798.
9. Sternberg P Jr, de Juan E Jr, Michels RG. Penetrating ocular injuries in young patients: initial injuries and visual results. *Retina* 1984;4:5.
10. Duke-Elder SS, MacFaul PA. Mechanical injuries. In: *Duke-Elder System of Ophthalmology.* Vol. XIV. Part 1. St. Louis: CV Mosby; 1972.
11. Humayun MU, de al Cruz Z, Maguire A, et al. Intraocular cilia: report of six cases 6 weeks to 32 years duration. *Arch Ophthalmol* 1993;111:1396.
12. Sneed SR, Weingeist TA. Management of siderosis bulbi due to a retained iron-containing intraocular foreign body. *Ophthalmology* 1990;97:375.
13. Boldt HC, Pulido JS, Blodi CF, et al. Rural endophthalmitis. *Ophthalmology* 1989;96:1722.
14. Rubsamen PE, Cousins SW, Winward KE, Byrne SF. Diagnostic ultrasound and pars plana vitrectomy in penetrating ocular trauma. *Ophthalmology* 1994;101:809.
15. Nouby-Mahmoud G, Silverman RH, Coleman DJ. Using high-frequency ultrasound to characterize intraocular foreign bodies. *Ophthalmic Surg* 1993;24:94.
16. Smiddy W, Contact lenses for visual rehabilitation after corneal laceration repair. *Ophthalmology* 1989;96:293.
17. Crock GW, Janakiraman P, Reddy P. Intraocular magnet of Parel. *Br J Ophthalmol* 1986;70:879.
18. McCuen BW, Hickingbotham D. A new retractable micromagnet for intraocular foreign body removal. *Arch Ophthalmol* 1989;107:1819.
19. Parel JM, Machemer R. Diamond-coated all purpose foreign body forceps. *Am J Ophthalmol* 1981; 91:267.
20. Brinton GS, Aaberg TM, Parver LM, Fowler CJ. Penetrating eye injuries related to assault. *Arch Ophthalmol* 1992;110:849.
21. Slusher MM, Greven CM, Yu DD. Posterior chamber intraocular lens implantation combined with lensectomy-vitrectomy and intraretinal foreign body removal. *Arch Ophthalmol* 1992;110:127.
22. Slusher MM. Intraretinal foreign bodies. Management and observations. *Retina* 1990;(suppl 1):50.
23. Sternberg P Jr, de Juan E Jr, Green WR, et al. Ocular BB injuries. *Ophthalmology* 1984;91:1269.
24. Delaney WV Jr. Presumed ocular chalcosis: a reversible maculopathy. *Ann Ophthalmol* 1975;14: 378.
25. McCaslin MF. An improved hand electromagnet for eye surgery. *Trans Am Ophthalmol Soc* 1958; 56:571.
26. Bronson NR. Practical characteristics of ophthalmic magnets. *Arch Ophthalmol* 1968;79:22.
27. Joondeph BC, Flynn HW Jr. Management of subretinal foreign bodies with a cannulated extrusion needle. *Am J Ophthalmol* 1990;110:250.

Management of Ocular Injuries and Emergencies,
edited by Mathew W. MacCumber.
Lippincott–Raven Publishers, Philadelphia © 1998.

22

Traumatic Maculopathies

Mathew W. MacCumber, Thomas B. Connor, Jr., and Neil M. Bressler

Retina Service, Department of Ophthalmology, Rush Medical College, Chicago, Illinois 60612; Department of Ophthalmology, Wilmer Eye Institute, The Johns Hopkins University School of Medicine, Baltimore, Maryland 21287; and Vitreoretinal Section, Retina Service, Medical College of Wisconsin, Milwaukee, Wisconsin 53226

Basic Considerations 320
    Retinal Vascular Injuries 320 · Direct Blunt Injuries 320 · Retinal Burns (Photic Injury) 320
Purtscher's Retinopathy 321
    Diagnosis 321 · Management 321
Valsalva Retinopathy 321
    Diagnosis 322 · Management 322
Terson's Syndrome 322
    Diagnosis 322 · Management 322
Shaken Baby Syndrome 322
    Diagnosis 323 · Management 323
Central Retinal Artery Occlusion 323
    Diagnosis 323 · Management 323
Commotio Retinae (Berlin's Edema) 324
    Diagnosis 324 · Management 324
Retinal Pigment Epithelial Contusion 324
    Diagnosis 324 · Management 325
Choroidal Rupture 325
    Diagnosis 325 · Management 326 · Procedure: Photocoagulation of Choroidal Neovascularization 326
Traumatic Macular Hole 327
    Diagnosis 327 · Management 328
Retinal Burns 328
    Diagnosis 329 · Management 330

BASIC CONSIDERATIONS

Apart from direct injuries from severe penetrating trauma or traumatic retinal detachment (see Chapters 15 and 20), the posterior pole is susceptible to three broad types of trauma: retinal vascular injuries, direct blunt injuries, and retinal burns.

Retinal Vascular Injuries

Retinal vascular disruption can occur via sudden changes in blood flow or coagulation caused by injuries distant to the globes. Features noted include Purtscher's retinopathy, Valsalva retinopathy, retinal artery occlusion secondary to emboli (see Chapter 23), Terson's syndrome, and the shaken baby syndrome.

Direct Blunt Injuries

Blunt injuries to the globe can injure the posterior pole through tractional forces induced by globe compression and expansion or increased intraocular pressure. Such injuries include commotio retinae, retinal pigment epithelial (RPE) contusion, choroidal rupture, traumatic macular hole, central retinal artery occlusion secondary to increased intraocular pressure (see Chapter 23), and traumatic optic neuropathy (see Chapter 24). Whiplash-like movements of the head can produce retinal vascular injury (see Shaken Baby Syndrome below) or tractional retinal injuries (see Traumatic Macular Hole below).

Retinal Burns (Photic Injury)

Photic injury is caused by the special light-focusing and -absorbing characteristics of the eye.

The examining physician must have a high level of suspicion to look for injuries of the posterior pole to decrease the chance that a diagnosis will be missed. Several different types of injury can exist in the same eye (e.g., commotio retinae and traumatic macular hole). Associated injuries that interfere with the ocular media (e.g., hyphema, cataract, or vitreous hemorrhage) may prevent the examiner from visualizing the damaged retina and choroid. When the media are not clear, ultrasonography, computed tomography, or magnetic resonance imaging may aid in diagnosis in the acute setting (see Chapter 5). Regular follow-up examinations are critical to diagnose injuries initially missed because of examination difficulties (e.g., media opacity, ecchymotic lids) or to diagnose complications that develop after the initial visit (e.g., choroidal neovascularization [CNV] at a previous site of choroidal rupture).

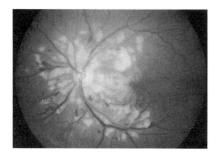

FIG. 22–1. Purtscher's retinopathy. (Courtesy of Dr. K. Packo.) *For a color representation of this figure, please see the color insert facing p. 256.*

PURTSCHER'S RETINOPATHY

Purtscher's retinopathy is the uncommon finding of posterior pole whitening and hemorrhages that has been described in association with a number of conditions, including head, chest, or long-bone trauma (Fig. 22–1) (1). Retinal whitening is recognized to be due to ischemia. Several proposed mechanisms include (a) granulocyte aggregation and leukoemboli secondary to complement (C5a) activation (2), (b) fat embolization in long-bone fractures, (c) air embolization in compressive chest injuries, and (d) venous reflux or vasospasm in response to increased a sudden increase in venous pressure.

Diagnosis

1. May be unilateral or more commonly bilateral; visual acuity 20/20 to counting fingers and may progress over 1 to 2 days. Dense scotomas and a relative afferent pupillary defect may be present.
2. Clinical findings include marked generalized retinal edema, peripapillary superficial retinal whitening (probably secondary to ischemia), multiple cotton-wool spots, preretinal or intraretinal hemorrhages often along major vessels, and disk edema.

Management

1. Vision may return to normal or visual loss may be permanent.
2. No treatment is known to alter clinical course.
3. Rule out nontraumatic causes of Purtscher's retinopathy, including acute pancreatitis, lupus erythematosus, dermatomyositis, scleroderma, amniotic fluid embolism during pregnancy or childbirth, and cardiac left ventricular aneurysm (3).

VALSALVA RETINOPATHY

Valsalva retinopathy is caused by a sudden increase in intrathoracic pressure that increases intravenous pressure within the eye.

Diagnosis

1. A history may be given of heavy lifting, straining at stool, sexual activity, coughing, or vomiting.
2. Superficial intraretinal hemorrhages may be seen bilaterally.
3. Visual loss is caused by hemorrhagic detachment of the internal limiting membrane, breakthrough vitreous hemorrhage, or subretinal hemorrhage.

Management

1. Visual acuity usually returns to normal over days to months depending on the extent of retinal hemorrhage.
2. After waiting several months, vitrectomy may be necessary for nonclearing vitreous hemorrhage (see Chapter 20).

TERSON'S SYNDROME

Simultaneous vitreous and intracranial hemorrhages are known as Terson's syndrome. Intracranial hemorrhage of any etiology is believed to cause an acute increase in intraocular venous pressure with rupture of papillary and retinal vessels.

Diagnosis

There is simultaneous vitreous and intracranial hemorrhages without other cause of vitreous hemorrhage.

Management

1. Rule out retinal detachment, choroidal hemorrhage, or other concurrent ocular injury by a thorough examination and ultrasound.
2. In a child, see Shaken Baby Syndrome below and Chapter 4.
3. Immediate referral to neurosurgery service.
4. Visual recovery may be hastened by vitrectomy; however, visual outcome appears similar if hemorrhage is allowed to clear without surgery (4).
5. Once vitreous hemorrhage has cleared, closely examine the retina for epiretinal membrane (a common development in these patients) or other abnormality that may limit final visual acuity.

SHAKEN BABY SYNDROME

Ophthalmic findings are found in 30% to 40% of abused children and can result from direct head or ocular trauma, chest injuries, suffocation or body shaking (see Chapter 4) (5).

Diagnosis

1. Caused by a coup-contrecoup mechanism similar to whiplash injury.
2. Mild to severe preretinal, intraretinal, and subretinal hemorrhages, cotton-wool spots, and disk edema with or without external signs of ocular trauma (6).
3. May be associated with intracranial hemorrhage.
4. Other signs of trauma/child abuse such as bruising, fractures, and burns are often present.

Management

1. See Chapter 4.
2. Dense vitreous hemorrhage not clearing within the first month after the injury should be removed by specialized vitrectomy to prevent deprivation amplyopia (7).

CENTRAL RETINAL ARTERY OCCLUSION

A central retinal artery occlusion (CRAO) is uncommonly caused by trauma. Prolonged compression of the globe occluding the central retinal artery can be caused by external pressure on the eyelids or from severe orbital swelling such as from orbital hemorrhage. One scenario is the face-down patient without eye protection undergoing lumbar spine surgery. Fat emboli from long-bone fractures can cause central or branch retinal arterial occlusion hours to days after the original injury.

Animal studies have suggested that irreversible retinal damage occurs after 90 to 100 minutes of occlusion (8).

Diagnosis

1. Narrow arterioles, optic disk pallor, and segmentation of the blood column may be seen.
2. Diffuse retinal whitening with macula cherry-red spot occurs several hours after the occlusion.
3. In the case of long-bone fractures, arteriolar fat emboli in addition to cotton-wool spots and retinal hemorrhages may be seen (1).

Management

1. Acute management is similar to that for nontraumatic CRAO or branch retinal artery occlusion from other forms of emboli (see Chapter 23).
2. In the case of orbital hemorrhage, see Chapter 9.

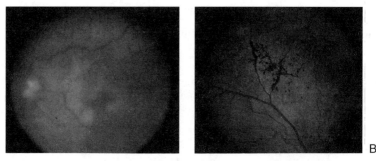

FIG. 22–2. A: Commotio retinae (Berlin's edema). *For a color representation of this figure, please see the color insert facing p. 256.* **B:** Traumatic retinopathy years after blunt injury.

COMMOTIO RETINAE (BERLIN'S EDEMA)

Commotio retinae is likely due to shearing of photoreceptor outer segments as demonstrated in the model of Sipperly, Quigley, and Gass (9). It may be associated with edema of the outer plexiform and nuclear retinal layer and subretinal fluid. The macula may contain cystoid spaces that may coalesce and degenerate to form a macular hole.

Diagnosis

1. Commotio retinae is a common finding after blunt injury to the globe.
2. Commotio retinae is characterized by gray-white opacification of the deep sensory retina involving the macula and/or peripheral retina (Fig. 22–2A).
3. Visual acuity may be 20/20 to 20/400, which usually, but not always, returns to baseline.
4. Be observant for a traumatic macular hole or underlying choroidal rupture.

Management

1. No treatment is indicated.
2. Patients should be followed for several days to weeks until vision stabilizes.
3. With time, bone spicule pigmentation can occur (Fig. 22–2B).

RETINAL PIGMENT EPITHELIAL CONTUSION

Diagnosis

1. Blunt trauma can cause functional damage in a localized area of RPE, resulting in an overlying serous retinal detachment.
2. Creamy discoloration of the RPE is seen within 48 hours of the injury followed by progressive depigmentation (10).

3. Fluorescein angiography demonstrates progressive, patchy hyperfluorescence of the RPE (10).
4. Visual acuity is only affected if the fovea is directly involved.

Management

1. No specific treatment is indicated.
2. Follow patient until serous retinal detachment is resolved.

CHOROIDAL RUPTURE

Diagnosis

1. Direct ruptures occur at the site of contusive impact, usually in periphery and adjacent to ora serrata (see Chorioretinitis Sclopeteria, Chapter 20).
2. Indirect ruptures are usually in the posterior pole, often crescent-shaped and oriented concentric to the optic disk and in the macula (Figs. 22–3A and 22–4D). Inelasticity of Bruch's membrane results in tears typically of the RPE layer, Bruch's membrane, and the choriocapillaris. The retina and large choroidal vessels usually remain intact. Visual acuity is often worse than 20/200 (11).
3. Initially only suprachoroidal, sub-RPE, subretinal, or vitreous hemorrhage may be seen.
4. As hemorrhage clears over days to months, a yellowish scar is seen at the level of Bruch's membrane.
5. Patients with pseudoxanthoma elasticum or other causes of fragile connective tissues are at especially high risk of choroidal rupture.

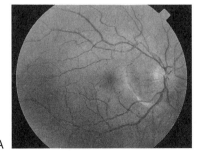 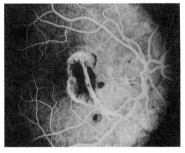

A   B

FIG. 22–3. A: CNV secondary to choroidal rupture. Choroidal neovascular membrane was identified 3 weeks after the injury. *For a color representation of this figure, please see the color insert facing p. 256.* **B:** Fluorescein angiography demonstrates the choroidal neovascular membrane. (Courtesy of Dr. B. McCuen.)

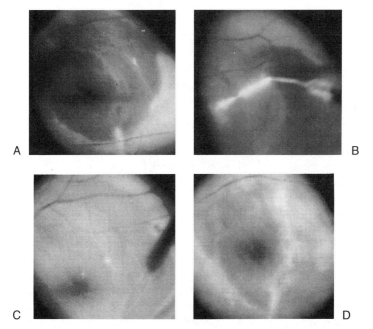

FIG. 22–4. A: Submacular hemorrhage secondary to choroidal rupture. **B:** Subretinal injection of 25 μg/0.1 ml tissue plasminogen activator (tPA). **C:** Lysis of clot 15 minutes later. **D:** Choroidal rupture near fovea is shown after aspiration of the subretinal blood.

Management

1. Once the blood begins to clear, fluorescein angiography can demonstrate small choroidal ruptures. The rupture tends to be hypofluorescent in the early phase and hyperfluorescent in the late phase as the surrounding choriocapillaris leaks into it.
2. Sequential examination is required until the blood clears and then routinely thereafter to rule out CNV within the Bruch's membrane scar (Fig. 22–3A and B).
3. CNV can occur within months to years after the injury, resulting in serous or hemorrhagic retinal detachment (12).
4. Laser photocoagulation is believed to be helpful in preserving vision when well-defined CNV occurs. Treatment is similar to that used CNV due to other causes (procedure below).
5. Vitrectomy with aspiration of the subretinal blood during the first 10 days after injury may prevent subretinal fibrosis and improve visual outcome if choroidal rupture does not pass near the foveal center (Fig. 22–4A through D).

Procedure: Photocoagulation of Choroidal Neovascularization

1. Consider retrobulbar block.
2. Define CNV with fluorescein angiography. Consider postponing treatment if extensive hemorrhage remains.

3. Dye yellow, argon green, or krypton red, 0.2 to 0.5 seconds, 100- to 200-micron spot size, sufficient power to cause chalk white spot.
4. Initially outline the border of the treatment area based on fluorescein angiogram, then fill in.
5. Obtain posttreatment photograph to rule out untreated area.
6. Follow up in 2 to 4 weeks with repeat fluorescein angiography to rule out a recurrence. If recurrence occurs, consider retreatment if not in foveal center. If no recurrence, repeat fluorescein angiography every 3 to 4 months during first year (when risk of recurrence is greatest).
7. Educate the patient to contact an ophthalmologist promptly for new symptoms of visual distortion or loss of vision which may indicate a recurrence.

TRAUMATIC MACULAR HOLE

The fovea is susceptible to traumatic injury because it is extremely thin, has high metabolic demand, and is particularly adherent to the posterior vitreous. Postcontusion necrosis can result in macular edema and macular cyst formation. Over months to years, rupture of the inner layer of the cyst would produce a lamellar hole, whereas rupture of both layers would result in a full-thickness hole. Contrecoup vitreous traction can cause an acute lamellar or full-thickness macular hole (Fig. 22–5).

Diagnosis

1. In acute full-thickness or lamellar macular holes, a premacular operculum may be seen.
2. The size of the macular hole varies, but the margins are usually sharp and regular.
3. Differentiation of a lamellar and full-thickness traumatic macular hole is aided by the following typical characteristics:

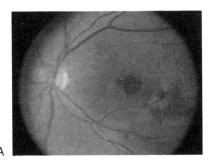 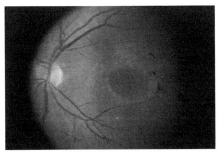

A   B

FIG. 22–5. A: Traumatic macular hole. **B:** Same eye, 1 year later, the hole has markedly enlarged. (Courtesy of Dr. B. McCuen)

Lamellar macular hole	Full-thickness macular hole
Acuity better than 20/60	Acuity 20/60 to 20/200
No cuff of fluid	Cuff of subretinal fluid
No central scotoma (Watzke–Allen sign negative)	Central scotoma (Watzke–Allen sign positive)
±Window defect by fluorescein angiography (Aaberg's sign)	+Window defect by fluorescein angiography (Aaberg's sign)

4. Progression to a larger retinal detachment after traumatic macular hole occurs in at most 1% to 2% (13).

Management

1. Patients should be followed initially because traumatic full-thickness macular holes may close spontaneously with variable improvement in visual acuity.
2. The role of macular hole surgery has not been defined for traumatic macular holes. However, vitrectomy could be beneficial for holes with substantial surrounding cuffs of subretinal fluid that do not spontaneously close over a few months (as indicated for idiopathic macular holes).*
3. Progression of the cuff of fluid to large retinal detachment would be an indication for pneumatic retinopexy or vitrectomy with fluid-gas exchange (15).
4. No surgical intervention is required for lamellar macular holes.

RETINAL BURNS

Visible and near-infrared light is focused on the retina by the optics of the eye increasing the radiant exposure by as much as 100,000 times. Thus, a variety of high-intensity light sources can induce retinal injury, including the sun (16), solar eclipse (17), sunlamps, welding arcs (18), search lights, flares, short-circuiting electric current (19), and lasers used in the workplace (20,21) or military. Self-induced retinal burns occur occasionally in psychiatric patients (22) or those under the influence of psychotropic drugs (23) via gazing at intense light sources. In particular, new military applications of tactical lasers provide a new threat for accidental or intentional retinal burns (24). Prolonged exposure to ophthalmic instruments, including the intraocular fiberoptic light (25,26) and the operating microscope (27) can cause inadvertent retinal burns. Ophthalmic lasers can, of course, cause accidental photocoagulation when used improperly (27).

Light causes damage to the retina via three basic mechanisms (3):

1. Photochemical: caused by absorption by photoreceptor pigments, especially at blue end of the visible spectrum.
2. Photocoagulation: caused when light generates an elevation of temperature of greater than 10°F and coagulates retinal proteins.

---

*Vitreoretinal surgery for this condition is beyond the scope of this text. See text of Glaser (14).

3. Mechanical: caused by acoustic waves or gaseous formation after rapid tissue absorption of light.

Ocular pigmentation, clarity of the optical media, wavelength, irradiation power, body temperature, and other factors contribute to the extent of injury. Ultraviolet and mid- to far-infrared radiation are absorbed by the cornea and lens, usually sparing the retina, but may injure anterior structures (see Chapter 13). Macular xanthophyll provides some absorption of shorter wavelengths in the visual spectrum, and the choroid provides a heat-sink for absorption of longer wavelengths.

Diagnosis

Mild-to-Moderate Photic Maculopathy

1. History is usually given of exposure to a high-intensity light source. This history may be denied by some patients, such as by those who used psychotropic drugs.
2. Soon after exposure, patients may complain of central scotoma, chromatopsia, metamorphopsia, and headache.
3. Visual acuity is often in the range of 20/40 to 20/70.
4. Initially a yellow-white spot with a surrounding gray zone is seen in the foveolar area (Fig. 22–6). This fades in few days and is replaced by a reddish spot with a pigment halo. At about 2 weeks this fades and is replaced by a small (25 to 50 μm) reddish, sharply but irregularly circumscribed, faceted lamellar hole or depression that is permanent. Larger lesions with mottling of the RPE may be seen in more severe injuries (Fig. 22–6) (3).
5. Fluorescein angiography is usually normal or shows a window defect in the foveolar area.

Severe Photic Maculopathy

1. There is usually a history of severe focal light exposure such as from ophthalmic instruments or industrial or military lasers.

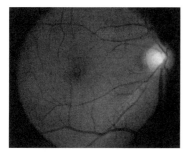

FIG. 22–6. Moderate photic maculopathy secondary to sungazing. (Courtesy of Dr. K. Packo.) *For a color representation of this figure, please see the color insert facing p. 256.*

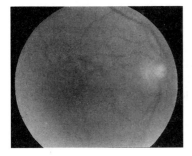

FIG. 22–7. Pigmentary changes seen several months after intense light exposure from an operating microscope filament during cataract extraction. (Courtesy of Dr. G. Jaffe.) *For a color representation of this figure, please see the insert facing p. 256.*

2. In exposure from ophthalmic instruments, lesions are usually paracentral and often cause permanent paracentral scotomas. Initially an irregular yellow-white deep retinal lesion is seen which stains intensely on fluorescein angiography. Over days to weeks it is replaced by mottled RPE with an associated window defect on fluorescein angiography (Fig. 22–7) (3).
3. Injury by laser photocoagulation can range from a yellow-white deep retinal lesion as described above to localized subretinal or overlying vitreous hemorrhage if a break in Bruch's membrane occurred. A permanent scotoma will be present at the site of the injury, but vision may improve as hemorrhage clears.

Prevention During Ocular Surgery

1. Reduce operating light intensity.
2. A yellow filter on the operating microscope can reduce shorter wavelength exposure.
3. Reduce the exposure time through shortening the operative time and covering the cornea when possible.
4. Avoid foveal exposure through tilting the microscope and globe.

Management

1. In milder injuries, visual acuity usually returns to 20/20 to 20/40 within 3 to 6 months.
2. No treatment is of proven value in mild to moderate injuries.
3. In severe photocoagulative injuries with breaks in Bruch's membrane and associated subretinal or vitreous hemorrhage, vitreoretinal surgery may be beneficial (15).

REFERENCES

1. Chuang EL, Miller S III, Kalina RE. Retinal lesions following long bone fractures. *Ophthalmology* 1985;92:370.

2. Blodi B, Johnson MW, Gass JDM, Fine SL, Joffe LM. Purtscher's-like retinopathy after childbirth. *Ophthalmology* 1990;97:1654.

3. Gass JDM. *Stereoscopic Atlas of Macular Disease: Diagnosis and Treatment.* 3rd ed. St. Louis: CV Mosby; 1987.

4. Schultz PN, Sobol WM, Weingeist TA. Long-term visual outcome in Terson's syndrome. *Ophthalmology* 1991;98:1814.

5. Harley RD. Ocular manifestations of child abuse. *J Pediatr Ophthalmol Strabismus* 1980;17:5.

6. Caffey J. The whiplash shaken infant syndrome: manual shaking by the extremities with whiplash-induced intracranial and intraocular bleedings, linked with residual permanent brain damage and mental retardation. *Pediatrics* 1974;54:396.

7. Ferrone PJ, de Juan E. Vitreous hemorrhage in infants. *Arch Ophthalmol* 1994;112:1185.

8. Hayreh SS, Kolder HE, Weingeist TA. Central retinal artery occlusion and retinal tolerance time. *Ophthalmology* 1980;87:75.

9. Sipperley JO, Quigley HA, Gass JDM. Traumatic retinopathy in primates: the explanation of commotio retinae. *Arch Ophthalmol* 1978;96:2267.

10. Friberg TR. Traumatic retinal pigment epithelial edema. *Am J Opthalmol* 1979;88:18.

11. Hart JCD, et al. Indirect choroidal tears at the posterior pole: a fluorescein angiographic and perimetric study. *Br J Ophthalmol* 1980;64:59.

12. Smith RE, Kelley JS, Harbin TS. Late macular complications of choroidal rupture. *Am J Ophthalmol* 1974;77:650.

13. Margherio RR, Schepens CL. Macular breaks: diagnosis, etiology and observations. *Am J Ophthalmol* 1972;74:219.

14. Glaser BM. Management of idiopathic macular holes. In: Ryan SJ, ed. *Retina.* Vol. 3. St. Louis: CV Mosby; 1994.

15. Benson WE. Vitrectomy. In: Tasman W, Jaeger EA, eds. *Clinical Ophthalmology.* Vol. 6. Philadelphia: Lippincott-Raven; 1995.

16. Gladstone GJ, Tasman W. Solar retinitis after minimal exposure. *Arch Ophthalmol* 1978;96:1368.

17. Cordes FC. Eclipse retinitis. *Am J Ophthalmol* 1948;31:101.

18. Naidoff MA, Sliney DH. Retinal injury from a welding arc. *Am J Ophthalmol* 1974;77:663.

19. Gardner TW, Ai E, Chrobak M, Shoch DE. Photic maculopathy secondary to short-circuiting of a high-tension electic current. *Ophthalmology* 1982;89:865.

20. Boldrey EE, Little HL, Flocks M, Vassiliadis A. Retinal injury due to industrial laser burns. *Ophthalmology* 1981;88:101.

21. Fowler BJ. Accidental industrial laser burn of macula. *Ann Ophthalmol* 1983;15:481.

22. Anaclerio AM, Wicker HS. Self-induced solar retinopathy by patients in a psychiatric hospital. *Am J Ophthalmol* 1970;69:731.

23. Fuller DG. Severe solar maculopathy associated with the use of lysergic acid diethylamide (LSD). *Am J Ophthalmol* 1976;81:413.

24. Field Manual 8-50 (FM 8-50). *Prevention and Medical Management of Laser Injuries.* Washington, DC: Department of the Army; 1990.

25. Fuller D, Machemer R, Knighton RW. Retinal damage produced by intraocular fiber optic light. *Am J Ophthalmol* 1978;85:519.

26. Meyers SM, Bonner RF. Retinal irradiance from vitrectomy endoilluminators. *Am J Ophthalmol* 1982;94:26.

27. Boldrey EE, Ho BT, Griffith FE. Retinal burns occurring at cataract extraction. *Ophthalmology* 1984;91:1297.

Management of Ocular Injuries and Emergencies,
edited by Mathew W. MacCumber.
Lippincott–Raven Publishers, Philadelphia © 1998.

23

Sudden Nontraumatic Visual Loss and Visual Disturbances

Mark J. Rivellese, Mathew W. MacCumber, and Andrew P. Schachat

Retina Service, Department of Ophthalmology, Rush Medical College, Chicago, Illinois 60612; and Department of Ophthalmology, Wilmer Eye Institute, The Johns Hopkins University School of Medicine, Baltimore, Maryland 21287

Basic Considerations   333
Visual Disorders Affecting the Retina and Choroid   334
    Amaurosis Fugax   334 · Retinal Artery Occlusion (RAO)   335
    Central Retinal Vein Occlusion   338 · Branch Retinal Vein Occlusion   339
    Choroidal Neovascularization   340 · Central Serous Chorioretinopathy   341
    Rhegmatogenous Retinal Detachment   342 · Idiopathic Macular Hole   344
    Intraocular Tumor   344 · Migraine   345 · Erythropsia   346
Disorders Affecting the Vitreous   347
    Floaters and Flashing Lights: Posterior Vitreous Detachment   347
    Spontaneous Vitreous Hemorrhage   348

BASIC CONSIDERATIONS

Sudden visual disturbances may be caused by an abnormality at any point in the visual pathway. Therefore, a complete ophthalmic examination is critical and must include visual acuity, visual field and pupillary testing, slit-lamp examination, and ophthalmoscopy. A careful history must be taken in addition to an examination to determined whether the visual loss was transient or permanent, and whether one or both eyes were affected.

Anterior segment causes of sudden visual loss not associated with trauma are many, including, for example, dry eye and other tear film or corneal irregularities (see Chapter 13), anterior uveitis (see Chapter 11), rapidly progressive diabetic cataract, and angle-closure glaucoma (see Chapter 17).

This chapter addresses nontraumatic disorders that affect the retina, choroid, and vitreous. Inflammatory conditions affecting the retina and choroid are reviewed in Chapter 11.

Proliferative diabetic retinopathy, in addition to causing vitreous hemorrhage, may present with sudden visual loss due to involvement of the macula by ischemia or tractional retinal detachment (1) or vision loss associated with optic neuropathy (so-called diabetic papillopathy).

Visual disturbances associated with disorders of the optic nerve or central nervous system are discussed in Chapter 24.

As a guide to the patient with vision loss, the examiner should consider the following five possibilities. Each is followed, parenthetically, by the major clue on the examination and an example:

1. Refractive error (vision improves with pinhole; myopia).
2. Media opacity (inadequate ophthalmoscopic view despite pupil dilation; cataract).
3. Macular disease (abnormal appearance on ophthalmoscopy; macular edema).
4. Optic nerve disease (relative afferent pupillary defect; abnormal appearance on ophthalmoscopy; disk swelling).
5. Other causes, e.g. functional vision loss (see Chapter 29), nystagmus, bilateral occipital lobe disease, etc. The first four causes represent the overwhelming majority.

VISUAL DISORDERS AFFECTING THE RETINA AND CHOROID

Amaurosis Fugax

Amaurosis fugax, Latin for "fleeting blindness," is transient monocular visual loss lasting seconds to minutes. The most common cause is retinal emboli, and it usually occurs in older patients with atherosclerosis. In such cases, it is a form of transient ischemic attack. The most common cause in younger patients is vasospasm. These patients may have an autoimmune predisposition or ocular migraine.

Diagnosis

1. Patients often describe a "curtain of darkness" falling over the eye, with resolution like a "clearing fog." Occasionally, patients describe a moving point of light; this may represent the movement of an embolus through the retinal circulation.
2. Careful retinal examination should be performed to identify emboli. Cholesterol emboli, or Hollenhorst plaques, are shiny, golden crystals that frequently arise from carotid plaques. Calcific emboli are gray-white in appearance and frequently originate from cardiac valvular lesions. Fibrin-platelet emboli, which are elongated and cream colored, are rarely seen.

Management

1. The above symptoms in an older patient or a younger patient with predisposing cardiovascular disease demands immediate referral for complete cardiovascular

workup, including carotid Doppler, echocardiography, and consideration of electrocardiography (EKG). Five to ten percent of patients with amaurosis fugax may experience a major stroke within 1 month.

2. In younger patients with recurrent attacks who do not have migraine as a cause, workup for an autoimmune predisposition or coagulopathy should be considered. Female patients should be asked if they use oral contraceptives. Testing may include erythrocyte sedimentation rate (ESR), complete blood count, anticardiolipin antibody, antiphospholipid antibodies, prothrombin time (PT), partial thromboplastin time (PTT), rapid plasma reagin (RPR) and fluorescent treponal antibody absorption (FTA-Abs), protein S, and protein C. A definitive diagnosis is infrequently made, and the exact relationship between abnormal laboratory values is in many cases not certain.

Retinal Artery Occlusion (RAO)

Central retinal artery occlusion (CRAO) and branch retinal artery occlusion (BRAO) are causes of severe monocular vision loss that are potentially reversible if treatment is provided in a timely fashion. Animal studies have suggested that irreversible retinal damage occurs after 90 to 100 minutes of occlusion (2). However, anecdotal reports suggest that at least partial improvement in visual acuity can be achieved after several hours. The treating physician should act quickly first to make the diagnosis and then deliver treatment. It should be emphasized that although many ophthalmologists treat patients with acute CRAO/BRAO, there is no clear evidence that treatment is preferable to doing nothing. Treatment is often undertaken on the assumption that complications are infrequent in this severe situation, so the risk of treatment seems warranted.

Many cases of RAO are caused by emboli. CRAO is occasionally caused by trauma (see also Chapter 22). Other uncommon causes include coagulopathy or autoimmune predisposition, oral contraceptives, sickle cell disease, systemic lupus erythematosus, giant cell arteritis (see Chapter 24), migraine, hypotension, and optic nerve drusen.

Diagnosis

1. Mean age at presentation is early 60s. There may be a history of amaurosis fugax.
2. Patients relate a history of sudden visual loss over seconds or new visual loss noticed after awakening. In CRAO, 90% of patients present with visual acuity of counting fingers or worse.
3. After visual acuity, intraocular pressure, and pupillary response are checked, dilating drops should be given immediately and ophthalmoscopy attempted.
4. Narrow arterioles, optic disk pallor, and segmentation of the blood column may be seen. Emboli are seen in about 20% of cases (see Amaurosis Fugax above).
5. Diffuse whitening of the affected retina occurs several hours after the occlusion.

In CRAO, a cherry-red spot is usually seen in the foveolar area (where the retina is thinner).

6. About 20% of patients have retained perfusion of the macula via a cilioretinal artery (Fig. 23–1). In such cases, visual outcome usually is still less than 20/100.

Management

1. If RAO is present for less than 24 hours and believed to have an embolic cause, treatment should begin as soon as the diagnosis is made. The goal of treatment is to promote migration of the embolus downstream and thus reverse the occlusion.

2. Begin ocular massage transiently to elevate and then decrease intraocular pressure. This is performed by pressing on the globe for 10 to 15 seconds and then releasing. The patient may perform this until anterior chamber paracentesis can be performed.

3. Anterior chamber paracentesis can be performed to abruptly lower intraocular pressure (3). Anterior chamber paracentesis should only be performed by someone with experience. Given the low rate of marked benefit, it is not likely that the risk should be accepted by a nonophthalmologist.

4. Give topical beta-blocker, apraclonidine, and/or carbonic anhydrase inhibitor (CAI) to maintain low IOP. Consider intravenous or oral CAI (e.g., acetazolamide).

5. Deliver 95% oxygen/5% carbon dioxide mixture via face mask for 24 hours if clinical response to treatment is observed. This mixture promotes the dilation of retinal vessels but is of unproven benefit and is rarely used today.

6. Early results demonstrate a possible benefit of intravenous thrombolytic therapy (4). However, the risks are significant and the results are equivocal.

7. Begin workup for systemic cause. Patients have been routinely admitted to our hospital for evaluation by neurology or internal medicine. In an older patient, or

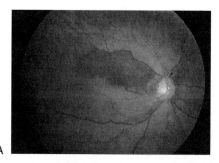 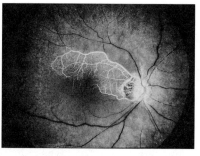

A   B

FIG. 23–1. A: Central retinal artery occlusions (CRAO) with retained superior macular perfusion by a cilioretinal artery. *For a color representation of this figure, please see the color insert facing p. 256.* **B:** Fluorescein angiography demonstrates the CRAO and retained perfusion of the cilioretinal artery. (Courtesy of Dr. L. Abrams.)

in a younger patient with predisposing cardiovascular disease, complete cardiovascular workup including carotid Doppler, echocardiography, and EKG should be considered.

8. In younger patients, examine optic disk for optic nerve head drusen or prepapillary loop. Ask about use of oral contraceptives and intravenous drugs. Consider an autoimmune predisposition or coagulopathy. Testing may include an ESR, complete blood count, anticardiolipin antibody, antiphospholipid antibodies, PT, PTT, and VDRL. In African Americans and patients of Mediterranean descent, hemoglobin electrophoresis should be performed.

9. Observe patient for development of iris neovascularization (NVI) or neovascular glaucoma (NVG). NVG occurs in about 10% of patients with CRAO.

Procedure: Anterior Chamber Paracentesis

1. Inform patient of the potential risks of the procedure, including cataract and endophthalmitis. Obtain written consent.

2. Anesthetize the eye with topical anesthetic (e.g., proparacaine hydrochloride). Use a cotton tip applicator to deliver a high concentration to the site of entry.

3. Prepare eye with topical 5% Betadine solution and antibiotic drop. Place a sterile lid speculum.

4. Place a 27- or 30-gauge needle on the end of a tuberculin (TB) syringe. If no assistant is available, remove the plunger.

5. Position the patient comfortably at the slit lamp (or operating microscope). Enter the anterior chamber so the needle tip is over the iris (Fig. 23–2). If penetration is difficult, entry can be made first with a no. 11 Bard-Parker blade. In aphakic eyes, be careful not to engage prolapsed vitreous. Allow 15 seconds for fluid egress. An assistant can slowly withdraw the plunger so the anterior chamber mildly shallows and 0.1 to 0.2 cc of fluid is removed.

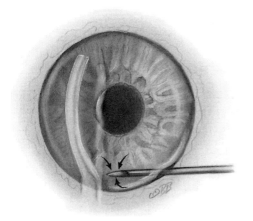

FIG. 23–2. Anterior chamber paracentesis.

6. Remove needle and speculum and deliver another antibiotic drop.
7. Check intraocular pressure; it should be 5 mm Hg or less.

Central Retinal Vein Occlusion

Diagnosis

1. Patients most commonly present with sudden vision loss in the affected eye. Patients also may complain of transient obscurations of vision lasting seconds to minutes over days to weeks. If decreased vision is not appreciated or medical attention not requested, central retinal vein occlusion (CRVO) can present with pain secondary to neovascular glaucoma ("90 day glaucoma").
2. Mean age at presentation is mid- to late 60s; however, it can occur in young adults. About 60% of individuals have systemic hypertension (5). About 10% have open-angle glaucoma (5).
3. Ophthalmoscopic examination shows intraretinal hemorrhages in all four quadrants. The retinal veins are often tortuous and engorged (compared with the unaffected eye), and the optic disk may be edematous. There are usually no spontaneous venous pulsations on the disk (significant if present in the unaffected eye).
4. CRVO may be "ischemic" or "perfused." Ischemic CRVO presents with worse visual acuity (generally less than 20/200) and more intraretinal hemorrhages ("blood and thunder" appearance). Greater than 10 disk areas of nonperfusion on fluorescein angiography predicts 60% chance of subsequent development of NVI (5).
5. Simultaneous cilioretinal artery occlusion occurs in a small percentage of eyes. In these cases visual potential is poor.

Management

1. Intraocular pressure should be checked and careful examination made for iris and angle neovascularization (NVI and NVA, respectively). The opposite eye should be examined for evidence of open-angle glaucoma and bilateral CRVO.
2. If simultaneous bilateral CRVO is present, workup should include complete blood count and measurement of blood viscosity. For older patients with CRVO, because of the high rate of hypertension and possibly increased frequency of diabetes, confirm that the patient sees a family physician or internist periodically. However, no special workup for unilateral CRVO is necessary or advised.
3. Further workup of CRVO in younger individuals has not been found to be beneficial (6).
4. Undilated and dilated examination and gonioscopy should be performed initially at monthly intervals to identify NVI or NVA. Risk of anterior segment neovascularization is about 60% in ischemic CRVO and about 3% in perfused CRVO (7). About 16% of perfused CRVO convert to ischemic CRVO within 4

months (5). Pan-retinal photocoagulation (PRP) is beneficial in preserving eyes with anterior segment neovascularization. However, if follow-up is reliable, one should wait until neovascularization develops before applying treatment (8).

5. Laser photocoagulation for persistent macular edema is, in general, of no benefit (8). In perfused CRVO, laser treatment to create a retinochoroidal anastomosis has shown benefit in selected patients (9).

Branch Retinal Vein Occlusion

Diagnosis

1. Branch retinal vein occlusion (BRVO) usually presents with the sudden onset of loss of vision or a scotoma in the affected eye.
2. Ophthalmoscopy shows intraretinal hemorrhages and cotton-wool spots in the affected quadrant(s) (Fig. 23–3). Macular edema is generally present if the BRVO occurred in a temporal quadrant.
3. Multiple cardiovascular risk factors (e.g., systemic hypertension) have been weakly correlated with BRVO (10).

Management

1. Large areas of ischemia (greater than five disk areas) predict a higher risk of retinal or disc neovascularization. However, initial fluorescein angiography is usually not helpful due to the number of intraretinal hemorrhages. Patients should be observed initially at regular intervals (every 1 to 2 months).
2. If neovascularization develops, scatter photocoagulation in the affected quadrant is beneficial in preventing severe visual loss secondary to vitreous hemorrhage (11).
3. If perfused macular edema is present at 3 to 4 months and visual acuity is worse than 20/40, visual outcome is improved by macular grid photocoagulation (12).

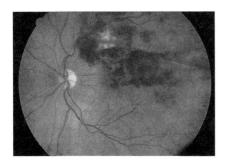

FIG. 23–3. Acute superotemporal branch retinal vein occlusion. (Courtesy of Dr. D. Finkelstein.) *For a color representation of this figure, please see the color insert facing p. 256.*

Choroidal Neovascularization

There are multiple causes of choroidal neovascularization (CNV). In older patients, the most likely cause is age-related macular degeneration (AMD). In younger patients, the most common cause is ocular histoplasmosis syndrome (OHS). The OHS is most prevalent in endemic areas such as the Mississippi valley. Other causes of CNV include high myopia, choroidal rupture (see Chapter 22), other inflammatory conditions such as multifocal choroiditis, and idiopathic conditions.

Diagnosis

1. Because most conditions that predispose to CNV are bilateral and chronic and often result in recurrent CNV, many patients are aware that they are at risk. This is particularly true for AMD.
2. Patients who present emergently with CNV often complain of distortion in vision in the affected eye. They may experience sudden or gradual loss of central vision.
3. Careful ophthalmoscopic examination with a slit lamp and fundus lens is necessary to identify macular changes suggestive of CNV. The retina and/or retinal pigment epithelium is usually elevated, there may be a grayish membrane visible, and there is often subretinal fluid and hemorrhage (Fig. 23–4*A*). Other changes predisposing to CNV are commonly seen, for example, drusen and pigmentary changes in AMD or peripheral punched out lesions and peripapillary atrophy in OHS.
4. The opposite eye should also be carefully examined for evidence of CNV.

Management

1. Prompt fluorescein angiography is critical for diagnosis of CNV and to determine if it is treatable. If the foveal area is threatened, as is often the case if patients present emergently, fluorescein angiography and treatment should not be delayed beyond a number of days. Transit of the affected macula and late views of both maculas should be requested. On fluorescein angiography, CNV usually stains early and leaks brightly in the mid- to late transit views (Fig. 23–4*B* and *C*).
2. CNV may be considered treatable or not treatable based on its size, its definition on fluorescein angiography, its location, the location of associated subretinal hemorrhage, and its predisposing cause. Recommendations for laser photocoagulation have been better defined by the Macular Photocoagulation Study (13,14). The indication for surgical management is currently under study (15). Experimental therapies such as photodynamic therapy, pharmacotherapy, and radiation are being actively pursued.
3. If indicated, laser photocoagulation should be performed by those experienced in the technique, particularly if the CNV threatens or involves the foveal area.

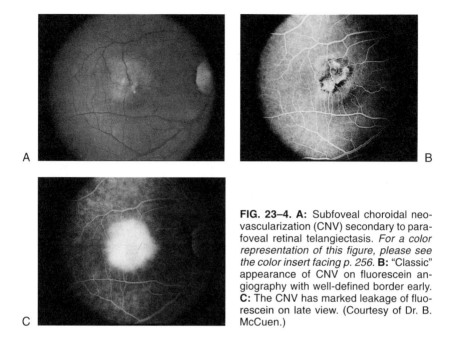

FIG. 23–4. A: Subfoveal choroidal neovascularization (CNV) secondary to parafoveal retinal telangiectasis. *For a color representation of this figure, please see the color insert facing p. 256.* **B:** "Classic" appearance of CNV on fluorescein angiography with well-defined border early. **C:** The CNV has marked leakage of fluorescein on late view. (Courtesy of Dr. B. McCuen.)

Procedure: Photocoagulation of Choroidal Neovascularization

1. Consider retrobulbar block, particularly for juxtafoveal membranes.
2. Define CNV with fluorescein angiography. Consider postponing treatment if extensive hemorrhage remains.
3. Dye yellow, argon green, or krypton red, 0.2 to 0.5 seconds, 200-micron spot size, sufficient intensity to cause chalk white spot.
4. Initially outline the border of the treatment area based on fluorescein angiogram, then fill in.
5. Obtain posttreatment photograph to rule out untreated area.
6. Follow up in 2 to 4 weeks with repeat fluorescein angiography to rule out persistence. If persistent CNV, consider retreatment. If no persistence, repeat fluorescein angiography every 3 to 4 months during first year.
7. Educate patient in contacting an ophthalmologist promptly for new symptoms of visual distortion or loss of vision which may indicate a recurrence.

Central Serous Chorioretinopathy

Diagnosis

1. Central serous chorioretinopathy (CSR) classically presents in middle-aged men with type A personality.

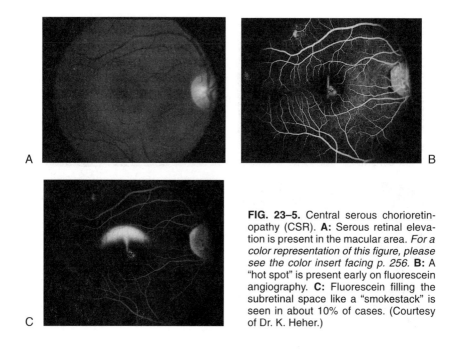

A

B

C

FIG. 23–5. Central serous chorioretin-opathy (CSR). **A:** Serous retinal eleva-tion is present in the macular area. *For a color representation of this figure, please see the color insert facing p. 256.* **B:** A "hot spot" is present early on fluorescein angiography. **C:** Fluorescein filling the subretinal space like a "smokestack" is seen in about 10% of cases. (Courtesy of Dr. K. Heher.)

2. Patients usually complain of distortion or micropsia in the affected eye. The condition may be bilateral and recurrent.
3. Ophthalmoscopy shows retinal elevation in the macular area (Fig. 23–5*A*). Oc-casionally subretinal fluid extends inferiorly outside the macula. There may be a whitish subretinal deposit believed to be fibrin.
4. Fluorescein angiography should be performed, particularly to rule out CNV. Typ-ically, one or more focal sites of dye leakage are identified (Fig. 23–5*B* and *C*).

Management

1. No treatment is indicated initially because CSR usually resolves spontaneously. Visual acuity usually returns, although complete resolution may take months.
2. If subretinal fluid does not resolve spontaneously or CSR is recurrent, focal laser photocoagulation may be indicated (16).

Rhegmatogenous Retinal Detachment

Diagnosis

1. Patients usually complain of a "shadow" or "curtain" across the visual field of the affected eye. They may have noticed flashing lights or floaters if a predis-posing posterior vitreous detachment (PVD) had occurred. Visual acuity is nor-

mal or reduced, consistent with vitreous opacity (pigment, blood) if macula is attached. Visual acuity is markedly reduced, 20/200 or worse, if the foveal center is detached.
2. Dilated fundus examination may show pigment clumps within the vitreous cavity ("tobacco dust"), vitreous hemorrhage, and/or a Weiss ring (the latter indicative of PVD). If bullously elevated, the detached retina has a corrugated appearance (Fig. 23–6*A* and *B*) and moves with eye movement. A magnified view may be necessary to identify whether the macula is detached.
3. Ophthalmoscopy should include depressed examination of both eyes to identify all retinal tears. Retinal tears may range from a size too small be visualized (often in aphakic or pseudophakic retinal detachments) to giant retinal tears (greater than 90 degrees; Fig. 23–6*C*).

Management

1. Detailed discussion of the management of retinal detachment is beyond the scope of this chapter. For further discussion of retinal detachment see Chapter 20.
2. Vitreoretinal consultation should be obtained as soon as possible because faster treatment predicts better outcome, particularly when the macula is still attached. However, in general, surgical management can be postponed to the following day even for macula-on detachments (see Chapter 6).

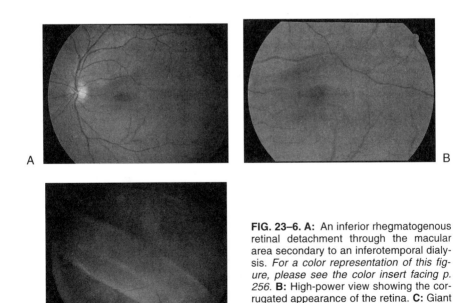

A

B

C

FIG. 23–6. A: An inferior rhegmatogenous retinal detachment through the macular area secondary to an inferotemporal dialysis. *For a color representation of this figure, please see the color insert facing p. 256.* **B:** High-power view showing the corrugated appearance of the retina. **C:** Giant retinal tear; the superior retina has flapped over obscuring the macula.

Idiopathic Macular Hole

Idiopathic macular hole rarely presents emergently; however, it is presented here because it is relatively common and should not be missed on ophthalmoscopic examination.

Diagnosis

1. Acuity is usually 20/60 to 20/200 for a full-thickness hole, better for an impending (stage I) macular hole. The patient may describe a central area of distortion (impending hole) or scotoma (full-thickness hole).
2. A full-thickness hole has a sharp margin and surrounding cuff of fluid in the foveolar area; a preretinal operculum may be present. When a narrow slit-lamp beam is shined across a full-thickness hole, attentive patients usually report that they see a complete break in the beam (Watzke-Allen sign). A yellow spot or ring in the foveolar area may represent an impending macular hole.
3. Fluorescein angiography would demonstrate a window defect for a full-thickness hole (Aaberg's sign) and may be normal for an impending hole.

Management

1. A patient with impending hole should be re-examined within 3 to 6 months because of about 50% progress to a full-thickness macular hole. Vitrectomy and fluid-gas exchange at this stage are under study.
2. Vitrectomy and fluid-gas exchange may be of benefit for full-thickness idiopathic macular holes (17).

Intraocular Tumor

Intraocular tumors are insidious in their growth and are thus an uncommon cause of sudden loss of vision, although vision may decrease quickly associated with hemorrhage or macular detachment. It is critical that they be accurately diagnosed and not confused with other conditions that may have a similar appearance.

Diagnosis

1. Intraocular tumors may be found incidently on routine examination. Presenting symptoms include decreased vision, visual field defects, and photopsias. Decreased vision may be caused by tumor involvement of the fovea, exudative retinal detachment, or tumor compression of the lens with cataract formation (18).
2. A detailed history should be obtained with special emphasis on previous malignancies.
3. Extensive examination of the adnexa, anterior, and posterior segments should

be performed on both eyes. Binocular indirect ophthalmoscopy is the most important clinical method of diagnosing fundus tumors (19).

4. Ultrasound is particularly useful in eyes with opaque media and when differentiating fluid masses such as subretinal hemorrhage or choroidal effusion from solid tumors. Choroidal melanomas have low to moderate internal reflectivity on A-scan, whereas highly vascular masses have high internal reflectivity.

5. Magnetic resonance imaging (MRI) can be valuable when vitreous hemorrhage obscures the view or when ultrasonography does not differentiate subretinal blood from solid tumor (20). In most cases, if there is access to an experienced ultrasonographer, there is little benefit to computed tomography or MRI.

Management

The management of intraocular tumors is largely dependent on the type and location of the tumor and is beyond the scope of this text. The initial management of intraocular tumors should include the appropriate referral for systemic evaluation whether the lesion is metastatic or primary. For an extensive discussion of ocular tumors, the reader is referred elsewhere (21).

Migraine

Visual complaints are frequent among recurrent headache sufferers. The complaint of recurrent headache and visual symptoms should alert the physician to the possibility of migraine. The new classification for migraine consists of two main categories: migraine without aura and migraine with aura. Migraine without aura includes what was previously termed "common migraine." Migraine with aura includes the classic and complicated categories of the previous classification system. The terms "ophthalmoplegic migraine" and "retinal migraine" are still used in the present system (22). Migraine also may follow ocular surgery and should be in the differential diagnosis of atypical postoperative pain and nausea (23).

Diagnosis

1. The typical migraine sufferer is a woman whose headaches began in adolescence or young adulthood. The typical headache is described as unilateral, pulsating, and associated with nausea and photophobia. Bifrontal or generalized pressure is less common but not unheard of. There may be aggravating factors such as physical exertion, stress, or certain foods.

2. Visual symptoms in the form of scintillating scotomas are the most common sensory complaint accompanying migraine with aura. The scintillating scotoma may be described as a small gray spot starting centrally and expanding toward the periphery with bright zigzag flashes. The aura phase typically lasts 15 to 60 minutes (24).

3. Retinal migraine is uncommon but is in the differential diagnosis for transient monocular loss of vision.
4. Most migraines can be diagnosed by history alone. Patients usually have a history of headache dating back to adolescence. The frequency, position, quality, severity, and associated symptoms such as nausea and vomiting as well as focal neurologic symptoms should be elucidated in the history. Elucidation of aggravating and ameliorating factors also may be helpful. For example, migraine sufferers will usually seek a quiet dark place or sleep to calm the headache.
5. The diagnosis of migraine should not be made on the first attack. A single severe or unremitting headache should clue the physician to an organic cause. Further diagnostic studies such as neuroimaging should be considered when there is no history of headache, the headache is atypical from previous episodes, or there are new focal neurologic deficits. Organic disease also should be ruled out in the presence of altered mental status, poor vision, fever, stiff neck, or papilledema.

Management

There are two types of pharmacologic treatment for migraine: abortive for an acute attack and prophylactic.

Drugs number 1 through 4 below may be used to abort a migraine attack.

1. Nonsteroidal anti-inflammatory drugs (NSAIDs): naprosyn 325 to 750 mg or ibuprofen 800 mg orally in a one-time dose. Bulbital and caffeine are often added if NSAIDS are unsuccessful.
2. Ergotamine and dihydroergotamine are alkaloid alpha adrenergic blockers. The average oral dose of ergotamine is 2 to 3 mg. Excessive dosing will cause vomiting. Caution should be used in patients with hypertension, angina, and renal failure.
3. Sumatriptan is a selective 5-HT1 receptor agonist. It may be used orally or subcutaneously by injection. The average adult dose is 25 to 100 mg orally or in a 6-mg subcutaneous injection. Sumatriptan should be avoided in ischemic heart disease, Printzmetal's angina, and vertebrobasilar migraine (24).
4. Metaclopramide 10 mg intravenously can abort a migraine attack (23). Metaclopramide 10 mg orally or promethazine 25 to -50 mg (oral or suppository form) are useful to control nausea.
5. Prophylactic therapy may include an oral beta-blocker, amitriptyline, or calcium channel blocker.

Erythropsia

Erythropsia literally means "seeing red." In aphakic eyes this condition was originally described by Duke-Elder (25). It also has been described in pseudophakic eyes that have been implanted with intraocular lenses that do not filter ultraviolet radiation. Erythropsia is a phenomenon experienced by some patients who are aphakic or pseudophakic and are exposed to prolonged bright light. It is believed to be caused by bleaching of the blue cones in the macula, leaving predominantly a red-green population. Therefore, patients temporarily see red or pink under scotopic conditions (26). In phakic patients, the crystalline lens acts as a filter to ultraviolet radiation.

Diagnosis

1. There should be a history of prolonged exposure to bright light or ultraviolet radiation.
2. Previous lens extraction (aphakic or pseudophakic).
3. A thorough examination with dilation should be performed to rule out vitreous hemorrhage or other retinal pathology.

Management

1. Erythropsia is usually a temporary condition and needs no treatment.
2. Ultraviolet protection may prevent further episodes (sunglasses or glasses with ultraviolet filters).
3. Secondary intraocular lens implantation with an ultraviolet filter is an alternative.

DISORDERS AFFECTING THE VITREOUS

Floaters and Flashing Lights: Posterior Vitreous Detachment

Spontaneous PVD occurs with increasing frequency from middle to older age. Younger individuals with moderate to high myopia also may experience a PVD correlating with the severity of the myopia. About 3% to 5% of individuals with an acute PVD develop a retinal break, so it is a prime risk factor for rhegmatogenous retinal detachment.

Diagnosis

1. Patients note the sudden onset of flashing lights and/or a new floater in their central field of vision.
2. The anterior vitreous cavity should first be inspected for pigmented cells or pigment clumps (tobacco dust); this indicates an increased frequency of a retinal break in the phakic eye. The vitreous also should be examined for acute vitreous hemorrhage.
3. The vitreous cavity should be examined for inflammatory cells. Extensive white cells signify a vitritis and not acute PVD. Evidence of vitritis requires more extensive workup for infectious, uveitic, or neoplastic cause.
4. A dilated retinal examination must be performed. A partial or complete Weiss ring suspended in the vitreous cavity identified by magnified examination of the posterior pole is the only definite sign of posterior vitreous detachment. A peripheral

retinal examination with indirect ophthalmoscopy and depression or mirrored contact lens must be performed to identify retinal breaks or detachment.

5. If vitreous hemorrhage prevents complete ophthalmoscopic evaluation of the retinal periphery, see below under Spontaneous Vitreous Hemorrhage.

Management

1. All retinal breaks with persistent traction (e.g., flap tears) and breaks with small areas of surrounding subretinal fluid should be considered for treatment with cryotherapy or laser (see Chapter 20). Breaks not associated with traction (e.g., operculated holes, atrophic holes) have a lower incidence of subsequent retinal detachment; treatment can be applied but is of more limited value. If retinal detachment is identified, see above and Chapter 20.

2. Follow-up dilated retinal examination with depression should be performed at about 1 month to 6 weeks after the onset of symptoms because the PVD can extend, resulting in a new retinal break.

3. The patient should be counseled that new floaters or increased flashing requires an examination as soon as possible (e.g., within 24 hours). Loss of visual acuity or visual field requires an immediate follow-up because this likely represents a retinal detachment.

Spontaneous Vitreous Hemorrhage

Diagnosis

1. Blood is seen preretinally or collected within the vitreous cavity. Red blood cells may be seen in the anterior vitreous cavity by slit-lamp microscopy. With large vitreous hemorrhage the normally red-orange–colored "red reflex" is replaced by a bright or dark red reflex or no reflex at all.

2. The most common cause is proliferative diabetic retinopathy. Other causes include other proliferative retinopathies (e.g., sickle retinopathy, ischemic retinal vein occlusion), acute retinal vein occlusion, acute posterior vitreous detachment with avulsed or torn retinal blood vessel, breakthrough subretinal hemorrhage from choroidal neovascularization, and Terson's syndrome. See also Vitreous Hemorrhage Secondary to Trauma (Chapter 20).

3. Simultaneous vitreous and intracranial hemorrhages comprise Terson's syndrome. Intracranial hemorrhage of any etiology is believed to cause an acute increase in intraocular venous pressure, with rupture of papillary and retinal vessels (see Chapter 22).

Management

1. Careful ophthalmoscopic examination must be performed in an attempt to identify the source of the hemorrhage. Peripheral depression or examination with a Goldmann three-mirror lens should be used to identify associated retinal

breaks, particularly if there is no history of a proliferative retinopathy. If the view is at all limited, ultrasound should be performed (see Chapter 5).
2. Retinal breaks should be treated with laser or cryotherapy (see Chapter 20). Occasionally, ultrasound can be used to guide cryotherapy of poorly visualized retinal breaks (27). A limited period of bedrest with elevation of the head for 24 hours may allow gravitational settling of the hemorrhage to permit ophthalmoscopic view of the retina. Significant vitreous hemorrhage with associated retinal detachment is an indication for early vitrectomy (see Chapter 20).
3. If untreated or incompletely treated active proliferative diabetic retinopathy is identified, PRP should be performed. If the view is too limited for the application of adequate treatment, cryotherapy or vitrectomy may be indicated (1).

Procedure: Pan-Retinal Photocoagulation for Proliferative Diabetic Retinopathy

1. Consider retrobulbar block.
2. Place Rodenstock panfunduscopic, Goldmann three-mirror, or other lens for peripheral fundus viewing.
3. Argon green or krypton red, 0.05 to 0.1 seconds, 500-micron spot size (Goldmann) or 250-micron spot size (Rodenstock), sufficient power to cause gray-white spot.
4. Cover retina outside the temporal arcades and nasal to optic disk (outside macular area) maintaining spots one spot-width apart. Treat inferior fundus first if this is not obscured by vitreous hemorrhage.
5. Be careful to avoid macular area. Lower the power setting if moving to a clearer area from an area partially blocked by vitreous hemorrhage to avoid overly "hot" burns.

4. In non-diabetic individuals of African or Mediterranean descent, a sickle preparation and hemoglobin electrophoresis should be considered. If proliferative sickle retinopathy is identified, laser photocoagulation surrounding the causative neovascular seafan has been recommended (28).
5. If a retinal tear is suspected as the source of the vitreous hemorrhage (e.g., in an individual without a history of retinovascular disease), then weekly examination as the hemorrhage clears is initially required to locate the tear or diagnose an early retinal detachment. Most hemorrhages from other causes are followed for at least 1 month, by which time repeat examination should be performed. Timing of vitrectomy should be based on its cause (e.g., diabetes mellitus type 1), the status of the fellow eye, the patient's occupation, children at risk of amblyopia, and patient anxiety.

REFERENCES

1. Benson WE, Tasman W, Duane TD. Diabetes mellitus and the eye. In: Tasman W, Jaeger EA, eds. *Clinical Ophthalmology.* Vol. 3 Philadelphia: Lippincott-Raven; 1995.

2. Hayreh SS, Kolder HE, Weingeist TA. Central retinal artery occlusion and retinal tolerance time. *Ophthalmology* 1980;87:75.
3. Chen JC, Cheema D. Repeated anterior chamber paracentesis for the treatment of central retinal artery occlusion. *Can J Ophthalmol* 1994;29:207.
4. Schmidt D, Shumacher M, Wakhloo AK. Microcatheter urokinase infusion in central retinal artery occlusion. *Am J Ophthalmol* 1992;113:429.
5. Central Vein Occlusion Study Group. Baseline and early natural history report. The Central Vein Occlusion Study. *Arch Ophthalmol* 1993;111:1087.
6. Fong ACO, Schatz H. Central retinal vein occlusion in young adults. *Surv Ophthalmol* 1993;37:393.
7. Hayreh SS, Rojas P, Podhajsky P, et al. Ocular neovascularization with retinal vascular occlusion. III: Incidence of ocular neovascularization with retinal vein occlusion. *Ophthalmology* 1983;90:488.
8. Central Vein Occlusion Study Group. A randomized clinical trail of early panretinal photocoagulation for ischemic central vein occlusion. The Central Vein Occlusion Study N Report. *Ophthalmology* 1995;102:1434.
9. McAllister IL, Constable IS. Laser-induced chorioretinal venous anastomosis for treatment of non-ischemic central retinal vein occlusion. *Arch Ophthalmol* 1995;113:456.
10. Orth DH, Patz A. Retinal branch vein occlusion. *Surv Ophthalmol* 1978;22:357.
11. Branch Vein Occlusion Study Group. Argon laser scatter photocoagulation for prevention of neovascularization and vitreous hemorrhage in branch vein occlusion. *Arch Ophthalmol* 1986;104:34.
12. Branch Vein Occlusion Study Group. Argon laser photocoagulation for macular edema in branch vein occlusion. *Am J Ophthalmol* 1984;98:271.
13. Elman MJ, Fine SL. Exudative age-related macular degeneration. In: Ryan SJ, ed. *Retina.* Vol. 2. St. Louis: CV Mosby; 1994:1103–1141.
14. Hawkins BS, Alexander J, Schachat AP. Ocular histoplasmosis. In: Ryan SJ, ed. *Retina.* Vol. 2. St. Louis: CV Mosby; 1994:1661–1675.
15. Lambert HM, Capone A, Aaberg TM, et al. Surgical excision of subfoveal neovascular membranes in age-related macular degeneration. *Am J Ophthalmol* 1992;113:257.
16. Samy CN, Gragoudas ES. Laser photocoagulation treatment of central serous chorioretinopathy. *Int Ophthalmol Clin* 1994;34:109.
17. Glaser BM. Management of idiopathic macular holes. In: Ryan SJ, ed. *Retina.* Vol. 3. St. Louis: CV Mosby; 1994:2379–2384.
18. Mukai S, Gragoudas ES. Diagnosis of choroidal melanoma. In: Albert DM, Jakobiec FA, eds. *Principles and Practice of Ophthalmology.* Vol. 5. Philadelphia: WB Saunders; 1994:3209.
19. Tolentino FI, Schepens CL, Freeman HM. *Vitreoretinal Disorders: Diagnosis and Management.* Philadelphia: WB Saunders; 1976.
20. DePotter P, Shields JA, Shields CL. *MRI of the Eye and Orbit.* Philadelphia: JB Lippincott; 1995:97.
21. Schachat A. Tumors. In: Ryan SJ, ed. *Retina.* Vol. I. St. Louis: CV Mosby; 1994:517–808.
22. Solomon S. Migraine diagnosis and clinical symptomatology. *Headache* 1994;34(suppl):8.
23. MacCumber MW, Jaffe GJ, McCuen BM II. Treatment of migraine headache after ocular surgery with intravenous metoclopromide hydrochloride. *Am J Ophthalmol* 1996;121:96.
24. Silberstein SD, Lipton RB. Overview of diagnosis and treatment of migraine. *Neurology* 1994;44(suppl):S6.
25. Duke-Elder S, ed. Ophthalmic optics and refraction. In: *System of Ophthalmology.* Vol. 5. St. Louis: CV Mosby; 1970:381.
26. Lawrence HM, Reynolds TR. Erythropsial phototoxicity associated with nonultraviolet-filtering intraocular lenses. *J Cataract Refract Surg* 1989;15:571.
27. DiBernardo C, Blodi B, Byrne SF. Echographic evaluation of retinal tears in patients with spontaneous vitreous hemorrhage. *Arch Ophthalmol* 1992;110:511.
28. Jampol LM, Farber M, Rabb MF, Serjeant G. An update on techniques of photocoagulation treatment of proliferative sickle cell retinopathy. *Eye* 1991;5:260.

Management of Ocular Injuries and Emergencies,
edited by Mathew W. MacCumber.
Lippincott–Raven Publishers, Philadelphia © 1998.

24

Disorders of the Optic Nerve and Afferent Visual System

John B. Kerrison and Neil R. Miller

Malcolm-Grow Medical Center, Andrews Air Force Base, Maryland 20762-6600 and Department of Ophthalmology, Wilmer Eye Institute, The Johns Hopkins University School of Medicine, Baltimore, Maryland 21287

Basic Considerations 352
　History 352 · Examination 352
Traumatic Optic Neuropathy: Direct and Indirect 353
　Diagnosis 354 · Management 354
Nonarteritic Ischemic Optic Neuropathy 355
　Diagnosis 355 · Management 356
Arteritic Ischemic Optic Neuropathy: Giant Cell Arteritis 356
　Diagnosis 357 · Management 358
Optic Neuritis 358
　Diagnosis 359 · Management 360
Leber Hereditary Optic Neuropathy 360
　Diagnosis 361 · Management 361
Pseudotumor Cerebri 361
　Diagnosis 361 · Management 362
Toxic/Metabolic Optic Neuropathy 362
　Diagnosis 362 · Management 363
Compressive Optic Neuropathy 363
　Diagnosis 363 · Management 363
Trauma to the Optic Chiasm 364
　Diagnosis 364 · Management 364
Optic Tract Trauma 364
　Diagnosis 364 · Management 365
Trauma to the Lateral Geniculate Body 365
　Diagnosis 365 · Management 365
Retrogeniculate Trauma and Cortical Blindness 365
　Diagnosis 366 · Management 366

BASIC CONSIDERATIONS

Emergent disorders of the optic nerve and afferent visual system often present with marked visual loss. However, detailed neuro-ophthalmic examination is necessary because other important clinical findings may be subtle. In the setting of blunt or penetrating head trauma, performing a complete neuro-ophthalmic evaluation may be difficult because associated neurologic and systemic injuries often make both the examination and the interpretation of findings complicated. Nevertheless, it is important that such an evaluation be as accurate and complete as possible because subsequent management decisions may be based on initial findings.

The neuro-ophthalmologic evaluation ideally should be conducted in an ophthalmic examination area, but a bedside evaluation must suffice in many instances. Certain aspects of the history and examination are of particular importance in the neuro-ophthalmic evaluation (see also Chapter 3).

History

The history should include the previous best-corrected visual acuity, history of amblyopia, optic atrophy, and inherited color deficit.

Examination

Visual acuity: near card with numbers, letters, "illiterate E," finger counting, or finger mimicking.

Visual fields: using confrontation techniques; amsler grid testing.

Motility: alignment, fixation, comitance or incomitance of strabismus, ductions and versions, saccades, pursuit, random movements, vestibulo-ocular reflex, forced ductions, Bell's phenomenon, optokinetic nystagmus, and caloric responses.

Pupils: size and reactivity to light and near stimulation. Remember that anisocoria is never caused by a defect in the afferent portion of the pupillomotor pathway. Test for a relative afferent pupillary defect (RAPD) using a swinging flashlight test. If one of the pupils is dilated and nonreactive or poorly reactive because of injury to the iris or the oculomotor (third) nerve, one can still test for an RAPD using a reverse method. Instead of observing the reaction of each pupil to light stimulation as the light is swung from one eye to the other, observe only the reactive pupil when swinging the light to the eye back and forth from one eye to the other. If there is an RAPD in the eye with the dilated, poorly reactive pupil, the pupil of the contralateral eye will redilate when the light is swung from that eye to the affected eye. Recall that an RAPD is not necessarily present in patients with bilateral optic neuropathies, even when there is marked asymmetry of visual sensory function. In such cases, however, both pupils may react sluggishly. The pupillary examination is of major importance in patients with head trauma because it may be the only means of objective evaluation of visual sensory function in such patients.

Other tests of afferent function: relative brightness, color vision testing, and red desaturation.

Trigeminal and facial nerve function: corneal reflex, sensation to light, touch and sharp object, and facial asymmetry.

Slit-lamp biomicroscopy: a small sphincter tear or iridodialysis may be noted and explain a dilated or an irregular, poorly reactive pupil. Vermiform movements or sector paralysis of the sphincter may indicate damage to the ciliary ganglion or short posterior ciliary nerves.

Ophthalmoscopy: optic disk swelling, retinal or vitreous hemorrhages. Do not dilate the pupils in patients who are comatose or are being prepared for surgery. Communicate with the primary physician before dilating and inform other caregivers verbally and through the chart. A note may be posted above the patient's bed. Use only short-acting agents, such as 0.5% tropicamide, to dilate, and be sure to dilate both eyes.

TRAUMATIC OPTIC NEUROPATHY: DIRECT AND INDIRECT

Optic nerve trauma is classified as direct, in which an object has penetrated the orbit and injured the optic nerve (Fig. 24–1), or indirect, in which the optic neuropathy has developed in the setting of closed head trauma (1). Indirect traumatic optic neuropathy (TON) is generally subdivided into an anterior and a posterior (retrobulbar) type. Anterior TON results from damage to the intraocular or anterior orbital portions of the optic nerve. It may occur when the globe is suddenly rotated or pulled forward, resulting in tearing at the lamina cribosa and leading to hemorrhage at the disk or avulsion in some cases (the condition is also known as "optic nerve avulsion". The optic disk is invariably swollen in this condition, which may result from blunt forehead trauma or when a finger is accidentally poked in the eye (2,3). Posterior TON results from damage to the posterior orbital, intracanalicular, or intracranial portions of the optic nerve. In such cases, there is loss of vision that initially is unassociated with ophthalmoscopic evidence of injury to the optic nerve and which also may be unassociated with external evidence of injury to the eye or orbit.

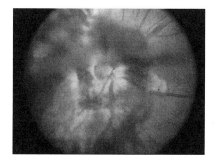

FIG. 24–1. Direct traumatic optic neuropathy. This man lost all vision in this eye when an automobile antenna entered his right orbit. There is a depression in the area of the optic disk, and hemorrhage emanates from it. Visual acuity remained at no light perception. (Courtesy of Dr. T. Deutsch.) *For a color representation of this figure, please see the color insert facing p. 256.*

Diagnosis

1. Signs of an optic neuropathy are present, including an RAPD, sluggish pupil(s), decreased relative brightness, red desaturation, and dyschromatopsia that cannot be explained by retinal findings, such as a submacular hemorrhage. Visual acuity usually is reduced, although it may be relatively preserved, and a visual field defect is present.
2. In anterior TON, the optic nerve appears swollen, and it may be surrounded by flame-shaped hemorrhages. The retinal veins are often somewhat dilated. The appearance thus may mimic that of a central retinal vein occlusion. In some cases, the retina may be white and edematous from an associated central retinal artery occlusion.
3. In posterior TON, the optic nerve head appears normal. Optic disk pallor will not appear for 4 to 5 weeks.
4. Computed tomography (CT) of the orbits with axial and coronal thin cuts may demonstrate a retained orbital foreign body, canal fracture, optic nerve hemorrhage, subperiosteal hematoma compressing the optic nerve, or avulsion of the optic nerve. CT scanning in patients with an anterior TON invariably shows diffuse enlargement of the orbital portion of the optic nerve. In some cases, changes consistent with blood can be detected within the optic nerve sheath or within the swollen nerve itself.
5. Carefully examine the fellow eye to rule out damage to the optic chiasm or contralateral optic nerve.

Management

1. Consider immediate hospitalization.
2. Patients with anterior TON may require immediate optic nerve sheath decompression. Treatment with high-dose corticosteroids, given intravenously (i.v.), has been recommended for indirect posterior TON; however, some patients may improve without therapy. Also consider high-dose i.v. corticosteroids for selected cases of both direct posterior TON and indirect anterior TON. The regimen used in a multi-centered prospective study of optic nerve trauma is an i.v. methylprednisolone loading dose of 30 mg/kg over 15 minutes followed by 5.4 mg/kg/hour for 47 hours. No taper is used. An H_2-blocker, such as ranitidine 150 mg orally twice a day, may be added.
3. Consider immediate treatment of any surgical lesion such as an orbital foreign body, hematoma, or canal fracture impinging on the optic nerve. Optic nerve fenestration has been performed for intra-sheath optic nerve hematoma.
4. If visual loss occurs after an interval of intact vision, if visual loss is progressive, or if vision initially improves and then worsens, optic canal decompression should be performed. Thus, correct documentation of initial visual acuity is important. Otolaryngologists or neurosurgeons perform optic canal decompression in most centers.

5. Optic canal decompression combined with high dose intravenous corticosteroids is the initial approach to indirect posterior traumatic optic neuropathy in some centers.
6. No light perception is not necessarily a contraindication to treatment.
7. Comatose patients with evidence of TON generally should not undergo optic canal decompression or optic nerve sheath fenestration because they may have reasonably good visual function even though an RAPD may be present. Should surgery be performed and the patient ultimately be found to be blind in the affected eye, the possibility of damage to the nerve during surgery could be raised. The exception to this recommendation would be the patient in whom there is a completely amaurotic pupil (i.e., isocoric pupils, one of which is completely unreactive to light stimulation but that reacts consensually). In such a case, one can safely assume that the eye is completely blind.

NONARTERITIC ISCHEMIC OPTIC NEUROPATHY

Ischemic optic neuropathy (ION) is characterized by a monocular loss of vision that is acute, painless, and not infrequently permanent. A relative afferent pupillary defect is invariably present, and the visual field loss is typically arcuate or altitudinal. When associated with optic disk swelling, it is called "anterior ischemic optic neuropathy" (AION). When no optic disk swelling is present, the ischemia is presumed to involve retrobulbar optic nerve and is called "posterior ischemic optic neuropathy" (PION). Most commonly, AION is idiopathic (nonarteritic) or due to giant cell arteritis (GCA) (arteritic). Other associated conditions include systemic lupus erythematosus, polyarteritis nodosa, syphilis, papilledema, malignant hypertension, hypotension, cataract extraction, optic disk drusen, or migraine. Despite its relatively frequent occurrence, the etiology of idiopathic AION is not well defined. Fluorescein angiography may demonstrate areas of optic nerve hypoperfusion, and optic nerves with small cups appear to be at greater risk.

Diagnosis

1. Patients present with sudden, monocular, and painless vision loss. Patients are typically more than 45 years of age and have an underlying systemic vasculopathy. Obtain a detailed history of the onset of visual loss with particular questioning as to the presence of systemic symptoms.
2. Test for dyschromatopsia and a relative afferent pupillary defect. Confrontation visual fields and formal perimetry should be performed. Altitudinal, arcuate, or central visual field defects may be observed.
3. Examine the optic nerve and retina for disk swelling, pallor, narrowed arteries, and peripapillary hemorrhages. The presence of cotton-wool spots suggests arteritic AION. Lack of disk swelling indicates a retrobulbar optic neuropathy. Examination of the fellow eye is extremely important in helping to distinguish arteritic from nonarteritic AION. A large cup suggests arteritic AION. A small cup is consistent with idiopathic AION, although it does not rule out the possibility of GCA.

4. If a retrobulbar optic neuropathy is present, the patient should be evaluated for underlying systemic vascular disease, such as arteriosclerotic carotid artery disease or GCA. Less likely possibilities include herpes zoster, connective tissue disorders, painless retrobulbar optic neuritis, or an intracranial mass. Perform neuroimaging in these patients.

5. If AION is thought to be present, one must distinguish between arteritic and nonarteritic (see below) forms by clinical features and laboratory tests. Patients with idiopathic AION are usually between 45 and 65 years of age, have no systemic symptoms of GCA, and have a small physiologic optic cup. Patients with arteritic AION are typically more than 60 years of age and usually have systemic symptoms, such as headache, myalgias, and arthralgias. They have an average size physiologic optic cup and may have signs of retinal ischemia such as cotton-wool spots. A fluorescein angiogram may show choroidal ischemia in patients with GCA.

6. Obtain an erythrocyte sedimentation rate (ESR). A guideline for upper limits of normal: male = ½ × age; female = ½ × (age − 10). In idiopathic AION, the ESR should be normal unless there is another reason for it to be elevated. General medical evaluation should assess for evidence of cardiovascular disease, diabetes mellitus, and hypertension. If ESR is elevated or systemic symptoms are present, begin arteritic ion workup and management.

Management

1. There is no proven therapy for idiopathic AION; however, approximately 40% of patients will have some improvement in vision within 6 months (4).

2. The majority of patients with idiopathic AION will have a stable visual acuity of 20/60 or better. The recurrence risk for another event in the same eye is 2% to 4% and in the fellow eye is 20% to 30%.

3. The occurrence of idiopathic posterior ION is so rare that the prognosis for vision in the affected and fellow eye is unknown.

4. Patients with idiopathic AION are at risk for developing subsequent cardiovascular or cerebrovascular events. Thus, all patients should be evaluated by their internist on a regular basis.

5. Aspirin has been suggested as a means of reducing the risk of an attack in the fellow eye.

ARTERITIC ISCHEMIC OPTIC NEUROPATHY: GIANT CELL ARTERITIS

Giant cell arteritis is a systemic necrotizing vasculitis primarily affecting cranial arteries originating from the aortic arch. Patients are typically more than 55 years of age and are at risk for permanent vision loss, most commonly from anterior ischemic optic neuropathy, unless the disease is recognized and treated. Other causes of vision loss include central retinal artery occlusion, branch retinal artery occlusion, choroidal ischemia, retrobulbar ischemic optic neuropathy, and ischemia of the chiasm and retrochiasmal visual pathway.

Diagnosis

1. Visual symptoms include sudden, painless unilateral visual loss that may become bilateral in hours to days. Patients will often complain of transient blurring of vision (amaurosis fugax) or double vision hours or days before vision loss.
2. Systemic manifestations include headache, jaw claudication, scalp tenderness, myalgias, arthralgias, anorexia, weight loss, or fever. Patients must be questioned specifically for the presence of these symptoms. The medical history also should include questions about cardiovascular disease, hypertension, and diabetes mellitus.
3. Findings on ophthalmic examination include decreased visual acuity (usually profound), a relative afferent pupillary defect with unilateral or asymmetric optic neuropathy, color vision loss, decreased brightness, an altitudinal visual field defect, and a swollen optic disk with peripapillary hemorrhages and cotton-wool spots (Fig. 24–2). Examine the fellow optic nerve head carefully with attention to the cup-to-disk ratio because a normal physiologic cup is suggestive of arteritic ischemic optic neuropathy. Abduction weakness may be present from a sixth nerve palsy or ischemia to the lateral rectus muscle.

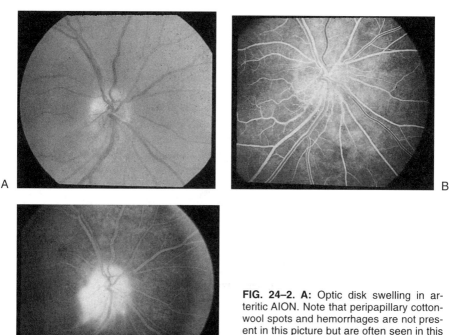

A

B

C

FIG. 24–2. A: Optic disk swelling in arteritic AION. Note that peripapillary cotton-wool spots and hemorrhages are not present in this picture but are often seen in this setting. **B:** Fluorescein angiography demonstrates irregular optic nerve head filling. **C:** Staining of the inferior nerve head (Courtesy of Dr. W.R. Green)

4. Other findings include scalp tenderness with a palpable, nonpulsatile, and often tender temporal artery.

5. Differential diagnosis of acute vision loss includes nonarteritic ischemic optic neuropathy, central retinal artery occlusion, central retinal vein occlusion, and optic neuritis.

6. If the patient is over 60 years of age with AION, stat westergren ESR should be drawn even if systemic symptoms are not present. Although the ESR does not have to be elevated in GCA, a general guideline for upper limits of normal will vary with age and sex as follows: male = ½ × age; female = ½ × (age − 10).

7. Perform a temporal artery biopsy. This should be performed within 10 to 14 days of starting steroids. Preferentially biopsy tender branches of the superficial temporal artery. Patients in whom GCA is strongly suspected who have a negative unilateral biopsy result should undergo biopsy of the contralateral vessel. Some advocate a bilateral, simultaneous biopsy as the initial procedure, but we have not found it helpful.

Management

1. If the ESR is elevated, begin oral steroids whether or not systemic symptoms are present (prednisone 60 to 100 mg/day orally). In patients with systemic symptoms, recent vision loss, and elevated ESR, consider hospital admission for temporal artery biopsy and a short course of i.v. steroids (methylprednisolone 1 g/day for 3 days) followed by oral steroids because i.v. methylprednisolone may reduce the risk of vision loss in the fellow eye (5). Patients usually experience improvement in their symptoms within 24 to 72 hours. Consider antiulcer prophylaxis with an H_2-blocker.

2. In patients with vision loss, elevated ESR, and negative biopsy results when GCA is strongly suspected, examine via biopsy the opposite temporal artery if not already done or consider occipital artery biopsy. Otherwise, consider workup for another etiology.

3. When biopsy result is positive, continue steroids and refer to internist or family practice physician. It is important that the patient and primary physician understand that although GCA may be self-limited, it may last 1 to 2 years. Steroids should be tapered slowly, and the ESR should be monitored for elevation after each dosage adjustment.

4. If the ESR is normal and biopsy result is negative, stop steroids.

OPTIC NEURITIS

Patients with acute optic neuritis are typically white women in the third or fourth decade of life. Patients typically present with unilateral, acute-onset, and painful vision loss. Management is based on the results of the multicenter Optic Neuritis Treatment Trial (ONTT) and influences the risk of developing future neurologic events. In about 25% of patients with multiple sclerosis (MS), acute optic neuritis is the initial manifestation.

Diagnosis

1. Presenting symptoms include blurred vision, a blank spot (scotoma), or flashes of light (photopsias). Ocular or orbital pain, often exacerbated by eye movements, is common, being present in 92% of patients in the ONTT. Patients may have Uhthoff's symptom, a worsening of vision with exercise or increase in body temperature.

2. Obtain a complete history with a detailed neurologic review of symptoms, including questions about incontinence, weakness, paresthesias, numbness, diplopia, Lhermitte's sign (tingling feeling in the back with passive neck flexion), ataxia, vertigo, and oscillopsia.

3. Median initial visual acuity is 20/80, but ranges from 20/20 to no light perception. Examine for dyschromatopsia, a relative afferent pupillary defect, nystagmus, and ocular misalignment. An RAPD will not be present with a bilateral optic neuropathy. Visual field testing should be performed and may demonstrate a variety of defects: central, cecocentral, arcuate, altitudinal, nasal step, diffuse depression, or even a hemianopia.

4. Ophthalmoscopy demonstrates optic disk swelling in about one-third of patients, retinal hemorrhages in 6%, vitreous cells in 3%, and retinal exudates in 2% (Fig. 24–3). The presence of a macular star indicates a diagnosis of neuroretinitis, should prompt a workup for inflammatory etiologies, and carries a good prognosis. The presence of vitreous cells should also prompt a workup for inflammatory and infiltrative disorders. The workup should include a lumbar puncture.

5. The etiology of optic neuritis includes idiopathic, MS, viral infections, contiguous inflammation of the sinuses or meninges, bacterial infections (tuberculosis, syphilis, or lyme disease), inflammatory disorders (sarcoidosis), and infiltrative disorders (leukemia).

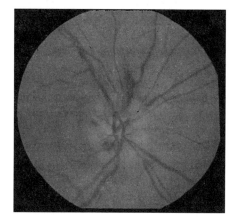

FIG. 24–3. Optic disk swelling in optic neuritis. In patients with optic neuritis, disk swelling is seen in approximately 33% and peripapillary hemorrhages in 6%. (Courtesy of Dr. W.R. Green.) *For a color representation of this figure, please see the color insert facing p. 256.*

6. The differential diagnosis includes papilledema, neuroretinitis, ischemic optic neuropathy, compressive optic neuropathy, leber hereditary optic neuropathy, toxic/metabolic optic neuropathy.

7. In patients with typical features of an isolated optic neuritis, ancillary testing (chest x-ray, FTA, ANA) yields little or no clinically useful information. MRI may rarely demonstrate a compressive optic neuropathy; however, it is generally obtained for prognostic rather than diagnostic purposes. Those patients with signal abnormalities suggestive of MS experience future neurologic events on follow-up more often than do those without signal abnormalities. These patients should receive intravenous steroids.

8. Atypical features including no pain, insidious onset, simultaneous bilateral onset, or vitreous cells should prompt ancillary testing including complete blood count, FTA, ANA, PPD, ESR, chest x-ray, and lyme testing. Lumbar puncture and MRI of the brain should be performed.

Management

1. The ONTT demonstrated that treatment with corticosteroids, whether oral or i.v., did not affect visual outcome; however, high-dose i.v. methylprednisolone hastened visual recovery. Oral corticosteroids increased the rate of optic neuritis attacks. Intravenous corticosteroids reduced the rate of new neurologic events, particularly in patients with abnormal MRI scans. Based on these data, we recommend patients be treated with i.v. methylprednisolone (1 g/day for 3 days) followed by oral prednisone (1 mg/kg/day for 11 days) with a quick taper over 2 days.

2. A discussion of the risk of MS should accompany a discussion of the potential disability of MS. A 15-year prospective study of 60 patients in New England presenting with uncomplicated optic neuritis indicated that 74% of women and 34% of men developed MS (6). Although the course of MS may be variable, a retrospective study of the population of Rochester, Minnesota, indicated that 74% of patients with MS survived 25 years compared with 86% of the general population, and at the end of 25 years, one-third of surviving patients were still working and two thirds were still ambulatory (7).

LEBER HEREDITARY OPTIC NEUROPATHY

Leber hereditary optic neuropathy (LHON) is a bilateral, maternally inherited optic neuropathy most often characterized by painless, rapidly progressive vision loss in both eyes simultaneously or one eye followed within a few days or weeks by vision loss in the fellow eye. This mitochondrial genetic disease is primarily due to mutations at nucleotide positions 3460, 11778, and 14484. Men are more commonly affected than women, and although vision loss typically occurs in a patient's 20s, it may become manifest as early as the first decade and as late as seventh decade of life.

Diagnosis

1. Patients present with rapidly progressive vision loss, dyschromatopsia, and a central or cecocentral visual field defect.
2. Question patient for a family history of vision loss in maternal relatives.
3. Fundus examination discloses apparent disk swelling, optic nerve hyperemia, and peripapillary telangiectasia in some patients. In other patients, the optic nerves may appear normal.
4. Obtain blood sample for DNA testing.

Management

1. There is no proven therapy for LHON; however, some patients may have spontaneous improvement in vision.
2. Genetic counseling should be offered. Men do not pass the mutation to their offspring, but women do.
3. Consider cardiology evaluation because some patients may have conduction defects.

PSEUDOTUMOR CEREBRI

Pseudotumor cerebri is an idiopathic disorder characterized by normal neuroimaging, elevated intracranial pressure, and normal cerebrospinal fluid composition. Patients are typically female, presenting with intractable headaches and bilateral optic nerve swelling. Associations include obesity, pregnancy, and various medications (oral contraceptives, tetracycline, nalidixic acid, steroids, and vitamin A). Dural venous sinus thrombosis may present with similar findings, particularly in nonobese women or men.

Diagnosis

1. Symptoms include chronic headache, usually worse in the morning and with straining, diplopia, pulsatile tinnitus, nausea/vomiting, and transient visual obscurations, particularly when changing positions (e.g., lying to sitting, sitting to standing).
2. Visual acuity and color vision are typically normal unless papilledema is long-standing or associated with macular hemorrhages and exudates. Obtain kinetic visual fields to evaluate for visual field constriction and static fields to look for reduction in sensitivity and small arcuate defects.
3. Evaluate ocular motility because some patients may have abduction weakness due to abducens nerve dysfunction.
4. Bilateral optic disk swelling is present but may be asymmetric (Fig. 24–4). Evaluate for spontaneous venous pulsations that are absent with increased intracranial pressure. Consider the possibility of pseudopapilledema due to optic nerve drusen. An ultrasound is helpful in distinguishing echogenic buried optic

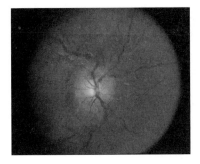

FIG. 24–4. Optic disk swelling in papilledema. True papilledema is distinguished from pseudo-papilledema by the presence of associated blurring of the peripapillary nerve fiber layer, vascular engorgement, peripapillary hemorrhages, cotton-wool spots, and lack of spontaneous venous pulsations. *For a color representation of this figure, please see the color insert facing p. 256.*

nerve head drusen (papilledema) and subarachnoid fluid (a positive 30-degree test/papilledema). Cotton-wool spots and hemorrhages associated with optic nerve swelling may suggest malignant hypertension or diabetes mellitus, prompting blood pressure and blood glucose evaluation.

5. Obtain immediate neuroimaging to rule out a space-occupying lesion, preferably MRI evaluating for dural venous sinus thrombosis.
6. Obtain a lumbar puncture (LP), evaluating opening pressure and cerebrospinal fluid composition.

Management

1. Indications for treatment include intractable headache, severe disk swelling without loss of vision, and vision loss.
2. Weight loss in obese patients is beneficial. Refer patient to dietitian.
3. Discontinue medications that may be contributing.
4. Diuretics help lower intracranial pressure. Most physicians titrate patients to maximally tolerated doses of acetazolamide, beginning with 250 mg orally four times daily or 500 mg sequels orally twice daily.
5. Optic nerve decompression or lumboperitoneal shunt may benefit some patients who cannot tolerate diuretics, who progress despite medical therapy, or who have optic neuropathy at the time of presentation.

TOXIC/METABOLIC OPTIC NEUROPATHY

Patients present with bilateral optic neuropathy of painless, insidious onset in the setting of tobacco/alcohol abuse, pernicious anemia, malnutrition, or chronic medications (chloramphenicol, ethambutol, and isoniazid).

Diagnosis

1. Question patient regarding substance abuse, particularly tobacco and alcohol, or chronic use of the above mentioned medications.

2. Visual acuity may range from 20/30 to 20/200 associated with dyschromatopsia and central or cecocentral visual field defects.
3. Ophthalmoscopy should demonstrate disk pallor with atrophy of the papillomacular bundle.
4. Genetic testing for LHON should be performed.
5. Test for serum B_{12} and red blood cell folate. If B_{12} is low, refer to internist for evaluation for pernicious anemia.

Management

1. Discontinue any medication possibly having a toxic effect.
2. Refer to substance abuse counselor as indicated.
3. Thiamine 100 mg orally twice daily.
4. Folate 0.1 mg orally daily.
5. Multivitamin orally daily.
6. Vitamin B_{12} 1,000 μg intramuscularly monthly for pernicous anemia.

COMPRESSIVE OPTIC NEUROPATHY

Although patients typically present with unilateral, insidious, and painless vision loss, the vision loss is occasionally noticed acutely. Tumors may compress the optic nerve intraorbitally, within the optic canal, or intracranially. Differential diagnosis includes optic nerve sheath meningioma, suprasellar meningioma, pituitary adenoma, optic nerve glioma, and aneurysm.

Diagnosis

1. Perform complete ophthalmic examination with attention to evidence of optic neuropathy (dyschromatopsia, RAPD). Perform exophthalmometry and visual field testing. Assess the visual field in the fellow eye to check for an anterior chiasmal syndrome.
2. Examine for evidence of optic disk swelling or pallor. Lesions in the orbit apex, optic canal, or suprasellar cistern do not typically cause disk swelling. Optociliary shunt vessels may be present with orbital tumors that slowly compress the optic nerve central retinal vein, leading to the shunting of venous blood from the retinal to the choroidal circulation.
3. Neuroimaging.

Management

Management depends on the size, location, and type of tumor as well as the state of health and age of the patient. Refer to an ophthalmologist specializing in orbital tumors and/or a neurosurgeon.

TRAUMA TO THE OPTIC CHIASM

Damage to the chiasm may occur from both penetrating and closed head trauma (8). Such injuries are severe and usually associated with loss of consciousness. Splitting of the chiasm in the central sagittal plane may occur. Because of the severity of the trauma, chiasmal syndromes caused by trauma may not be recognized initially. Be aware that pre-existing lesions, such as pituitary tumors, may produce loss of vision from pituitary apoplexy after minor head trauma. With delayed loss, consider compression from a hematoma, meningitis, adhesive arachnoiditis, or hydrocephalus.

Diagnosis

1. Bitemporal field defects are present, including complete and incomplete hemianopias, quadrantanopias, and hemianopic scotomas.
2. An RAPD is not present in a traumatic optic chiasmal syndrome unless an optic neuropathy or retinopathy also is present.
3. Visual acuity is preserved with traumatic splitting of the chiasm, as long as the optic nerves have not also been injured.
4. Optic nerves initially appear normal, but atrophy may be noted after several weeks.
5. Although fractures are better seen with CT, MRI is better for specifically examining the chiasm.

Management

1. For the unusual patient who presents acutely, no specific treatment has been advocated; however, it would seem reasonable to treat patients with incomplete bitemporal field defects with high-dose i.v. corticosteroids. For the more common patient who presents weeks to months after an injury, there is no treatment. Evaluation at a low vision center may help to assist the patient in subsequent visual functioning.
2. Penetrating objects in the region of the optic chiasm, such as poles or sticks, should be removed in the operating room by a multi-disciplinary team that is prepared for surgical intervention (9).

OPTIC TRACT TRAUMA

Damage to the optic tract usually occurs in association with severe head injuries and only rarely occurs as an isolated finding. Thus, most cases are seen weeks to months after the initial trauma.

Diagnosis

1. Both complete and incomplete homonymous visual field defects may occur, and both types may be scotomatous. Incomplete defects are usually incongruous but

may be congruous in rare cases. All defects are contralateral to the side of the lesion.

2. An RAPD is always present on the side contralateral to the damaged tract (on the side of the field defect) when the visual field defect is complete or nearly complete, unless there is an associated ipsilateral optic neuropathy.
3. Visual acuity is normal in both eyes, unless there is an associated traumatic optic neuropathy or there was pre-existing visual loss.
4. Both optic nerves initially appear normal, but hemianopic retinal and optic atrophy eventually occurs several weeks later in permanent cases. In such cases, there is typical "bow tie" or "band" atrophy in the eye contralateral to the damaged tract because of loss of crossed axons from ganglion cells nasal to the fovea. The eye ipsilateral to the damaged optic tract shows more diffuse atrophy from damage to uncrossed axons from ganglion cells temporal to the fovea.

Management

1. No specific treatment recommendations, but a low vision consultation may benefit the patient.
2. Although CT may be more readily obtainable in the acute setting, the study of choice for looking at the optic tract is an MRI, obtained before and after i.v. injection with gadolinium-DTPA or a similar paramagnetic contrast agent.

TRAUMA TO THE LATERAL GENICULATE BODY

Such damage is rare and almost never isolated. Nevertheless, damage to the lateral geniculate body produces characteristic visual field defects.

Diagnosis

1. A complete homonymous hemianopia may be present, but most patients have either an extremely incongruous homonymous hemianopic defect or a homonymous horizontal sector anopia.
2. Visual acuity is normal, unless there has been concomitant damage to the optic nerves or retinas, or if there was pre-existing visual loss from another cause.
3. The optic nerves initially appear normal, but they become pale within 4 to 6 weeks.

Management

1. There is no specific treatment for this condition.
2. A low vision consultation may benefit the patient.

RETROGENICULATE TRAUMA AND CORTICAL BLINDNESS

Damage to the optic radiations may occur in the temporal and parietal lobes from penetrating or closed head trauma. In such cases, substantial nonvisual neurologic deficits, such as aphasia, hemiparesis, hemisensory loss, and coma, are often present. Delayed onset of symptoms suggests an epidural or subdural hematoma. In contradistinction, blindness without evidence of neurologic dysfunction other than confusion may occur from damage to the occipital lobes from a concussive blow. Vision recovers spontaneously after a few hours in some patients (10). In others, however, there is permanent blindness.

Diagnosis

1. Damage to the optic radiations produces homonymous hemianopic or quadrantanopic defects. If the lesion is in the temporal lobe, superior quadrantanopsias or defects denser above the horizontal mid-line are the rule. Such defects are usually congruous. Incongruity suggests concomitant damage to the ipsilateral underlying optic tract. If the lesion is in the parietal lobe, inferior quadrantanopsias or defects denser below the horizontal mid-line may be produced. Lesions damaging the radiations in either the temporal or parietal lobe can produce a complete homonymous hemianopia.
2. Patients with unilateral damage to the parietal lobe that produces a homonymous hemianopia invariably show an asymmetric response to optokinetic testing with a drum or tape. When the tape is moved or the drum is rotated toward the side of the lesion, the resultant nystagmus is disordered and abnormal, compared with a relatively normal nystagmus induced when the tape is moved or the drum is rotated toward the side opposite the lesion.
3. Unilateral damage to the occipital lobe may produce a homonymous hemianopic or quadrantanopic defect that is exquisitely congruous and that may be scotomatous. There is often macular sparing. The peripheral temporal field or crescent in the eye contralateral to the lesion may be spared as it is represented monocularly in the anterior aspect of the visual cortex which often goes undamaged.
4. Bilateral damage to the occipital lobes produces bilateral homonymous defects that usually are associated with macular sparing. Such damage, particularly when diffuse, also may produce reduced visual acuity in both eyes. When the damage is extremely severe, there is cortical blindness, in which a patient experiences complete loss of all visual sensation. Such patients may exhibit Anton's syndrome, the denial of visual loss in the setting of blindness. This condition occurs most often in patients with occipital lobe damage, although it occasionally may be seen in other settings of bilateral blindness.
5. Normal pupillary reflexes are present and may initially cause the physician to question whether the visual loss is organic.

Management

1. No specific treatment recommendations are made, but a low vision consultation may benefit the patient.

2. Although CT may be more readily obtainable in the acute setting, the study of choice for looking at the retrogeniculate pathways is an MRI with gadolinium-DTPA or a similar paramagnetic contrast agent.

REFERENCES

1. Lessel S. Indirect optic nerve trauma. *Arch Ophthalmol* 1989;107:382–386.
2. Hillman JS, Myska V, Nissim S. Complete avulsion of the optic nerve: a clinical, angiographic, and electrodiagnostic study. *Br J Ophthal* 1975;59:503–509.
3. Park JH, Frenkel M, Dobbie JG, Choromokos E. Evulsion of the optic nerve. *Am J Ophthalmol* 1971;72:969–971.
4. Ischemic Optic Neuropathy Decompression Trial Research Group. Optic nerve decompression surgery for nonarteritic anterior ischemic optic neuropathy (NAION) is not effective and may be harmful: results of the Ischemic Optic Neuropathy Decompression Trial. *JAMA* 1995;273:625–632.
5. Liu GT, Glaser JS, Schatz NJ, Smith JL. Visual morbidity in giant cell arteritis. Clinical characteristics and prognosis for vision. *Ophthalmology* 1994;101:1779–1785.
6. Rizzo JF 3rd, Lessell S. Risk of developing multiple sclerosis after uncomplicated optic neuritis: a longterm prospective study. *Neurology* 1988;38:185–190.
7. Percy AK, Nobrega FT, Okazaki H, Glatter E, Kurland LT. Multiple sclerosis in Rochester, Minn. *Arch Neurol* 1971;25:105–111.
8. Savino PJ, Glaser JS, Schatz NJ. Traumatic chiasmal syndrome. *Neurology* 1980;30:963–970.
9. Michon JJ, Miller NR. Management of combined penetrating orbital and intracranial trauma. *Arch Ophthalmol* 1993;111:438–439.
10. Grennblatt SH. Posttraumatic transient cerebral blindness. *JAMA* 1973;225:1073–1076.

Management of Ocular Injuries and Emergencies,
edited by Mathew W. MacCumber.
Lippincott–Raven Publishers, Philadelphia ©1998.

25

Traumatic and Other Acute Disorders of Eye Movements and Pupils

John B. Kerrison and Neil R. Miller

Malcolm-Grow Medical Center, Andrews Air Force Base, Maryland 20762-6600 and Department of Ophthalmology, Wilmer Eye Institute, The Johns Hopkins University School of Medicine, Baltimore, Maryland 21287

Ocular Motor Nerve Palsies   369
  Third (Oculomotor) Nerve Palsy   369 · Fourth (Trochlear) Nerve Palsy   372
  Sixth (Abducens) Nerve Palsy   375 · Multiple Ocular Motor Nerve
  Palsies   376
Myasthenia Gravis   377
  Diagnosis   377 · Management   378
Supranuclear Lesions After Trauma   379
  Gaze Palsy   379 · Skew Deviation   379 · Internuclear Ophthalmoplegia   380
  Nystagmus   380 · Ocular Movements in Coma   381
Accommodation Insufficiency   381
  Diagnosis   381 · Management   382
Anisocoria   382
  Diagnosis   382 · Management   383
Horner's Syndrome   383
  Diagnosis   384 · Management   385

OCULAR MOTOR NERVE PALSIES

Ocular motor nerve palsies after trauma usually present in an acute-care setting. In addition, the sudden onset of diplopia without antecedent trauma is alarming enough to the patient to bring them into an urgent-care setting. Findings may be limited to the eyes. In addition to trauma, underlying etiologies of ocular motor nerve palsies include ischemia, compression, congenital, and inflammation.

Third (Oculomotor) Nerve Palsy

Careful motility and pupillary examination as well as examination for other neurologic deficits are critical in the evaluation of a patient with a third-nerve palsy. A complete third-nerve palsy refers to full ptosis with no third-nerve motility function. Incomplete third-nerve palsies retain some third-nerve lid or extraocular muscle motility. The pupil may or may not be involved in a third-nerve palsy whether complete or incomplete. Divisional third-nerve palsies may be superior or inferior.

Traumatic third-nerve palsies are usually associated with multiple cranial nerve palsies due to severe skull fracture. The nerve may be lacerated or rendered ischemic from impairment of its blood supply. However, isolated third-nerve palsies may arise in the setting of a frontal blow to the head. The palsy is usually complete, and the pupil is usually involved, being dilated and nonreactive or poorly reactive. Although the damage may occur in the brain stem, either at the site of the oculomotor nucleus or fascicle, the most common site of injury is in the subarachnoid space where the nerve enters the dura lateral to the posterior clinoid process. Shearing at this level as well as compression from a hematoma may occur.

Third-nerve palsy, complete with pupil involvement, may be due to cerebral swelling with herniation of the hippocampal gyrus over the ridge of the dura between the free edge of the tentorium and the clivus. Patients are virtually always obtunded or comatose. In this setting, pupillary dilation is the first sign of cerebral edema. Rarely, one may observe pupillary dilation contralateral to the herniation or a pupil-sparing traumatic third-nerve palsy.

After injury to the oculomotor nerve at any point along its path, a syndrome of oculomotor synkinesis or aberrant regeneration may develop beginning about 9 weeks after the trauma. Aberrant regeneration also may be seen with compressive lesions but not typically with ischemia or inflammation. After nerve injury, fibers within the oculomotor nerve that originally innervated specific extraocular muscles reinnervate the iris sphincter or different extraocular muscles supplied by the same nerve. The levator palpebrae superioris and the iris sphincter are the most common muscles affected in this setting. As a consequence one may see the lid elevate during attempted depression (pseudo-Graefe sign) or adduction of the eye; pupillary constriction, usually segmental, with elevation, depression, or adduction; or globe retraction on attempted vertical movement.

Compressive lesions such as tumor or aneurysm, particularly posterior communicating artery aneurysm, may present with a pupil-involved, complete third-nerve palsy. Less commonly, aneurysms may present with some sparing of muscle function and without pupil involvement only to become a pupil-involved, complete third-nerve palsy with time. Although aneurysmal third-nerve palsies are typically painful, the presence or character of pain is not a useful diagnostic tool because ischemic third-nerve palsies are often painful. The absence of pain in the setting of pupil-involved, complete third-nerve palsy makes the diagnosis of aneurysm less likely but still possible.

Ischemia due to small vessel occlusion may lead to a complete or incomplete pupil-sparing third-nerve palsy. These patients usually have long-standing diabetes or hypertension. They begin to resolve by 2 months and are not associated with aberrant regeneration.

Inflammation may lead to third-nerve palsy. Causes include giant cell arteritis, herpes zoster, sarcoidosis, and Tolosa-Hunt syndrome, which is an acute inflammation of the superior orbital fissure/anterior cavernous sinus that is a diagnosis of exclusion.

Leukemic infiltration is a rare cause of isolated third-nerve palsy. Congenital third-nerve palsies are rare and unlikely to present in an acute setting.

Diagnosis

1. The patient may not complain of diplopia because of unilateral ptosis; however, when the ptotic eyelid is held open, the patient usually will have oblique diplopia.
2. A dilated unreactive or poorly reactive pupil may be present and is a key diagnostic feature.
3. Limited or absent elevation, depression, and adduction are present with intorsion, exotropia, and hypotropia due to functioning superior oblique and lateral rectus muscles. Test superior oblique muscle function in the setting of a third-nerve palsy by looking for intorsion of globe on attempted downgaze when the eye is abducted. Observation of intorsion is most easily accomplished by looking at the limbal vessels. Some traumatic third nerve palsies have a divisional pattern:
   • Superior-division palsy: ptosis and impaired upgaze.
   • Inferior-division palsy: dilated, unreactive pupil associated with impaired depression and adduction.
   With oculomotor palsy at the level of the oculomotor nucleus, findings are usually bilateral, particularly as regards ptosis and upward gaze, although one may have symmetric ptosis and upgaze palsy with unilateral complete third-nerve palsy.
4. Complete neuro-ophthalmic examination should be performed to determine if the third-nerve palsy is isolated.
5. In the setting of trauma, neuroimaging should be performed. In addition, neuroimaging should include immediate computed tomography, looking for subarachnoid hemorrhage, or magnetic resonance imaging (MRI)/magnetic resonance angiography (MRA) for the following:
   • Pupil-involved (complete or incomplete) third-nerve palsy: If there is no pain, neuroimaging should still be performed. If negative for a compressive lesion, medical workup for underlying systemic vasculopathy (erythrocyte sedimentation rate [ESR], glucose) and lumbar puncture (LP) should be performed.
   • Pupil-sparing third-nerve palsy in the following circumstances: incomplete, shows no improvement after 2 months, occurs in a young person without long-standing diabetes or hypertension, or is associated with another cranial nerve or neurologic abnormality.
   In some instances, MRA may miss small (less than 2 mm) aneurysms. When suspicion is high for aneurysm despite a negative MRA, cerebral angiography may be indicated.

Patients with pupil-sparing complete third-nerve palsies should undergo a Tensilon testing for myasthenia gravis and a general medical evaluation that includes fasting blood sugar and ESR (in patients more than 55 years of age).

6. With history of third-nerve palsy, evaluate for signs of aberrant regeneration (secondary aberrant regeneration). If the patient has signs of aberrant regeneration with no prior history of third-nerve palsy (primary aberrant regeneration), evaluate for cavernous sinus tumor or aneurysm. Also evaluate for these possibilities when trauma seems disproportionate to findings.

Management

1. Patch the eye if the patient is having double vision. Double vision may not be problematic until ptosis starts to improve. In children, be wary of occlusion amblyopia developing during the period of complete ptosis or being induced by occlusion of the eye for diplopia. Follow such patients closely and consider alternate eye patching.

2. Recovery after trauma may not begin for weeks to months and is usually complete after 1 year, although late recovery has been reported (1). Recovery from ischemic insult should begin by 2 months. If not, perform neuroimaging.

3. Patients should be followed for 6 to 12 months before considering definitive treatment with surgery. Realignment in primary position is the goal and may be accomplished with chemodenervation (2), surgery, or both (3). The more severe the palsy and the less recovery of function, the less likely that surgery will be successful. Patients who develop partial recovery with or without secondary aberrant regeneration may achieve better results after surgery (4).

Fourth (Trochlear) Nerve Palsy

Trauma is one of the most common causes of fourth-nerve palsy, accounting for approximately 30% in most series (5). Although fourth-nerve palsies typically occur after severe head trauma, they may occur after fairly minimal trauma that is unassociated with loss of consciousness. Unless other neurologic signs are present, the lesion cannot be precisely localized to the nucleus, fascicle, or subarachnoid space. Approximately 38% of cases are bilateral, and these patients are more likely to have experienced loss of consciousness than patients with unilateral palsies (6). Spontaneous resolution occurs in 65% of unilateral palsies and 25% of bilateral palsies.

Diagnosis

1. Complaints include binocular vertical diplopia, image tilting, asthenopia, and neck strain.

2. Causes of vertical binocular diplopia in addition to fourth-nerve palsy include third-nerve palsy, myasthenia gravis, thyroid eye disease, orbital tumor, orbital

inflammatory pseudotumor, and skew deviation, which is usually associated with other neurologic findings.

3. Look at old photographs for prior head tilt, suggesting a pre-existing, possibly congenital fourth-nerve palsy.

4. Perform cover-uncover testing with prisms to measure the amount of deviation in primary gaze, upgaze, downgaze, right gaze, left gaze, right head tilt, and left head tilt. Double Maddox rod testing as well as assessment for ocular fundus torsion should be performed. Red glass testing demonstrates diplopia that is greatest on downgaze and gaze opposite from the involved muscle, although this is variable, depending on the degree of secondary superior rectus contracture and inferior oblique overaction. The three-step test is key to diagnosis of fourth-nerve palsy/superior oblique paresis but is unreliable when the patient is tested in the supine position (Fig. 25–1). Remember that the reason for the hypertropia on head tilt is that the superior rectus muscle normally intorts (as does the superior oblique muscle) and elevates (as opposed to the superior oblique muscle) the eye. In patients with a superior oblique palsy, there is variable extorsion of the affected eye. When the head is tilted to the side of the lesion, the extorsion increases, causing the brain to try to reduce the extorsion by stimulat-

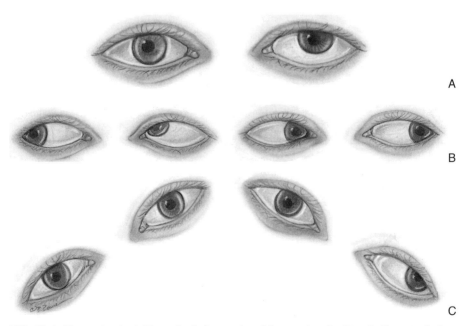

FIG. 25–1. Three-step test. Example: Left superior oblique palsy. **A:** Step 1: Hypertropia is present in primary gaze on the side of superior oblique paresis. **B:** Step 2: Hypertropia increases on gaze to the opposite side of superior oblique paresis. **C:** Step 3: Hypertropia increases on head tilt to the same side of superior oblique paresis.

ing both the ipsilateral superior oblique and superior rectus muscles. Because the superior oblique muscle is paretic, the only muscle that is activated is the superior rectus, producing some degree of intorsion but also increased elevation of the eye. The pre-existing hypertropia caused by paralysis of the superior oblique muscle thus is increased by the action of the superior rectus muscle.

5. A V pattern in excess of 25 prism diopters, excyclotorsion of greater than 10 degrees in primary position, a right hypertropia in left gaze and a left hypertropia in right gaze (alternating hypertropia), a right hypertropia on right head tilt and a left hypertropia on left head tilt, and head trauma severe enough to cause loss of consciousness all suggest bilateral fourth-nerve palsies.

   With unilateral palsies:
   - Large hypertropia in primary position
   - Predominately vertical diplopia
   - Compensatory head tilt to obtain fusion in some cases
   - Positive three-step head tilt test

   With bilateral palsies:
   - Small hypertropia in primary gaze alternating on right and left gaze
   - A large V pattern esotropia with excyclotorsion that is frequently bilateral
   - Compensatory head posture characterized by a chin down, face forward position, allowing fusion in upgaze

   Remember that many bilateral fourth-nerve palsies may be extremely subtle.

6. Complete neuro-ophthalmic examination should be performed to determine if the fourth-nerve palsy is isolated.

7. CT or MRI should be performed as part of the workup in the acute trauma setting. We do not routinely perform neuroimaging in patients with a distant history of trauma who present with isolated fourth-nerve palsy. Neuroimaging should be obtained when the fourth-nerve palsy is not isolated (associated with other cranial nerve or neurologic deficit) or occurs in children.

8. A general medical workup should be performed on patients with isolated fourth-nerve palsy. This should include fasting blood sugar and ESR (in patients more than 55 years of age). These patients should be observed for improvement. If there is no improvement after 2 months or worsening, neuroimaging should be performed.

Management

1. Patch eye if the patient is having double vision, although if patient is a child, one must be careful not to induce occlusion amblyopia. In such cases, one may have to patch the eyes alternately.

2. Small deviations (less than 10 prism diopters) may be treated with vertical prisms.

3. Strabismus surgery is generally recommended in patients who show no improvement or who incompletely improve and then are stable for 6 to 12 months.

Surgery may be performed for torsional component, vertical component, or both.

Sixth (Abducens) Nerve Palsy

Trauma is a common cause of sixth nerve palsy, which usually is unilateral but may be bilateral. The site of injury is not at the abducens nucleus because, in such a case one would observe a horizontal gaze palsy from damage to both abducens motor neurons and internuclear neurons that connect the abducens nucleus with the contralateral medial rectus subnucleus, and thus subserve horizontal conjugate gaze. The site of injury may be the fascicle of the sixth nerve, although this is rare and usually associated with profound brain stem neurologic deficits. As is the case with the third nerve, the most common site of damage to the sixth nerve is in the subarachnoid space, particularly where it penetrates the dura of the petrous bone. The sixth nerve also may be injured as it passes through the petrous bone, particularly when there is a basal skull fracture. Sixth-nerve palsies also have been described in patients placed in halo-pelvic traction after trauma (7).

Other etiologies of sixth-nerve palsy include ischemia in the setting of diabetes or hypertension, increased intracranial pressure, giant cell arteritis, sarcoidosis, multiple sclerosis, compression by tumor or aneurysm, and cerebrovascular accident.

Diagnosis

1. Complaints include binocular horizontal diplopia that is worse at distance, as well as lateral gaze to the side of the abduction weakness.
2. Causes of horizontal binocular diplopia in addition to sixth nerve palsy include myasthenia gravis, thyroid eye disease, orbital tumor, orbital inflammatory pseudotumor, and convergence insufficiency.
3. Findings include esotropia with abduction weakness and uncrossed diplopia on red glass testing. Red glass testing is a simple bedside test that can aid in the diagnosis of a sixth-nerve palsy. Place a red glass or Maddox rod over the right eye (by convention) and have the patient observe the light from a penlight or similar light source. Ask the patient whether the red image is to the right (uncrossed diplopia) or left (crossed diplopia) of the white image. If the diplopia is uncrossed, this establishes the esotropia nature of the strabismus. Then ask the patient if the diplopia is worse on left gaze or right gaze. This establishes the side of the palsy.
4. Carefully evaluate for the presence of other cranial neuropathies, particularly third, fourth, fifth, seventh, and eighth nerve palsies. Complete neuro-ophthalmic examination including exophthalmometry and examination of the optic disks should be performed.
5. CT or MRI should be performed as part of the workup in the setting of acute trauma. We do not routinely perform neuroimaging in patients who present with

isolated sixth nerve palsy. Neuroimaging should be obtained when the sixth nerve palsy is painful, occurs in children, occurs in the setting of cancer, shows no improvement after 2 months, or is not isolated (associated with other cranial nerve or neurologic deficit).

6. A Tensilon test should be performed when myasthenia gravis is suspected (see below). A general medical workup should be performed on patients with isolated sixth-nerve palsy. This should include fasting blood sugar and ESR (in patients more than 55 years of age). These patients should be followed for improvement. If there is no improvement after 2 months or worsening, neuroimaging should be performed.

Management

1. Patch eye if the patient is experiencing double vision; however, if the patient is a child, be wary of producing occlusion amblyopia. In such cases, the patient must be observed closely, and alternate eye patching may be required.
2. Small deviations (less than 10 prism diopters) may be treated with horizontal prisms.
3. Strabismus surgery, chemodenervation using botulinum toxin, or both are generally recommended in patients who show no improvement or partially improve and then remain stable for 6 to 12 months.

Multiple Ocular Motor Nerve Palsies

Multiple ocular motor nerve palsies often occur with trauma, particularly when there are penetrating wounds of the orbit that reach the superior orbital fissure. Cavernous sinus lesions, such as aneurysms, tumors, and carotid-cavernous sinus fistulae, also may produce such palsies (see Chapter 26). When other cranial nerves such as the fifth or seventh nerve are damaged, one must be vigilant about ensuring that the eye is properly lubricated and protected.

Diagnosis

1. Limitation of eye movement corresponding to a combination of third-, fourth-, and sixth-nerve palsy. In the setting of third-nerve palsy, test the fourth by asking the patient to look down while the eye is abducted. If the fourth nerve is functioning, one sees intorsion of the globe. This is seen best by observing the limbal vessels.
2. Impaired corneal sensation or numbness in the cutaneous distribution of the trigeminal nerve may be present.
3. Ptosis or lagophthalmos may be present, as may be weakness of the face.
4. Horner's syndrome (postganglionic) from damage to the oculosympathetic pathways or a fixed dilated pupil from damage to the oculomotor nerve, ciliary ganglion, or short posterior ciliary nerves may be present.

5. The differential diagnosis is broad: aneurysm; cavernous sinus/sphenoidal tumor (metastasis, pituitary adenoma, apoplexy, meningioma, craniopharyngioma); Tolosa-Hunt syndrome; meningitis (carcinomatous, infectious); carotid-cavernous sinus fistula; orbital tumor; orbital cellulitis; orbital inflammatory pseudotumor; mucormycosis; herpes zoster; sarcoidosis, vasculitis, nasopharyngeal carcinoma; opthalmoplegic migraine; brain stem lesion (tumor, ischemia); Guillian-Barré (Fisher variant); myasthenia gravis (normal pupils).
6. CT and/or MRI of the sinuses, orbit, and brain should be performed.
7. Further workup should be performed based on the results of clinical suspicion and neuroimaging and may include LP, angiography, biopsy, chest radiography, Tensilon testing, etc.

Management

1. Ensure proper lubrication and protection of the globe. For patients with neuroparalytic keratopathy from seventh-nerve palsy, trigeminal neuropathy, or both, a patch made from household plastic wrap may be helpful. A temporary chemical tarsorrhaphy using botulinum toxin or glue may be helpful in some cases. In others, a permanent surgical tarsorrhaphy may be necessary.
2. Long-term management may include ptosis repair, repair of lagophthalmos, or strabismus surgery.
3. Treat the underlying condition.

MYASTHENIA GRAVIS

Myasthenia gravis is an autoimmune, neuromuscular junction disorder caused by autoantibodies to postsynaptic acetylcholine receptors of skeletal muscle. Commonly involved muscles include the levator, extraocular muscles, orbicularis oculi, triceps, quadriceps, and tongue. Patients present with complaints of drooping eyelid(s), double vision, weakness of facial muscles, and generalized weakness. Pupil abnormalities are not present. Ocular muscles are initially affected in up to 70% of patients. Fifty to eighty percent of patients who present with isolated ocular involvement develop generalized involvement within 2 years. Ten percent of patients have thymomas.

Diagnosis

1. Symptoms include fluctuating ptosis, double vision, and weakness that worsens through the day. Patients may have a history of thyroid disease, diabetes, or cancer.
2. Key neuro-ophthalmic findings include ptosis with poor levator function, strabismus, and facial weakness. No pupil abnormalities or proptosis are present.
   • Ptosis should be measured by evaluating the margin-to-reflex distance. Sus-

tained upgaze may cause worsening of ptosis. Patients with apparent unilateral ptosis may have drooping of the contralateral eyelid when the ptotic eyelid is manually elevated. When patients look to primary position after looking downward for 20 to 30 seconds, one may see a characteristic twitch of the eyelid (Cogan's lid twitch).
- Patients may have ophthalmoparesis without ptosis resembling an ocular motor nerve palsy or intranuclear ophthalmoplegia. Measure the deviation.
- Test facial weakness by asking patient to close eyes tightly. Attempts to open the eyelids manually will show orbicularis weakness.

3. Myasthenia gravis should be considered in the differential diagnosis of any disorder with ptosis or strabismus. It may present in a variety of ways and should always be considered. The broad differential includes third-, fourth-, or sixth-nerve palsy; internuclear ophthalmoplegia (INO); thyroid eye disease; chronic progressive external ophthalmoplegia; Kearns-Sayre syndrome; Horner's syndrome; senile ptosis; orbital tumor; orbital inflammatory pseudotumor; myotonic dystrophy; Eaton-Lambert syndrome.

4. *A Tensilon test* may be performed to confirm the diagnosis. Inject 0.2 ml of edrophonium chloride (Tensilon) intravenously. Observe patient for a minute for systemic side effects of a cholinergic crisis, syncope, or breathing difficulty. If a patient experiences these symptoms, their vital signs should be monitored and atropine 0.4 mg administered intravenously. If the patient tolerates the initial dose, observe for improvement in ptosis of ophthalmoparesis. If the test is positive at this point, it may be terminated. If no improvement occurs, an additional 0.4 mg is administered while monitoring for systemic side effects and ocular response for another 2 minutes. If again there is no response, the final 0.4 mg is administered.

5. Alternatively, a pyridostigmine test may be administered. Pyridostigmine, in an adult dose of 1.5 mg mixed with 0.6 mg of atropine (in children, 0.04 mg pyridostigmine per kilogram not to exceed 1.5 mg) is administered by intramuscular deltoid injection. This is particularly useful in children and adults without ptosis. Ocular motility is assessed 30 to 45 minutes after injection.

6. Keep in mind that a falsely positive result may occur in a patient with an intracranial tumor. A negative test does not rule out myasthenia gravis.

7. Other tests that may support the diagnosis include acetylcholine receptor antibodies and single-fiber electromyography.

8. Additional testing that should be performed includes chest CT to evaluate for thymoma, thyroid function tests, serologic studies for collagen vascular disease, and pulmonary function studies.

Management

1. Patients are generally managed in consultation with a neurologist or internist.
2. Patients with difficulty swallowing or breathing should be hospitalized immediately to undergo plasmapharesis and possible intubation.
3. Some patients with ocular symptoms alone may not require systemic therapy.

4. Treatment is usually initiated with pyridostigmine at 60 mg orally four times daily and may be adjusted up to 120 mg orally every 3 hours according to their response. Be aware of possible cholinergic crisis.
5. Systemic steroids and possible immunosuppressive therapy may be required.
6. Thymomas should be surgically removed.
7. Surgery is occasionally performed for residual ptosis that is refractory to medical therapy.

SUPRANUCLEAR LESIONS AFTER TRAUMA

Gaze palsy, skew deviation, INO, or nystagmus may occur after trauma, ischemia, demyelination, inflammation, and compression, leading to damage to cerebral, cerebellar, and brain stem ocular motor pathways. In addition, one may observe eye movements in comatose patients that do not specifically localize to an area of injury. The ophthalmologist's role in these settings should be to aid the neurologist and neurosurgeon in interpreting the significance of the ocular motor findings.

Gaze Palsy

Impaired upgaze, usually bilateral but occasionally unilateral, may occur from bilateral thalamic lesions or from damage to the dorsal mid-brain. When bilateral paralysis of upgaze occurs, it may be associated with other evidence of dorsal mid-brain dysfunction, including eyelid retraction (Collier's sign), fixation instability, pupillary light-near dissociation, convergence-retraction nystagmus, and skew deviation. Many patients also have impairment of downward gaze in both eyes.

Lesions of the rostral mesencephalon may produce paralysis of downgaze. In some of these cases, skew deviation also may be present.

Horizontal gaze palsy may occur with unilateral lesions of the pons or frontal lobe. With pontine lesions, one observes deviation of both eyes toward the side opposite the lesion. The deviation can be overcome using oculocephalic testing (doll's head maneuver) in patients with lesions of the paramedian pontine formation but not in patients with lesions of the sixth-nerve nucleus. With frontal lobe lesions, the eyes deviate toward the side of an ablative lesion and away from the side of an irritative lesion. In most cases, the gaze palsy can be overcome using oculocephalic testing because the vestibulo-ocular reflex is intact.

Skew Deviation

Skew deviation is a vertical misalignment that may be incomitant or comitant but is not associated with torsion or cyclodeviation. It is caused by damage to a variety of brain-stem and cerebellar ocular motor structures and thus is diagnosed in part by the presence of other brain-stem and cerebellar neurologic deficits. When a skew deviation is associated with an INO, the hypertropic eye usually is on the side of the lesion. It is thought that skew deviation represents an imbalance of otolith inputs that ascend in the medial longitudinal fasciculus after crossing in the medulla.

Internuclear Ophthalmoplegia

Lesions of the medial longitudinal fasciculus cause a reduced velocity of adduction saccades that is usually associated with weakness of adduction that is ipsilateral to the lesion in unilateral cases. In some cases, the weakness of adduction is profound, and the affected eye cannot adduct beyond the mid-line. In other cases, however, there appears to be full adduction, but the velocity of saccades in the adducting eye is markedly less than the velocity of saccades in the simultaneously abducting eye. In all cases, horizontal jerk-type nystagmus is seen in the abducting eye when the patient attempts to look toward the side of adduction weakness. Both unilateral and bilateral INO can be detected more easily when an optokinetic drum is rotated or an optokinetic tape is moved toward the side opposite the presumed adduction weakness. The eyes initially pursue the moving objects on the drum or tape and then must refixate in the opposite direction, necessitating a saccade in the direction of adduction weakness.

A bilateral INO with a large exotropia has been referred to as a WEBINO (wall-eyed bilateral INO). This is thought to be due to a rostral lesion of the medial longitudinal fasciculi impinging on the medial rectus subnuclei of the oculomotor nucleus complex.

The combination of a gaze palsy with unilateral INO is referred to as a one-and-a-half syndrome and localizes the lesion to the upper pons, involving the sixth-nerve nucleus/paramedian pontine reticular formation and the ipsilateral medial longitudinal fasciculus. Patients have abduction and adduction weakness ipsilateral to the lesion and abduction weakness contralateral to the lesion. A vertical nystagmus may be present. The only horizontal movement is an adduction movement of the contralateral eye.

Nystagmus

Convergence-retraction nystagmus may be seen as part of a dorsal mid-brain syndrome. It usually is most apparent when the patient attempts to look quickly upward or during attempted convergence. It also can be induced using an optokinetic drum rotated downward or an optokinetic tape moved downward, in which case normal upward quick phases after slow downward phases are replaced by convergence and retraction. Dissociated nystagmus is seen in the abducting eye in an INO as noted above. Gaze-paretic nystagmus occurs when there is attempted eye movement in the direction of a paretic muscle. See-saw nystagmus consists of an alternating elevation and intorsion of one eye with depression and extorsion of the other. It has been seen after trauma to the rostral brain stem, thalamus, and optic chiasm. Manifest latent nystagmus may occur in patients with latent nystagmus who develop blindness in one eye.

Ocular Movements in Coma

Assessment of ocular movements in the comatose patient allows one to test the integrity of the brain stem and should include observation for spontaneous movements and vestibular testing (oculocephalic reflex or cold calorics).

Spontaneous movements include ocular bobbing, inverse ocular bobbing, and reverse ocular bobbing. Ocular bobbing consists of an intermittent, conjugate rapid downward movement of the eyes followed by a slow return to primary position and may be seen in pontine lesions. Inverse ocular bobbing (ocular dipping) consists of a slow downward movement of the eyes followed by a rapid return to primary gaze. Reverse ocular bobbing consists of a rapid deviation upward followed by a slow return to primary gaze.

If a patient is comatose or obtunded, and cervical trauma has been ruled out, test horizontal gaze using the oculocephalic reflex, where the head is gently turned to one side. This should induce a conjugate horizontal gaze in the opposite direction if the patient's vestibulo-ocular pathways are intact. If the patient is comatose or obtunded and cervical trauma has not been ruled out, test horizontal gaze using cold caloric testing. Irrigating each ear separately with 5 to 10 cc of ice water will cause movement of both eyes toward the irrigated ear of a patient with normal vestibular function. In an alert patient, irrigation with cold water causes nystagmus with the fast phase away from the irrigated ear and the slow phase toward the irrigated ear.

ACCOMMODATION INSUFFICIENCY

Patients who have sustained a cerebral concussion may later develop vague symptoms of difficulty focusing associated with pain around the face and eyes, particularly in the first few months after the injury. Most tests of accommodation are subjective, thus making the evaluation somewhat unreliable. One must also consider patients who are attempting secondary gain. A tonic pupil may occur after trauma leading to anisocoria and accommodation difficulty.

Diagnosis

1. Complaints include difficulty reading, asthenopia, brow ache, and burning eyes after trauma.
2. Look for increased near point of accommodation and decreased accommodation amplitude for age. Determine the near point of accommodation by bringing fine print closer until it blurs. Measure accommodation amplitude by gradually adding minus power to the best corrected distance refraction until the image blurs. Accommodation amplitude decreases with age according to the rule of 4s: accommodation amplitude = $4 \times 4 - (age/4)$.
3. Test accommodation using dynamic retinoscopy. The patient should be wearing the best correction for distance. Have the patient look at a small target held just

above the pinhole of the retinoscope. If the patient accommodates on the near target, the reflex should be neutralized. If the patient does not accommodate, "with" movement will be seen.

4. Patient should have isocoric pupils that react normally to both light and near stimulation.

Management

Although the condition may resolve spontaneously after a few months, reading glasses may alleviate the patient's symptoms.

ANISOCORIA

Patients may present in an acute-care setting with isolated pupillary dilation. Trauma may cause dilation of the pupil by several mechanisms, including direct damage to the iris sphincter, damage to the third nerve, or selective damage to the ciliary ganglion or short posterior ciliary nerves. In the setting of head trauma when the patient is obtunded, one may be concerned about uncal herniation.

With an otherwise unremarkable examination, the presence of anisocoria prompts the clinician to determine whether the pupillary asymmetry is due to uni-lateral dilation, unilateral constriction, or physiologic anisocoria. The differential diagnosis of pupillary dilation includes iris sphincter tear(s), Adie's tonic pupil, pharmacologic dilation (red top drops), ophthalmoplegic migraine, and third-nerve palsy. The differential diagnosis of unilateral pupillary constriction includes use of miotic drops (pilocarpine-green top), iritis, Horner's syndrome, long-standing Adie's tonic pupil, and Argyll-Robertson pupil in which typically both pupils are small, irregular, and react poorly to light but normally to convergence.

Diagnosis

1. Approach the patient with anisocoria by assessing pupil reactivity and whether the anisocoria is greater in dark or light. If anisocoria is greater in the light, the abnormal pupil is probably the larger pupil. If anisocoria is greater in the dark, the abnormal pupil is probably the smaller pupil.
2. If the pupils are briskly reactive and the degree of anisocoria is similar under both conditions, the patient has physiologic anisocoria.
3. If the pupils are briskly reactive but the degree of anisocoria is greater in dark-ness than in light, the abnormal pupil is the smaller pupil and the patient most likely has a traumatic Horner's syndrome. Such a patient should also have a variable ipsilateral ptosis.
4. If the degree of anisocoria is greater in the light than in darkness and the larger pupil is less reactive than the smaller one, there has been damage to the efferent arm of the pupillary light reflex. First, examine the affected eye at the slit lamp to look for damage to the pupillary sphincter or an irregular, slowly reacting

pupil consistent with damage to the ciliary ganglion or short posterior ciliary nerves.

5. Confirm an Adie's tonic pupil with instillation of two drops of 1/8% pilocarpine (by diluting a 1/2% or 1% solution) into each inferior cul-de-sac and observing the size of the pupils 30 to 45 minutes later. The tonic pupil should show denervation supersensitivity and usually constricts under these conditions, whereas most normal pupils show no constriction to dilute pilocarpine solution. It should be noted, however, that denervation supersensitivity usually is not present immediately after injury to the ciliary ganglion or short posterior ciliary nerves.

6. Pharmacologic dilation can be distinguished from the dilated pupil associated with a third-nerve palsy not only by the absence of other evidence of third-nerve dysfunction (i.e., ptosis, ophthalmoparesis) but also by placing two drops of 1% or 2% pilocarpine into each inferior cul-de-sac and observing the size of the pupils 30 to 45 minutes later. A normal pupil or one that is dilated because of third-nerve palsy will show substantial constriction in this setting, whereas a pupil that is pharmacologically dilated will show little or no constriction.

Management

Patients with traumatic mydriasis may feel more comfortable wearing dark glasses. Pilocarpine 1/2% may be used to constrict a tonic pupil in patients who are distressed about their appearance or who are bothered by glare. Glasses for near viewing may be helpful in some patients with a traumatic tonic pupil.

HORNER'S SYNDROME

Horner's syndrome consists of unilateral ptosis, miosis, and, in some cases, loss of sweating ability (anhidrosis). In addition, heterochromia and a slightly lower intraocular pressure may occur, particularly in long-standing cases Efferent sympathetic outflow to the pupil consists of a three-neuron arc. The first-order neuron descends from the hypothalamus to the intermediolateral gray matter of the lower cervical and upper thoracic spine. The second order neuron exits the spinal cord and ascends through the paraspinal ganglia to the superior cervical ganglion. The third-order neuron travels with the internal carotid artery through foramen lacerum, into the carotid canal, and then into the cavernous sinus, where it briefly joins with the sixth nerve before joining with the ophthalmic branch of the trigeminal nerve, which passes into the orbit to eventually reach the eye with the long posterior ciliary nerves.

Trauma accounts for approximately 4% of cases of Horner's syndrome (8). A third-order or postganglionic Horner's syndrome may be caused by trauma to the cavernous sinus. In such a case, invariably present is a sixth-nerve palsy and possibly other cranial nerve palsies. In such cases, a carotid-cavernous sinus fistula or a traumatic intracavernous aneurysm should be considered (see Chapter 26). A postganglionic Horner's syndrome also may occur in the setting of traumatic dissection of the internal carotid artery or basal skull fracture that includes the carotid canal. Other nontraumatic causes include headache syndromes such as cluster headache, migraine, Raeder's paratrigeminal neuralgia syndrome, herpes zoster, and cavernous sinus tumors. A second-order or preganglionic Horner's syndrome may occur from neck injury, proximal dissection of the internal carotid artery, and fracture-dislocation of the cervical spine. A first-order or central Horner's syndrome can occur from trauma to the brain stem or cervical spinal cord. In such cases, there are often other neurologic deficits that help localize the lesion. Patients with a lesion of the oculosympathetic pathway in the cervical spinal cord occasionally may present with an "alternating Horner's syndrome" that is characterized by alternating anisocoria and ptosis (9). Other nontraumatic causes of preganglionic Horner's syndrome include cerebrovascular accident, severe osteoarthritis, thoracic aneurysm, and tumor (intracranial tumor, apical lung tumor, thyroid tumor, and metastasis).

Diagnosis

1. In a patient with anisocoria after trauma, establish that the eye with the smaller pupil is the abnormal pupil by observing that the anisocoria is greater in the dark than in the light and that both pupils react normally to light.
2. Variable ptosis is present.
3. Confirm Horner's syndrome by instilling two drops of 10% cocaine in each inferior cul-de-sac, placing the drops first in the eye with the presumed Horner's syndrome so that if the patient begins to squeeze the eyes shut, one can be assured that the drops definitely went into the abnormal eye. Check the pupils after 45 minutes in a dark room. Cocaine blocks the reuptake of norepinephrine at the neuromuscular junction of the iris dilator muscle. Because a damaged oculosympathetic pathway results in a reduced amount of norepinephrine regardless of the location of the lesion, a Horner's pupil either will not dilate or will dilate poorly compared with a normally innervated pupil (i.e., in a patient with physiologic anisocoria).
4. Localize a lesion of the oculosympathetic pathway initially by other findings, such as the presence of brain stem or spinal cord signs, cranial neuropathies, etc. Pharmacologic localization may be performed to distinguish postganglionic from preganglionic and central lesions. This should be performed at least 24 hours after a cocaine test has been performed to allow the effects of cocaine to dissipate. Instill two drops of 1% hydroxyamphetamine (Paredrine) in each inferior cul-de-sac. Observe 45 minutes later in a dark room. Hydroxyamphetamine actively releases norepinephrine from the presynaptic terminal of the neuromuscular junction. Lesions of the third-order (postganglionic) neuron will result in loss of all norepinephrine at the neuromuscular junction. Thus, if the Horner's pupil does not dilate, the lesion localizes to the third-order neuron. If the Horner's pupil does dilate, there must still be norepinephrine (albeit in a re-

duced amount) at the neuromuscular junction, and the third-order neuron must be intact. The lesion thus localizes to the first- or second-order neuron.

5. With third-order neuron lesions, cavernous sinus neuroimaging should be performed. Consider MRI and either conventional arteriography or MRA, looking for carotid-cavernous sinus fistula, traumatic intracavernous aneurysm, dissection of the extracranial portion of the internal carotid artery, or other lesions. Patients with first- or second-order neuron lesions should also undergo neuroimaging of the brain stem, spinal cord, and neck region in addition to chest radiography.

Management

No ophthalmic treatment is indicated except for ptosis surgery in some instances.

REFERENCES

1. Golnik KC, Miller NR. Late recovery of function after oculomotor palsy. *Am J Ophthalmol* 1991; 111:566–570.
2. Saad N, Lee J. The role of botulinum toxin in third nerve palsy. *Aust N Z J Ophthalmol* 1992;20: 121–127.
3. Gottlob I, Catalano RA, Reinecke RD. Surgical management of oculomotor nerve palsy. *Am J Ophthalmol* 1991;111:71–76.
4. O'Donnell FE, del Monte M, Guyton DL. Simultaneous correction of blepharoptosis and exotropia in aberrant regeneration of the oculomotor nerve by strabismus surgery. *Ophthalmic Surg* 1980;11: 695.
5. Richards BW, Jones FR, Younge BR. Causes and prognosis in 4,278 cases of paralysis of the oculomotor, trochlear, and abducens cranial nerves. *Am J Ophthalmol* 1992;113:489–496.
6. Syndor CF, Seaber JH, Buckley EG. Traumatic superior oblique palsies. *Ophthalmology* 1982;89: 134–138.
7. Rozario RA, Stein BM. Complication of halo-pelvic traction: case report. *J Neurosurg* 1976;45: 71–718.
8. Maloney WF, Younge BR, Moyer NJ. Evaluation of causes and accuracy of pharmacologic localization in Horner's syndrome. *Am J Ophthalmol* 1980;90:394–402.
9. Zur PHB. Intermittent Horner's syndrome: recurrent alternate Horner's syndrome in cervical cord injury. *Ann Ophthalmol* 1975;7:955–962.

Management of Ocular Injuries and Emergencies,
edited by Mathew W. MacCumber.
Lippincott–Raven Publishers, Philadelphia ©1998.

26

Neurovascular Disorders: Carotid Cavernous Sinus Fistula, Cavernous Sinus Thrombosis, and Aneurysm

John B. Kerrison and Neil R. Miller

Malcolm-Grow Medical Center, Andrews Air Force Base, Maryland 20762-6600 and Department of Ophthalmology, Wilmer Eye Institute, The Johns Hopkins University School of Medicine, Baltimore, Maryland 21287

Carotid-Cavernous Sinus Fistula   387
　Diagnosis   388 · Management   388
Cavernous Sinus Thrombosis   389
　Diagnosis   389 · Management   389
Aneurysm   390
　Diagnosis   390 · Management   390

CAROTID-CAVERNOUS SINUS FISTULA

A carotid-cavernous sinus (CC) fistula is an abnormal communication between the cavernous sinus and the carotid artery. Most traumatic CC fistulas are direct fistulas that are characterized by a tear in the wall of the intracavernous portion of the internal carotid artery (1). Direct CC fistulas should be distinguished from dural CC fistulas, which are congenital arteriovenous malformations between the cavernous sinus and one or more extradural branches of the intracavernous portion of the internal carotid artery, the external carotid artery, or both, which develop spontaneously or in the setting of certain systemic diseases, such as hypertension. They are gradual in onset and may be mistaken for conjunctivitis or thyroid eye disease.

Traumatic, direct CC fistulas may be caused by penetrating or closed head injuries. The trauma may seem trivial or may be sufficiently severe to cause a basal skull fracture. Symptoms may arise immediately after the injury, arise within several hours, or be delayed days to weeks. Ocular manifestations develop primarily when the fistula drains anteriorly into the ophthalmic veins and are minimal when the drainage is posterior through the petrosal sinuses.

Diagnosis

1. Specifically question the patient about the following historical features: trauma, headache, diplopia, audible bruits, drooping eyelid, periorbital swelling, and periorbital numbness.
2. Clinical findings in this setting may be unilateral or bilateral and include decreased vision, relative afferent pupillary defect (RAPD), visual field defect, dyschromatopsia, orbital bruit, proptosis, pulsatile exophthalmos, decreased periorbital sensation, abnormal corneal reflex, ophthalmoparesis, Horner's syndrome, swelling of the eyelids, arterialization of conjunctival vessels, chemosis, exposure keratopathy, elevated intraocular pressure, dilated retinal veins, and retinal hemorrhages.
3. Ophthalmoparesis may be due to dysfunction of the extraocular muscles, ocular motor nerve dysfunction, or both. The abducens (sixth) nerve is most often affected because of its location within the body of the cavernous sinus.
4. Visual loss may be due to direct optic nerve trauma at the time of the injury in addition to exposure keratopathy, glaucoma, vitreous hemorrhage, and ischemic optic neuropathy.
5. Pneumotonography should be performed to measure the ocular pulse amplitude (OPA), the difference between the maximal and minimal intraocular pressure during the cardiac cycle. The OPA is higher in patients with CC fistulae, and a difference between eyes greater than 1.6 mm Hg is 100% sensitive and 93% specific for CC fistulae (2).
6. Color Doppler imaging will confirm both dilation of the superior ophthalmic vein on the side of the lesion (and often on the contralateral side as well) as well as reversal of flow in the vein.
7. Computed tomography, magnetic resonance imaging, and standard ultrasonography will confirm the dilation of one or both superior ophthalmic veins and may demonstrate enlargement of the cavernous sinus.
8. Arteriography with selective catheterization of both internal and external carotids on both sides is required to make the diagnosis.

Management

1. Direct fistulas usually can be closed with a detachable flow-guided latex balloon or platinum coils introduced through the ipsilateral carotid artery or, occasionally, through the ipsilateral inferior petrosal sinus or superior ophthalmic vein. Dural fistulas are often monitored because they may close spontaneously or after arteriography.
2. Effectiveness of treatment can be monitored with pneumotonometry, which will demonstrate a decrease in the ocular pulse amplitude, or with color Doppler imaging, which will demonstrate return of normal direction of flow in the superior ophthalmic vein. In most cases, however, a posttreatment arteriogram is needed to substantiate successful closure of the fistula.

3. Address exposure keratopathy with lubricants or moisture chamber. Diplopia can be managed with occlusion, prisms, or botulinum toxin injection until it either resolves or has been stable long enough for extraocular muscle surgery to be considered. Treat secondary glaucoma with topical beta-blocker.

CAVERNOUS SINUS THROMBOSIS

Thrombosis of the cavernous sinus may occur from the spread of infections from the face via anastomoses between the angular vein and the superior orbital vein. Infections also may spread from the mouth, throat, and sinuses. Less commonly, surgery, metastasis, local tumor, or trauma are the cause. Differential diagnosis includes orbital infection, orbital tumor, carotid-cavernous sinus fistula, and Tolosa-Hunt syndrome.

Diagnosis

1. Patients present with proptosis, chemosis, and ophthalmoplegia. Findings are often bilateral. Fever, nausea, vomiting, and altered mental status may be present.
2. Perform complete neuro-ophthalmic examination, including corneal sensation testing, motility examination, pupil examination, and exophthalmometry.
3. On external examination, evaluate for a potential facial source of infection that may be cultured.
4. Neuroimaging should be performed as soon as possible: CT or MRI scan of orbits, sinuses, and brain.
5. Perform three sets of blood cultures and culture any potential source of infection.

Management

1. The patient should be hospitalized and intravenous antibiotics initiated for potentially infectious cases. *Staphylococcus aureus* is a common pathogen. A suggested regimen includes: Clindamycin 600 mg intravenously (i.v.) every 8 hours (or vancomycin 1 g i.v. twice daily) and Ceftazidime 2 g i.v. every 12 hours. Readjust regimen depending on response to therapy and results of cultures. Consider infectious diseases specialist consultation.
2. For noninfectious cases, systemic anticoagulation should be performed with heparin followed by coumadin or aspirin. This should be done in consultation with an internist.
3. Exposure keratopathy and secondary glaucoma should be treated with topical lubricants and beta-blockers, respectively.
4. Intravenous fluid replacement may be required.

ANEURYSM

Aneurysms presenting with ocular findings most commonly arise along the posterior communicating artery leading to a complete third-nerve palsy. Traumatic aneurysms of particular importance to the ophthalmologist are those arising within the intracavernous portion of the internal carotid artery and from the ophthalmic arteries. Basilar artery aneurysms may cause eye findings from compression on the brain stem and cranial nerve palsy.

Most traumatic aneurysms are associated with severe injury and basal skull fractures. Traumatic intracavernous aneurysms, which may be bilateral, may produce progressive ophthalmoparesis and diplopia from compression and ischemia of one or more of the ocular motor nerves in the cavernous sinus. They also may cause loss of vision from superior expansion, with edema and hemorrhage around the optic nerve or compression of the nerve or ophthalmic artery (3). If the aneurysm expands into the sphenoid sinus and subsequently ruptures, it may cause epistaxis that can be fatal (4). The ophthalmic artery may develop a traumatic aneurysm in its intracranial, intracanalicular, or orbital portions. The aneurysm, in turn, may cause a compressive optic neuropathy or, if it is within the orbit and sufficiently large, pulsatile exophthalmos (5).

Diagnosis

1. Historical features include trauma, headache, blurry vision, diplopia, and numbness around the eye, and epistaxis.
2. Clinical findings include decreased visual acuity, RAPD, visual field defect, dyschromatopsia, proptosis, pulsatile exophthalmos, decreased periorbital sensation, abnormal corneal reflex, ophthalmoparesis, swelling of the eyelids, and optic atrophy.
3. Ophthalmoparesis is almost always caused by dysfunction of the ocular motor nerves.
4. Decreased vision may be caused by compression or ischemia of the ipsilateral optic nerve.
5. See Chapter 25 (Ocular Motor Nerve Palsies) for recommendations for imaging patients presenting with third-nerve palsy and possible aneurysm.
6. Arteriography with selective catheterization of the internal carotid artery is required to make the diagnosis.

Management

1. Treatment depends on location. Although some aneurysms may be clipped, others have a poorly defined neck and require excision with reanastomosis, trapping with bypass, and occlusion with bypass. In many cases, treatment can be performed using interventional neuroradiologic techniques.

2. Address exposure keratopathy with lubricants or a moisture chamber. Diplopia from ocular motor nerve paresis initially should be treated with occlusion, prism therapy, or botulinum toxin.

REFERENCES

1. Fleishman JA, Garfinkel RA, Beck RW. Advances in the treatment of carotid cavernous fistula. *Int Ophthalmol Clin* 1986;26:301–311.
2. Golnick KC, Miller NR. Diagnosis of cavernous sinus arteriovenous fistula by measurement of ocular pulse amplitude. *Ophthalmology* 1992;99:1146–1152.
3. Miller NR. *Walsh and Hoyt's Clinical Neuro-Ophthalmology.* 4th ed. Baltimore: Williams & Wilkins; 1991.
4. Chamber EP, Rosenbaum AE, Norman D, Newton TH. Traumatic aneurysm of cavernous internal carotid artery with secondary epistaxis. *Am J Neuroradiol* 1981;2:405–409.
5. Rhamat H, Abbassioun K, Amirjamshidi A. Pulsating unilateral exophthalmos due to traumatic aneurysm of the intraorbital ophthalmic artery: case report. *J Neurosurg* 1984;60:630–632.

Management of Ocular Injuries and Emergencies,
edited by Mathew W. MacCumber.
Lippincott–Raven Publishers, Philadelphia ©1998.

27

Selected Intraoperative and Postoperative Emergencies

Michael A. Johnson and John D. Gottsch

Scheie Eye Institute, Philadelphia, Pennsylvania 19104, and Department of Ophthalmology, Wilmer Eye Institute, The Johns Hopkins University Schoool of Medicine, Baltimore, Maryland 21287

Penetration of Globe During Retrobulbar Injection   393
  Diagnosis   394 · Management   394
Penetration of Globe During Strabismus Surgery   395
Retrobulbar Hemorrhage During Retrobulbar Injection   395
  Diagnosis   396 · Management   396
Expulsive Suprachoroidal Hemorrhage   397
Intraoperative Suprachoroidal Hemorrhage   397
  Diagnosis   397 · Management   397
Delayed-Onset Suprachoroidal Hemorrhage   398
  Diagnosis   398 · Management   399
Vitreous Loss   399
Dropped Cortical and Nuclear Lens Material During Cataract Extraction   400
Flat Anterior Chamber   401

This chapter reviews the management of several of the most serious emergencies that occur during or immediately after ophthalmic surgery.

PENETRATION OF GLOBE DURING RETROBULBAR INJECTION

Penetration of the globe during retrobulbar injection is a relatively rare event. The risk of penetration is increased with the use of long (greater than 1.5 inch), sharp needles (versus rounded needles) and with superior injection (1). In addition, myopic eyes (axial length greater than 26 mm), eyes with posterior staphylomas, prior scleral buckle procedures, and endophthalmic eyes are all associated with greater likelihood of penetration (2). In large series, rates for penetration with retrobulbar injection are reportedly less than 0.1% (0.075% in 4,000 patients) (3). Peribulbar injections (injections outside the muscle cone) are reportedly associated with slightly lower incidence (0.024%) (4). Penetration with local injection into the eyelids is a rare event, but when observed, proptosis has been a risk factor (5).

Precautions to prevent penetration of the globe should be practiced. For example, awareness of a given patient's anatomy is important. Long axial length or posterior staphyloma should alert the ophthalmologist to take great care with retrobulbar injection. Topical, peribulbar, or even general anesthesia are an alternative. If retrobulbar injection is attempted, we recommend a blunt 23-gauge needle no longer than 1.5 inches. This is thought to reduce the risk of penetration compared with that associated with long, sharp, 25-gauge needles, which are still in use (6). Moreover, the needle should not advance deeply into the muscle cone. The inferior orbital rim should always be palpated for orientation, and some investigators advocate lifting the eye with a finger during the inferior and temporal injection (7). The patient should never be advised to look up and in because this swings the optic nerve into the path of a retrobulbar needle (8). In addition, a surgeon or ophthalmologist should not alter his or her established routine for retrobulbar injection without thought and planning because a change in routine can lead to penetration.

Diagnosis

The two cardinal signs of a penetration are an abrupt softening (hypotony) and scleral infolding of the vitreous cavity (9,10). In addition, the patient may suddenly become restless and experience excruciating eye pain upon injection (1). Other signs include hemorrhage (usually vitreal), a common but variable finding, and loss of the red reflex.

Management

1. If anesthesia has been injected intraocularly and the intraocular pressure (IOP) is elevated, threatening central retinal perfusion, then an anterior chamber paracentesis is indicated. Retinal toxicity to the retina after intraocular injection of preservative-free retrobulbar anesthetic mixtures has not been recognized in the literature. Cases with lidocaine 2% with and without epinephrine and with or without hyaluronidase have been reviewed. When penetration is suspected, confirmation by direct visualization with indirect ophthalmoscopy through a fully dilated pupil is paramount. If a penetration site is observed, the surgery should be stopped and retinal consultation obtained.
2. Ultrasound, if available, can help assess for retinal pathology when unclear media precludes a view. If a retinal detachment, impending detachment, vitreous hemorrhage, or choroidal hemorrhage is present, it is left to the individual retinal surgeon to decide upon appropriate management: scleral buckling, vitrectomy, choroidal drainage, or laser application. The most common injury is a retinal break. This may be observed or treated with retinal photocoagulation. Most vitreoretinal surgeons lean toward treating such breakages. Recurrent retinal detachments after penetration varies from 16% to 43% in some series (7,11).

3. Long-term sequelae include retinal detachment, redetachment, epiretinal membrane formation, macular pucker, and proliferative vitreoretinopathy. If the fovea has not been injured and the optic nerve intact, a good visual prognosis can be expected (2,9).

PENETRATION OF GLOBE DURING STRABISMUS SURGERY

Penetration of the globe may occur rarely during strabismus surgery. The two most common times are during placement of a corneal traction suture or during scleral fixation of the muscles. This can be avoided by not pointing the needle toward the center of the eye and by loading the needle at the mid-point of its curvature. Both of these safeguards promote a tangential approach to the globe and reduce risk of penetration. If the anterior chamber is entered with the needle while passing a traction suture, surgery may continue if the wound is self-sealing. If the eye becomes hypotonus, the anterior chamber should be reformed, usually with balanced salt solution (BSS) and the surgery rescheduled. If the globe is perforated while attaching or disinserting muscles, the wound should be closed and a dilated funduscopic examination performed to assess for damage. The possibilities for damage are identical for those after penetration during retrobulbar injection and should be managed accordingly. Surgery can be continued if the eye is not hypotonus and there is no contraindicating trauma, such as a retinal detachment, vitreous hemorrhage, or hemorrhagic choroidal bleed.

If the globe becomes hypotonus, it should be reformed through the anterior chamber. Prompt vitreoretinal consultation should be obtained. Ultrasound can be used if the media are unclear. Choroidals can be assessed with transillumination or ultrasound.

Retinal breaks may be observed or treated. Laser photocoagulation is preferable to cryotherapy if it can be safely delivered. Treating retinal breaks requires careful follow-up.

Rarely, the globe may be ruptured during dissection for a muscle. This is much more likely to happen if there is scleromalacia or scar tissue from prior strabismus surgery or scleral buckling. Here again, the wound should be closed, the eye reformed with BSS, and intraocular damage assessed by direct visualization through a dilated pupil. A vitreoretinal consultation should be obtained. The strabismus surgery should be postponed.

RETROBULBAR HEMORRHAGE DURING RETROBULBAR INJECTION

Retrobulbar hemorrhage is most common after retrobulbar injections, occurring in the range of 1% to 2% after retrobulbar infiltrations of anesthetic agents (12–14). It is thought to occur at a higher rate in vasculopathic patients (i.e., those with hypertension and/or coronary artery disease) (15). In addition, retrobulbar hemorrhage is thought to be associated with chronic anticoagulation (15) (aspirin, coumadin, and nonsteroidal anti-inflammatory drugs [NSAIDs]). It is general principle to withhold anticoagulation before surgery if medically appropriate. Generally, aspirin should be withheld for 5 to 7 days, NSAIDs 3 to 5 days, and coumadin until a prothrombin time of at most 1.5 is reached.

Retrobulbar hemorrhage is thought to be secondary to laceration of the short ciliary arteries inside the muscle cone (16). Other arteries may be involved less commonly. Because the retrobulbar area is a closed, poorly compliant space, unabating hemorrhage resulting in an elevated orbital pressure and is transmitted to the eye, which in turn increases IOP. The IOP may become high enough to stop central retinal perfusion. However, this circumstance after hemorrhage associated with retrobulbar injection is reported as a rare eventuality (17).

The chance of lacerating the short ciliary artery can be minimized by avoiding positioning the eye up and nasally (16). Cadaver studies have shown that the ophthalmic artery and its branches are rotated near the path of an inferior and temporally inserted retrobulbar needle (18). It is probably safest to have the patient look down and temporally or simply straight ahead while performing a retrobulbar injection as one enters in the inferior and temporal quadrant of the orbit with the needle. In addition, we recommend that the retrobulbar needle be blunt and no longer than 1.5 inches in length.

Diagnosis

1. Retrobulbar hemorrhaging is heralded by the advent of proptosis, lid tightness, and resistance to retropulsion (15,16).
2. Diffuse subconjunctival hemorrhage with or without chemosis depending on whether or not the hemorrhage dissects anteriorly may be present.
3. Ecchymosis of the lids is another variable finding.

Management

1. Once a retrobulbar hemorrhage has been diagnosed, the IOP should be measured and the status of the central retinal artery should be ascertained with direct or indirect ophthalmoscopy (19). If the IOP is dangerously elevated or the central retinal artery pulsations appear compromised, a lateral canthotomy and cantholysis should be performed (see Chapter 9).
2. If the above maneuver fails to decrease the IOP, a paracentesis of the anterior chamber should be considered to reduce the unsalutary pressure gradient impeding central retinal artery flow (15,16,19).
3. It is wise to postpone surgery after a retrobulbar hemorrhage (15,16,19). Complications associated with continuing include excessive positive vitreous pressure, iris prolapse and vitreous loss, and even expulsive choroidal hemorrhage (13). These complications have transpired even after the surgeon has deemed a retrobulbar hemorrhage to be partial or minimal and elected to continue surgery (15,16,19). A partial or minimal hemorrhage is probably at a significant risk for

rebleeding, which can not only challenge the surgeon's skills but can result in a catastrophic visual outcome. Nevertheless, some investigators advocate continuing surgery if certain criteria are met (12–14). Postponement is generally advised. Surgery can be rescheduled in 2 to 4 weeks.
4. Monitoring the patient for at least a few hours after any retrobulbar hemorrhage is advised to check for additional hemorrhage and for the oculocardiac reflex, which may occur immediately or may be delayed (15).

EXPULSIVE SUPRACHOROIDAL HEMORRHAGE

Expulsive choroidal hemorrhage, the most feared and catastrophic complication of intraocular surgery, is fortunately a rare event. The largest retrospective studies place the incidence of expulsive hemorrhage during cataract surgery (extracapsular or phacoemulsification) in the range of 0.05% to 0.2% (14,15), 0.5% to 1% during penetrating keratoplasty (16,17), 0.15% to 0.7% during filtration surgery (16,19), and 0.41 % to 1.0% during vitreoretinal surgery (18,20). Delayed suprachoroidal hemorrhage may be as high as 2.0% after filtration surgery (21).

Risk factors for suprachoroidal hemorrhage include advanced age, vasculopathy (most commonly attributed to hypertension, atherosclerosis, and diabetes), glaucoma, aphakia, intraocular inflammation, vitreous loss, previous intraocular surgery, sudden change in IOP, myopia, and general anesthesia (22–25). Nevertheless, the exact mechanism of this potentially devastating complication is not well elucidated. It has become medical dogma that the source of the bleeding is likely the short posterior ciliary artery and possibly the long posterior ciliary arteries (26). The purported mechanisms for rupture of ciliary arterioles are numerous. For example, it is proposed that hypertension, atherosclerosis, and especially glaucoma (27) damage the ciliary arterioles. Glaucoma causing focal necrosis of the ciliary arterioles as they enter the suprachoroidal space was shown histopathologically in the classic work by Manshot of the Netherlands in 1955 (26). Arterioles thus weakened may rupture under the stress of surgery.

INTRAOPERATIVE SUPRACHOROIDAL HEMORRHAGE

Diagnosis

1. Expulsive hemorrhage is best managed if diagnosed early. The first evidence of suprachoroidal hemorrhage is often the patient complaining of ocular pain.
2. Initial signs include loss of red reflex, hardening of the globe, and anterior displacement of the lens diaphragm.

Management

1. It is paramount to suture the eye closed immediately to prevent expulsion of intraocular contents.

2. Forceps, clamps, and manual damming to plug the ocular wound during suturing may be needed. During penetrating keratoplasty, a temporary keratoprosthesis may be helpful. Even with early suspicion, it may be difficult to close the operative wound without iris, retinal, and vitreal prolapse. The entire intraocular contents may be expulsed before any intervention is possible.
3. Whether partial or complete prolapse of intraocular contents occurs, the only way to reposit the contents may be with immediate sclerotomy 4 to 10 mm posterior to the limbus (depending on the surgeon's preference) to decompress the hemorrhage and decrease the IOP.
4. In general, rhegmatogenous retinal detachment, central apposition of the retina, vitreous hemorrhage, vitreal incarceration to the wound, malignant elevation of IOP, and unremitting eye pain have been considered indications for secondary vitreoretinal intervention (28–31).

The timing of surgery is unresolved. Many believe that waiting 1 to 2 weeks for the suprachoroidal clotted blood to lyse is optimal so that repair of rhegmatogenous retinal detachment and vitrectomy can be combined with drainage of the suprachoroidal space. Installing the three ports used in modern pars plana vitreoretinal surgery cannot be safely performed until the suprachoroidal hemorrhage is drained; otherwise, entry into the posterior segment is hazardous and can result in iatrogenic damage to the anterior retina (32).

Despite heroic efforts, visual rehabilitation may be limited after a complete expulsive hemorrhage, with the end result being characterized by proliferative vitreoretinopathy or phthisis bulbi. However, occasional success has been reported (10,21).

DELAYED-ONSET SUPRACHOROIDAL HEMORRHAGE

Delayed suprachoroidal hemorrhage occurring in the postoperative period tends to be limited and is less catastrophic than expulsive hemorrhage. Glaucoma patients having undergone filtering surgery are probably at greatest risk, 2% (33,34). Most occur in the first postoperative 1 to 15 days (34). They are classically heralded by severe pain as the ciliary nerves are stretched beyond comfortable limits by the space-occupying effect of the bleed. Unless the sutures break, limited bleeds do not lead to ejection of intraocular contents. The IOP may be elevated secondary to anterior displacement of the iris-lens diaphragm or space-occupying effect of the bleed and may require aggressive medical management.

Diagnosis

1. The hemorrhage can be diagnosed by direct visualization with indirect ophthalmoscopy observing a dark brown dome of retina and choroid. When ultrasonography is not available, the diagnosis of hemorrhagic choroidals can be made by transillumination. A transilluminator is placed against the globe after being anes-

thetized with topical proparacaine. Next a 20-diopter lens is used with an indirect ophthalmoscope (light source off) to evaluate whether the choroidals transilluminate or not. If transillumination is present, either an effusion or detachment is present. If transillumination is blocked, then a hemorrhagic choroidal is likely.
2. Confirm diagnosis with ultrasonography (see Figs. 5-1 and 5-2).

Management

1. Generally, conservative management is possible with delayed choroidal hemorrhage when limited.
2. The visual prognosis is much more favorable than with intraoperative expulsive hemorrhage. From half to three fourths maintain preoperative visual acuity (15,35).

VITREOUS LOSS

Vitreous loss during cataract surgery is probably the second most significant complication after expulsive choroidal hemorrhage. However, modern surgical techniques have reduced its incidence, improved its management, and minimized its sequelae. In the early 20th century, ophthalmic surgeons expected a 10% to 12% rate of vitreous loss (36). Today's rates are generally held to be around 3% or less (37).

Iridodonesis, phacodonesis, history of vitreous loss in the contralateral eye, history of trauma, pseudoexfoliation syndrome, young patient, and high myopia are commonly reported risk factors. Phacodonesis, iridodonesis, and pseudoexfoliation imply weak lens zonules, and vitreous loss may result from zonular dialysis intraoperatively (38). Myopia is a risk factor secondary to scleral collapse and subsequent vitreous prolapse (37,39). Vitreous loss, especially during extracapsular cataract extraction, is associated with a small pupil (less than 6 mm), presumably secondary to poor visualization of the peripheral lens. Retrospective analysis shows a rate of vitreous loss to be 5.9% versus 2.8% when the pupil is less than 6 mm versus greater than 6 mm (40).

Perhaps the most significant measure that the surgeon can take to reduce the likelihood of vitreous loss is to soften the eye preoperatively with the use of digital pressure, super pinkie, or Honan balloon after the injection of retrobulbar anesthesia. Topical pressure drives free water out of the vitreous through the vitreous base and Schlemm's canal (41). Decreased vitreal volume reduces the likelihood of positive vitreous pressure. In addition, reduced vitreal volume means less chance of shallowing of the anterior chamber during capsulorhexis. Consequently, there will be a decreased likelihood of lateral extension and vitreal loss.

Decreased vitreal volume also means that the eye can accept more deformation from orbital pressure before the vitreous is pushed anterior. Increased orbital pressure may result from the retrobulbar injection of anesthetic or from a subclinical retrobulbar hemorrhage (37).

Digital, Honan, or super pinkie pressure should be applied for at least 5 minutes in order to achieve the adequate softening of the eye (42).

When vitreous loss is observed, an anterior vitrectomy should be performed before proceeding to the next step in the procedure. Attempting to retrieve a drooped nucleus through an anterior approach is not advised. A pars plana removal at the time or later by an experienced vitreal retinal surgeon is recommended. Observing vitreous strands adherent to a cellulose sponge, movement, or peaking of the pupil, especially when the iris is swept with a spatula, are definite signs of vitreous loss. The chief objective is to avoid vitreous wound incarceration and retinal detachment from vitreous traction. Wound incarceration can result in many untoward effects: epithelial downgrowth, bullous keratopathy, high degrees of astigmatism, endophthalmitis, iris prolapse, pupil irregularity, glaucoma, cystoid macular edema, and retinal detachment. Moreover, vitreous loss is thought to increase the chances of expulsive hemorrhage.

DROPPED CORTICAL AND NUCLEAR LENS MATERIAL DURING CATARACT EXTRACTION

Dropped cortex into the vitreous cavity is a relative indication for secondary vitreoretinal surgical retrieval. Small amounts of retained or dropped cortical lens material may be well tolerated by the eye. Short-term topical corticosteroid administration typically may be sufficient to manage any subsequent low-grade inflammation. The patient, however, may complain of floaters until the dropped cortex is resorbed (43).

The severity of the inflammation is a function of cortical load. Larger amounts induce inflammation unresponsive to topical or systemic corticosteroids and can result in evaluation of IOP and glaucoma. All patients with retained cortex should be closely monitored because a dangerous and sustained elevation of IOP may not occur for days to weeks postoperatively (43). Ultimately, the glaucoma can result in loss of vision if the definitive treatment, pars plana removal, is not performed in a timely manner (44).

Clinical experience and monitoring the patient will dictate medical versus surgical intervention. Dropped cortical material should not be considered a contraindication for intraocular lens (IOL) placement by the cataract surgeon. As long as the IOL can be adequately supported with, preferably, a 7-mm nonsilicone optic, subsequent pars plana removal is possible.

Dropped nuclear lens material, in contrast to dropped cortical material, is an indication for surgical removal by an experienced vitreoretinal surgeon. Nuclear lens fragments can incite inflammation, which occasionally results in severe elevation of IOP. In addition, the nuclear debris provides a scaffold for subsequent vitreal traction and possible retinal tear or detachment. Surgical retrieval is usually indicated within 24 to 36 hours (see Chapter 18 under Procedure: Pars Plana Lensectomy).

FLAT ANTERIOR CHAMBER

A shallow anterior chamber after anterior segment surgery should be assessed by evaluating two salient features: the relative depth of the anterior chamber and the IOP (too low or too high) (45). Spaeth introduced a widely accepted method for evaluating anterior chamber depth using three grades (46). Grade 1 is defined as peripheral iridocorneal touch only (Fig. 27–1A). Grade 2 indicates mid-peripheral touch (Fig. 27–1B). Grade 3 describes central corneal touch (Fig. 27–1C). The IOP should be assessed as inappropriately high or low by standard applanation methods.

When IOP is low and the anterior chamber is shallow, only a few possibilities exist: wound leak, choroidal detachment/effusion, ciliary body hyposecretion, or cyclodialysis cleft (45). Furthermore, only grade 3 shallowness is a medical urgency requiring action in 24 to 48 hours to prevent endothelial damage and peripheral anterior synechiae (45,47). However, synechiae may not form for a week or longer, especially if topical corticosteroids are given.

Hypotonus grade 3 anterior chamber depth should prompt a search for a wound leak with Seidel testing with 2% fluorescein. If a wound leak is diagnosed, then the surgery performed will dictate therapy. For penetrating keratoplasty, wound leak generally requires immediate operative repair. For cataract and filtering surgery, a pressure patch dressed with an antibiotic ointment will decrease flow through the wound as well as mechanically close the leak. Alternatively, a soft bandage contact lens can be used along with topical antibiotics (48). If unsuccessful, in 1 to 3 days surgical repair of the wound leak should be considered. Some authorities advocate

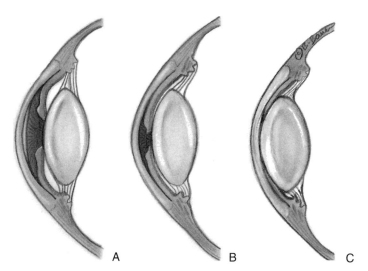

FIG. 27–1. A: Flattening of the anterior chamber. Grade 1 (peripheral iridocorneal touch only). **B:** Grade 2 (mid-peripheral touch). **C:** Grade 3 (central corneal touch).

a trial of sterile air or other gas to reform a grade 3 anterior chamber (49). It may be very difficult to reform a flat grade 3 chamber with air, especially at the slit lamp. A cataract wound can be surgically corrected with reformation of the anterior chamber with sterile viscoelastic, BSS, or air through a paracentesis track and then resuturing at physiologic IOP levels. Recent excitement in the therapeutic use of cyanoacrylate glues has developed (50). But application of glue to seal a wound leak requires special consent from the patient, is not U.S. Food and Drug Administration approved, and therefore is not very practical or widely used thus far, even among major academic centers. Leaking filtering conjunctival blebs after glaucoma procedures may be surgically repaired using suturing material on a tapered round needle.

If a hypotonus grade 3 anterior chamber presents without wound leak, then a choroidal effusion, hemorrhage, or detachment should be entertained (45,47) by direct visualization or by echography. The diagnosis of hemorrhagic choroidals is usually a giveaway because the patient will experience pain as the hemorrhage stretches the ciliary nerves. If the diagnosis is in question, echography can help. Short of ultrasound, a diagnosis can be made with a transilluminator placed on the globe or indirect ophthalmoscopy. A choroidal effusion or detachment will transilluminate, whereas a hemorrhage will block transillumination.

If a choroidal effusion, hemorrhage, or detachment is diagnosed, then the anterior chamber should be reformed and the patient placed on topical cycloplegia and aqueous suppression. Usually the choroidal effusion/detachment/hemorrhage will resolve with medical management as long as no other pathology is present (i.e., vitreous hemorrhage, retinal detachment). If despite medical therapy the situation arises in which (a) "kissing" choroidals are present and persist for greater than a week, (b) the anterior chamber remains shallow at grade 3 despite reformation, or (c) the threat of peripheral anterior synechiae looms, then surgical pars plana drainage is indicated (see Chapter 20). In these cases, the anterior chamber is usually reformed intraoperatively with sterile BSS, air, or viscoelastic to force fluid out of the suprachoroidal space and through the pars plana sclerotomies. If hemorrhagic choroidal detachment is suspected, then echography can be used to gauge the optimal drainage time because clot lysis typically occurs after a week to 14 days (51).

A cyclodialysis cleft also may be causative of a hypotonus grade 3 anterior chamber. Diagnosis with grade 3 shallowing may require reformation and gonioscopy in an operating room setting (52). Closure can be attempted with argon laser applications (53) or as a modified McCannel suture if the cleft is large (54) (see Chapter 18). Cyclodialysis clefts with grade 1 or 2 anterior chambers need to be closed only if they cause persistent macular edema and hypotony.

When IOP is high and the anterior chamber is shallow, the differential diagnosis is pupillary block, malignant glaucoma, and anterior rotation of the ciliary body by a hemorrhagic or serous choroidal detachment.

Again, only grade 3 shallowness is a medical urgency. This is unusual with pupillary block, which manifests itself with peripheral anterior shallowing. A peripheral iridotomy using argon or Nd:YAG laser can be diagnostic and therapeutic (see Chapter 17).

Rarely, malignant glaucoma (ciliary block, aqueous misdirection) may present with grade 3 shallowing. It is a diagnosis of exclusion. Pupillary block should be ruled out and the patient placed under cycloplegia (45,46). The exact mechanism is unknown. It may be caused by ciliary block or ciliary/anterior hyaloid apposition. However, perhaps the most compelling explanation has been promoted by Quigley. Two events are apparently causative: anterior displacement and compression of the vitreous. Cycloplegics are thought to help deepen the chamber by relaxing the ciliary ring, which also tightens the lens zonules, possibly acting to retard forward prolapse of vitreous (55).

Vitrectomy is usually required to relieve malignant glaucoma in the long term. However, a Nd:YAG laser application to the anterior hyaloid through a large peripheral iridectomy in a phakic patient or through the pupil in an aphakic or pseudophakic patient has been reported to be effective occasionally (56). Malignant glaucoma may return even after these measures. Close follow-up is advised.

Anterior rotation of the ciliary body by serous or hemorrhagic choroidal detachment may resolve with cycloplegia and corticosteroids (45,47). Serous choroidal detachment alone rarely results in grade 3 shallowness. However, hemorrhagic detachment may require pars plana drainage if the elevated IOP threatens central arterial perfusion or grade 3 shallowness threatens corneal endothelial cell loss or peripheral anterior synechiae formation (see Chapter 20). Moderate IOP elevation can be managed with aqueous suppressants (57).

REFERENCES

1. Albert DM, Jakobiec FA, eds. *Principles and Practice of Ophthalmology.* Vol. 5. Philadelphia: WB Saunders; 1994:2862.
2. Krupin T, Kolker A, eds. *Atlas of Complications in Ophthalmic Surgery.* London: Mosby Year Book; 1993:4.3.
3. Ramsay RC, Knuoblock WH. Ocular penetration following retrobulbar anesthesia for retinal detachment surgery. *Am J Ophthalmol* 19xx;86:61–64.
4. Kimble JA, Morris RE, Witherspoon CA, et al. Globe penetration form peribulbar injection. *Arch Ophthalmol* 1987;105:749.
5. Zaturansky B, Hyams. Penetration of the globe during the injection of local anesthesia. *Ophthalmol Surg* 1987;18:585–588.
6. Kimble J, Morris R, Witherspoon C, et al. Globe penetration from peribulbar injection. *Arch Ophthalmol* 1987;105:749.
7. Schneider M, Milstein D, Oyakawa R, et al. Ocular penetration from a retrobulbar injection. *Am J Ophthalmol* 19xx;106:35–40.
8. Unsold R, Satanley J, DeGroot J. The CT-topography of retrobulbar anesthesia: anatomic-clinical correlation of complications and suggestion of a modified technique. *Graefes Arch Clin Exp Ophthalmol* 1981;217:125–136.
9. Charlton J, Weinstein G, eds. *Ophthalmic Surgery Complications: Prevention and Management.* Philadelphia: JB Lippincott; 1995:100–101.
10. Jaffe NS, Jaffe MS, Jaffe GF, eds. *Cataract Surgery and Its Complications.* St. Louis: CV Mosby; 1990:40–41.
11. Zaturansky B, Hyams S. Ocular penetrations of the globe during the injection of local anesthesia. *Opthalmol Surg* 1987;18:585–588.

12. Hay A, Flynn M, Hoffman J, et al. Needle penetration of the globe during retrobulbar and peribulbar injections. *Ophthalmology* 1991;98:1017.
13. Cionni R, Osher R. Retrobulbar hemorrhage. *Ophthalmology* 1991;98:1154.
14. Morgan C, Schatz H, Vine A, et al. Ocular complications associated with retrobulbar injections. *Ophthalmology* 1988;95:660.
15. Krupin T, Kolker A, eds. *Atlas of Complications in Ophthalmic Surgery*. London: Mosby Year Book; 1993:1.10–1.11.
16. Albert D, Jakobiec F, eds. *Principles and Practice of Ophthalmology*. Philadelphia: WB Saunders; 1994:2861–2862, 3377–3378.
17. Krausher M, Seelenfreund M, Freilic D. Central retinal artery closure during orbital hemorrhage from retrobulbar injection. *Trans Am Acad Ophthalmol Otolaryngol* 1974;78:65–70..
18. Unsold R, Stanley J, DeGroot J. The CT-topography of retrobulbar anesthesia. *Graefes Arch Clin Exp Ophthalmol* 1981;217:125–136.
19. Charlton J, Weinstein G, eds. *Ophthalmic Surgery Complications: Prevention and Management*. Philadelphia: JB Lippincott; 1995:96.
20. Pfingst AO. Expulsive choroidal hemorrhage complicating cataract surgery. *South Med J* 1936;29:323.
21. Verhoeff FH. Scleral puncture for expulsive hemorrhage following sclerostomy-scleral puncture for postoperative separation of the choroid. *Ophthalmol Rec* 1915;24:55–59.
22. Straatsma BR, Khwang SG, Rajacich GM, et al. Cataract surgery after expulsive choroidal hemorrhage in the fellow eye. *Ophthalmol Surg* 17:400–403.
23. Taylor DM. Expulsive hemorrhage. *Am J Ophthalmol* 1978;78:961–966.
24. Guerriero PN, Met JA, et al. A case-controlstudy of risk factors for intraoperative suprachoroidal expulsive hemorrhage. *Ophthalmology* 1991;98:202–209.
25. Ingraham HJ, Donnerfeld ED, Perry HD. Massive suprachoroidal expulsive hemorrhage in penetrating keratoplasty. *Am J Ophthalmol* 1989;108:670–675.
26. Speaker M, Guerriero P, Met J, et al. A case-control study of risk factors for intraoperative suprachoroidal expulsive hemorrhage. *Ophthalmology* 1991;202–210.
27. Cantor LB, Katz LJ, Spaeth GL. Complications of surgery in glaucoma: suprachoroidal expulsive hemorrhage in glaucoma patients undergoing intraocular surgery. *Ophthalmology* 1985;1266–1270.
28. Lakhanpol V, Schocket SS, Elman MJ, Nirankau VS. A new modified vitreoretinal surgical approach in the management of massive suprachoroidal hemorrhage. *Ophthalmology* 1989;96:793–800.
29. Lambrou F Jr, Meredith TA, Kaplan HJ. Secondary surgical management of expulsive choroidal hemorrhage. *Arch Ophthalmol* 1987;105:1195–1198.
30. Berrocal JA. Adhesion of the retina secondary to large choroidal detachment as a cause of failure in retinal detachment surgery. *Mod Prob Ophthalmol* 1979;20:51–52.
31. Reynolds MG, Haemovici R, Flynn H Jr, et al. Suprachoroidal hemorhage—clinical features and results of secondary surgical management. *Ophthalmology* 1993;100:460–465.
32. Charlton J, Weinstein G, eds. *Ophthalmic Surgery Complications: Prevention and Management*. Philadelphia: JB Lippincott; 1995:403–405.
33. Ruderamn JM, Harbin T Jr, Campbell DG. Postoperative suprachoroidal hemorrhage following filtration procedures. *Arch Ophthalmol* 1986;104:201–205.
34. Givens K, Shields MB. Suprachoroidal hemorrhage after glaucoma filtering surgery. *Am J Ophthalmol* 1987;103:689–694.
35. Gressel MG, Parrish RK II, Heuer DK. Delayed expulsive suprachoroidal hemorrhage. *Arch Ophthalmol* 1984;102:1757.
36. Vail D. After-results of vitreous loss. *Am J Ophthalmol* 1965;59:573–586.
37. Jaffe NS, Jaffe MS, Jaffe GF, eds. *Cataract Surgery and Its Complications*. St. Louis: CV Mosby; 1990:342.
38. Skuta GL, Parrish RK, Hodapp E. Zonular dialysis during extracapsular cataract extraction in pseudoexfoliation syndrome. *Arch Ophthalmol* 1987;105:632–634.
39. Flieringa HJ. Procedure to prevent vitreous loss. *Am J Ophthalmol* 1953;36:1618–1619.
40. Guzek J, Holon M, Cutter J, et al. Risk factors for intraoperative complication in 1000 extracapsular cases. *Ophthalmology* 1987;94:461–466.
41. Francois J, Gdal-On M, Takiuki, Victoria-Tronco V. Ocular hypertension and message of the eyeball. *Ann Ophthalmol* 1973;5:645–662.

42. Kirsch R, Steinman W. Digital pressure: an important safeguard in cataract surgery. *Arch Ophthalmol* 1955;54:697–703.
43. Epstein DL. Diagnosis and management of lens induced glaucoma. *Opthalmology* 1982;89:3.
44. Postoperative endophthalmitis, Chapter 13. In: *Textbook of Ophthalmology, Lens and Cataract.* Vol. 3. 1992.
45. Krupin T, Kolker A, eds. *Atlas of Complications in Ophthalmic Surgery.* London: Mosby Year Book; 1993:3.9–3.15.
46. Spaeth G. *Ophthalmic Surgery: Principles and Practice.* 2nd ed. Philadelphia: WB Saunders; 1990:334–353.
47. Charleton J, Weinstein G, eds. *Ophthalmic Surgery Complications; Prevention and Management.* Philadelphia: JB Lippincott; 1995:155.
48. Blok M, et al. Use of megasoft bandage lens for treatment of complications after trabeculectomy. *Am J Ophthalmol* 1990;110:264–268.
49. Fourman S. Management of cornea-lens touch after surgery for glaucoma. *Ophthalmology* 1990; 97:424–428.
50. Zalta A, Wieder. Closure of leaking filtering blebs with cyanoacrylate tissue adhesive. *Br J Ophthalmol* 1991;75:170–173.
51. Ossoinig K. Standardized echography: basic principles, clinical applications and results. *Int Ophthalmol Clin* 1979;19:177–210.
52. Jaffe NS, Jaffe MS, Jaffe GF, eds. *Cataract Surgery and Its Complications.* St. Louis: CV Mosby; 1990:366–375.
53. Harbin T. Treatment of cyclodialysis clefts with argon laser photocoagulation. *Ophthalmology* 1982;89:1082–1083.
54. McCannel M. A retrievable suture idea for anterior uveal problems. *Ophthalmology Surg* 1976;7: 98–103.
55. Rice T, Michels R, Stark W, eds. *Rob & Smith's Ophthalmic Surgery.* St. Louis: CV Mosby; 1984: 205–206.
56. Epstein D, Steinert R, Puliafito C. Neodymium-YAG laser therapy to the anterior hyaloid in aphakic (ciliovitreal block) glaucoma. *Am J Ophthalmol* 1984;98:137–143.
57. Albert D, Jakobiec F, eds. *Principles and Practice of Ophthalmology.* Philadelphia: WB Saunders; 1994:1528–1539,1553–1554.

Management of Ocular Injuries and Emergencies,
edited by Mathew W. MacCumber.
Lippincott–Raven Publishers, Philadelphia © 1998.

28

Sympathetic Ophthalmia and Enucleation

Angelo P. Tanna and Nicholas T. Iliff

*Department of Ophthalmology, Wilmer Eye Institute, The Johns Hopkins University
School of Medicine, Baltimore, Maryland 21287*

Sympathetic Ophthalmia   407
   Diagnosis   408 · Differential Diagnosis   409 · Management   409
Enucleation   409
   Indications   410 · Implant Selection   410 · Postoperative Management   411
   Complications   412
Evisceration   413
   Indications   414 · Procedure Summary   414 · Postoperative
   Management   414

SYMPATHETIC OPHTHALMIA

Sympathetic ophthalmia (SO) is a rare disease defined as a bilateral granulomatous panuveitis that may occur days to decades after surgical or accidental penetrating ocular trauma. The eye that sustained the initial trauma is commonly referred to as the exciting eye, whereas the fellow eye is referred to as the sympathizing eye.

Although the mechanism is not fully understood, sympathetic ophthalmia is thought to be an autoimmune disease (1). As a result of surgery or penetrating ocular trauma, uveal or retinal autoantigens, normally sequestered in the eye, gain access to the regional lymphatics. It is thought that there is sensitization to these antigens, and subsequently an autoimmune reaction against tissues containing these antigens in both the exciting and sympathizing eyes. Although highly variable, the classic histopathologic picture is that of a diffuse uveal non-necrotizing granulomatous inflammation, usually with sparing of the choriocapillaris and retina (2).

The incidence of sympathetic ophthalmia has declined sharply as a result of improved microsurgical techniques in the management of penetrating ocular trauma and the appropriate early enucleation of sightless traumatized eyes (3). A Canadian-based study showed the frequency of SO to be 0.19% after accidental penetrating trauma and 0.007% after intraocular surgery (4).

SO has been reported in association with various surgical procedures, including evisceration, vitrectomy, cataract extraction, glaucoma-filtering procedures, retinal detachment surgery, and neodymium-YAG laser cyclocoagulation (5–7). In addition, SO also has been reported to occur after cyclocryotherapy (8). Uveal melanomas have been associated with SO, but almost always when associated with an occult perforation (9).

Diagnosis

1. The onset of disease is often insidious and typically occurs 2 weeks to 1 year after the initial trauma but has been reported to occur as early as 5 days to as late as 66 years after the initial insult (10). A recent review of 32 cases seen at the National Eye Institute showed that 25% of patients developed SO 3 or more years after the initial trauma (11). This figure, however, may be skewed as a result of referral bias.
2. Symptoms: Initially, there is often a worsening of inflammation in the exciting eye. There is bilateral pain, redness, photophobia, tearing, and blurred vision, especially at near.
3. Signs: There may be ciliary flush, a poorly reactive mid-dilated pupil, thickening of the iris, anterior chamber cell and flare, and vitritis in both eyes. The development of keratic precipitates, initially in the exciting eye, then in the sympathizing eye, is often seen.
4. On fundus examination, there may be papillitis, retinal edema, and perivasculitis. Yellow-white exudates beneath the retinal pigment epithelium (RPE) are referred to as Dalen-Fuch's nodules (Fig. 28–1). Peripherally, there may be areas of choroiditis. There may be multiple choroidal granulomas, which clinically resemble the lesions seen in acute posterior multifocal placoid pigment epitheliopathy (10).
5. There are no studies validating the previously used uveal pigment skin test in terms of sensitivity, specificity, or safety. The use of this test is currently not recommended in the diagnosis of SO.
6. Fluorescein angiography is often helpful. Multiple fluorescing dots are usually seen at the level of the RPE. Exudative detachments may be seen. This picture is similar to that of Harada's disease (10).

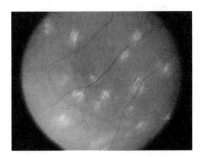

FIG. 28–1. Dalen-Fuch's nodules are seen as yellow-white exudates beneath the retinal pigment epithelium. (Courtesy of Dr. K. Packo.) *For a color representation of this figure, please see the color insert facing p. 256.*

Differential Diagnosis

1. Sympathetic irritation is similar to SO, but with a self-limited course and only mild inflammation in the sympathizing eye. Anterior chamber cells and flare are usually absent or minimal (10).
2. Phacoanaphylaxis may be associated with SO. Although usually unilateral, bilateral phacoanaphylaxis has been reported (12,13). Slit-lamp examination shows a ruptured lens capsule and lens fragments in the anterior chamber. Surgical removal of all lens material is curative.
3. Although similar in many regards, Vogt-Koyanagi-Harada syndrome is differentiated from SO by history because, by definition, the former cannot be diagnosed with a previous history of ocular trauma or surgery (14).
4. Infectious endophthalmitis and other potential causes of a bilateral granulomatous panuveitis, including syphilis and sarcoidosis, should be ruled out.

Management

1. The only methods of prevention of SO are careful microsurgical repair of all penetrating ocular wounds and enucleation, within 2 weeks, of eyes without useful vision that have sustained penetrating trauma. Early enucleation of the exciting eye after the development of SO is controversial, with some studies supporting early enucleation (9,15). However, one must bear in mind that the exciting eye may ultimately be the one with greater useful vision.
2. Systemic corticosteroid therapy with a gradual taper. We recommend prednisone 1.0 mg/kg/ day (most clinicians use prednisone with a starting dosage of 1.0 to 1.5 mg/kg/day, but some have recommended dosages as high as 2.0 mg/kg/day).
3. Topical steroid therapy with prednisolone acetate 1% every hour.
4. Periocular corticosteroids are generally not indicated if systemic therapy is used.
5. Cycloplegic agents such as atropine sulfate 1% three times daily.
6. Cytotoxic/immunosuppressive agents such as methotrexate, azathioprine, chlorambucil, or cyclosporine are effective alone or in combination with systemic corticosteroids and often allow a reduction of the prednisone dose. These are especially useful in refractory cases, in patients who fail to tolerate high-dose steroids due to unacceptable side effects, and in steroid-dependent patients requiring high doses of prednisone (16–18). Because these agents can have life-threatening side effects, they should be used only by experienced clinicians. Obtain early consultation with an internist for the management of long-term high-dose corticosteroids and/or immunosuppressive/cytotoxic therapy and their possible complications.

ENUCLEATION

Enucleation is the removal of the globe and anterior aspect of the optic nerve. The procedure is usually performed under general anesthesia but can be performed with a retrobulbar block and intravenous sedation, although patients may experience pain with transection of the optic nerve.

Indications

Enucleation can be considered in the management of a painful or cosmetically unacceptable blind eye or in the management of an intraocular malignancy. As a general rule, an eye that has sustained penetrating trauma and has no useful vision should be enucleated within 2 weeks of the initial injury to reduce the risk of the development of sympathetic ophthalmia. Primary enucleation in the setting of acute trauma should be considered only if the globe is irreparable with no light perception and if detailed preoperative discussion with the patient indicates acceptance of this approach.

Implant Selection

Implant selection is a critical step in anophthalmic socket reconstruction, especially in the setting of trauma. The benefits and disadvantages of using the various implants currently available must be carefully considered before undertaking enucleation.

The plastic sphere has the advantage of low extrusion and infection rates, low cost, and ease of insertion, but does not allow good motility of the prosthesis and is associated with a higher rate of migration. It is the implant of choice if there is a concern that the socket may be contaminated with microorganisms.

The hydroxyapatite implant has the advantage of very good motility after the completion of a series of procedures designed to couple the implant to the prosthesis. The implant is wrapped in donor sclera to which the rectus muscles are sutured. A six-month healing period is allowed before performing a technetium radionuclide scan to determine if fibrovascular ingrowth is complete. Once this is established, the patient is taken to the operating room to drill a hole in the implant, allowing the placement of a peg that can be coupled to the prosthesis.

The use of the hydroxyapatite implant is contraindicated in the setting of a potentially contaminated socket due to the risk of seeding the porous implant with microorganisms. Diabetes is also a relative contraindication because there may be a greater risk of infection. In addition, if the extraocular muscles have been damaged or there is extensive orbital or socket scarring, the major benefit of this implant, namely good motility, will not be realized. Implant exposure and extrusion have been reported, and occurs more frequently than with the plastic sphere. Clearly, the high cost of the implant, the need for donor sclera, the additional expense of an imaging study, the requirement of a second procedure, and emerging evidence of higher complication rates are drawbacks to the use of this implant. However, the improved prosthesis motility may outweigh these concerns in many patients.

The high-density porous polyethylene (Medpor) implant has the important advantage of a low risk of implant migration due to the roughness of its surface and fibrovascular ingrowth. There is an increased risk of infection over that seen with plastic spheres. At present, a system by which this implant can be fully integrated and mechanically coupled to the prosthesis is available but has not been well established. In light of the above-mentioned drawbacks of the hydroxyappatite implant, we favor the use of the Medpor implant in most cases.

Procedure: Enucleation with Insertion of Plastic Sphere or Medpor Implant

1. A-360 degree conjunctival peritomy at the limbus is performed. (Fig. 28–2*A*)
2. The four rectus muscles are each isolated in turn using a muscle hook. A double-armed 6-0 Vicryl suture is attached to each muscle near its insertion (Fig. 28–2*B*). The muscles are then excised from the globe using Westcott scissors (Fig. 28–2*C*).
3. The superior oblique tendon and inferior oblique muscle are then each isolated with muscle hooks and divided in a similar fashion. Clamping the inferior oblique muscle and cauterizing distal to the clamp minimizes bleeding.
4. A Foster tonsil snare is then placed around the optic nerve and pressed posterior to the globe 5 to 10 mm and tightened. An enucleation spoon can aid in breaking posterior adhesions and elevating the globe (Fig. 28–2*D*). The snare is slowly tightened over 5 minutes until the nerve is transected. The globe is then removed from the socket. Alternatively, a large curved hemostat may be used to clamp the optic nerve. After 5 minutes, curved enucleation scissors can be used to sever the optic nerve anterior to the hemostat. The end of the optic nerve can be cauterized, if desired.
5. Once meticulous hemostasis is achieved, the largest possible implant (up to 20 mm) should be placed in the socket. Insertion of Medpor implants is facilitated with an introducer. The superior and inferior rectus muscles and the medial and lateral rectus muscle are then sutured together anterior to the implant (Fig. 28–2*E*).
6. Tenon's capsule is approximated with interrupted 6-0 Vicryl sutures, burying the knots. Meticulous closure of this layer provides a significant barrier to implant extrusion (Fig. 28–2*F*).
7. Conjunctiva is closed with running 7-0 chromic cat gut (Fig. 28–2*F*).
8. Bupivacaine 0.75% is injected into the posterior orbit to aid in pain control.
9. A Parson's or Perry conformer is placed in the socket. Antibiotic ophthalmic ointment and a pressure dressing are applied.

Postoperative Management

Patients are generally admitted overnight after enucleation. After the effect of the local anesthetic diminishes, patients frequently complain of pain. Adequate analgesia is achieved with the use of oral or parenteral agents. On the first postoperative day, the pressure dressing is removed and the antibiotic ointment and pres-

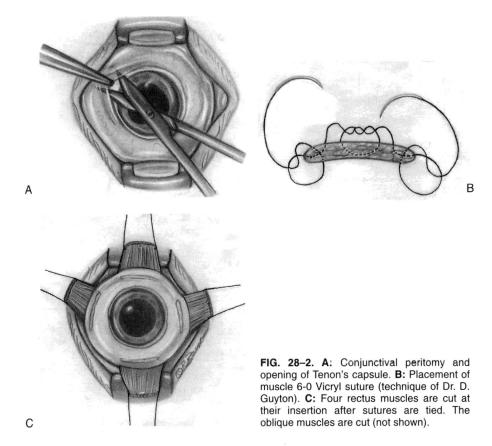

A

B

C

FIG. 28–2. A: Conjunctival peritomy and opening of Tenon's capsule. **B:** Placement of muscle 6-0 Vicryl suture (technique of Dr. D. Guyton). **C:** Four rectus muscles are cut at their insertion after sutures are tied. The oblique muscles are cut (not shown).

sure dressing are reapplied. The patient is discharged with instructions to replace the dressing and reapply antibiotic ointment on the third postoperative day. Thereafter, the patient replaces the dressing and reapplies ointment daily, until examined in the office 1 week after surgery. The antibiotic ointment is continued for a total of 3 weeks. Six weeks after surgery, a custom-designed prosthesis can be obtained and replaces the conformer. All patients should be instructed in the use of protective eyeware.

Complications

The incidence of complications is said to be higher when enucleation is performed in the setting of trauma. Orbital fractures that may accompany ocular trauma are associated with a higher risk of implant migration. The integrity of Tenon's capsule, the extraocular muscles, and the conjunctiva may be compromised, increasing the risk of implant extrusion. Contamination of the socket with

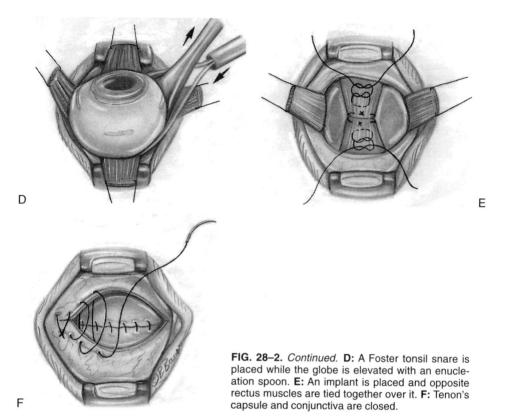

D

E

F

FIG. 28–2. *Continued.* **D:** A Foster tonsil snare is placed while the globe is elevated with an enucleation spoon. **E:** An implant is placed and opposite rectus muscles are tied together over it. **F:** Tenon's capsule and conjunctiva are closed.

microorganisms is also more likely to occur in the setting of trauma, increasing the risk of infection, especially if one of the porous implants is used.

Implant extrusion is best prevented by the imbrication of the extraocular muscles and the closure of Tenon's capsule as a separate layer. Early extrusion or exposure may sometimes be successfully managed with a donor scleral patch graft.

No implant should be used if there is significant risk of orbital infection. Wound infection is uncommon and should be treated with topical and systemic antibiotics after appropriate cultures are obtained. Rarely the implant must be removed.

Volume loss and associated superior sulcus deformities are best prevented by using a large implant placed posteriorly in the socket. Superior sulcus deformities can be corrected by changing the configuration of the prosthesis or by augmenting the orbital volume with a secondary implant (19).

EVISCERATION

Evisceration is the removal of the intraocular contents within the scleral shell, either with removal of or sparing of the cornea. Although controversial, some authorities believe that, despite the improved cosmesis, there is no indication for evisceration over enucleation in light of the possibility of sympathetic ophthalmia associated with the former. Evisceration is contraindicated in any setting in which an intraocular malignancy cannot be ruled out. In severely traumatized eyes, it may not be possible to preserve the sclera. Finally, in the blind, painful eye, evisceration and placement of an implant in the scleral shell is often associated with pain similar to that experienced before the procedure, often necessitating removal of the implant.

Indications

For the seriously ill patient with recalcitrant endophthalmitis who cannot be taken to the operating room, evisceration, without implant insertion, may be the surgical option of choice. The procedure can be performed at the bedside with a retrobulbar block.

Procedure Summary

1. The cornea is excised with a blade (19).
2. The intraocular contents are removed with an evisceration spoon.
3. The scleral shell is cleaned with a gauze sponge soaked in 70% alcohol, taking care to remove all visible uveal tissue.
4. The scleral shell is bathed with antibiotic solution and left open to drain.

Postoperative Management

The scleral shell contracts over a short time period, after which a prosthesis may be fitted. A secondary operation may be performed to insert an implant if volume augmentation is desired.

REFERENCES

1. Power WJ, Foster CS. Update on sympathetic ophthalmia. *Int Ophthalmol Clin* 1995;35:127–137.
2. Green WR. The uveal tract. In: Spencer WH, ed. *Ophthalmic Pathology: An Atlas and Textbook.* Philadelphia: WB Saunders; 1986:1913–1956.
3. Albert DM, Diaz-Rohena R. A histological review of sympathetic ophthalmia and its epidemiology. *Surv Ophthalmol* 1989;34:1–14.
4. Liddy BSL, Stuart J. Sympathetic ophthalmia in Canada. *Can J Ophthalmol* 1972;7:157–159.
5. Lam S, Tessler HH, Lan BL, Wilensky JT. High incidence of sympathetic ophthalmia after contact and noncontact neodymium:YAG cyclotherapy. *Ophthalmology* 1992;99:1818–1822.
6. Bechrakis NE, Muller-Stolzenburg NW, Helbig H, Foerster MH. Sympathetic ophthalmia following laser cyclocoagulation. *Arch Ophthalmol* 1994;112:80–84.
7. Lakhanpal V, Dogra MR, Jacobson MS. Sympathetic ophthalmia associated with anterior chamber intraocular lens implantation. *Ann Ophthalmol* 1991;23:139–143.
8. Harrison TJ. Sympathetic ophthalmia after cyclocryotherapy of neovascular glaucoma without ocular penetration. *Ophthalmic Surg* 1993;24:44–46.
9. Lubin JR, Albert DM, Weinstein M. Sixty-five years of sympathetic ophthalmia: a clinicopathological review of 105 cases (1913–1978). *Ophthalmology* 1980;87:109–121.

10. Rao NA. Sympathetic ophthalmia. In: Ryan SJ, ed. *Retina.* St. Louis: CV Mosby; 1994:1729–1735.
11. Chan CC, Roberge FG, Whitcup SM, Nussenblatt RB. 32 cases of sympathetic ophthalmia: a retrospective study at the National Eye Institute, Bethesda, Md, from 1982 to 1992. *Arch Ophthalmol* 1995;113:597–600.
12. Easom HA, Zimmerman LE. Sympathetic ophthalmia and bilateral phacoanaphylaxis: a clincopathologic correlation of the sympathogenic and sympathizing eyes. *Arch Ophthalmol* 1964;72: 9–15.
13. deVeer JA. Bilateral endophthalmitis phacoanaphylacta. *Arch Ophthalmol* 1953;49:607–632.
14. Snyder DA, Tessler HA. Vogt-Koyanagi-Harada syndrome. *Am J Ophthalmol* 1980;90:69–75.
15. Reynard M, Riffenburgh RS, Maes EF. Effect of corticosteroid treatment and enucleation on the visual prognosis of sympathetic ophthalmia. *Am J Ophthalmol* 1983;96:290–294.
16. Jennings T, Tessler HH. Twenty cases of sympathetic ophthalmia. *Br J Ophthalmol* 1989;73: 140–145.
17. Tessler HH, Jennings T. High-dose short-term chlorambucil for intractable sympathetic ophthalmia and Behcet's disease. *Br J Ophthalmol* 1990;74:353–357.
18. Nussenblatt RB, Palestine AG, Chan CC. Cyclosporin A therapy in the treatment of intraocular inflammatory disease resistant to systemic corticosteroids and cytotoxic agents. *Am J Ophthalmol* 1983;96:275–282.
19. Iliff CE, Iliff WJ, Iliff NT. Oculoplastic surgery. Philadelphia: WB Saunders; 1979:203–221.

Management of Ocular Injuries and Emergencies,
edited by Mathew W. MacCumber.
Lippincott–Raven Publishers, Philadelphia ©1998.

29

Nonorganic Visual Loss and Medical/Legal Considerations

J. B. Harlan, Jr., and Neil R. Miller

*Department of Ophthalmology, Wilmer Eye Institute, The Johns Hopkins University
School of Medicine, Baltimore, Maryland 21287*

Definitions and Terminology   417
   Malingering   417 · Psychogenic   417 · Münchausen's Syndrome   418
   General Considerations   418
Diagnostic Techniques   419
   Evaluation of Decreased Visual Acuity   419 · Monocular Diplopia   423
Management Issues   423
General Medical/Legal Considerations   424

DEFINITIONS AND TERMINOLOGY

Nonorganic visual disturbances may occur in the setting of malingering, psychogenic disorders, and Münchausen's syndrome (1).

Malingering

This may be defined as the deliberate and willful feigning of disease to achieve a desired end. The malingerer may produce complaints in an attempt to simulate nonexistent disease or may simply elaborate on or exaggerate pre-existing disease. Unlike psychogenic illness, the patient does not actually experience the specific symptoms (1,2).

Psychogenic

In psychogenic illness, the symptoms are truly experienced by the patient independent of volition yet have no foundation in real organic disease. The major categories are listed as follows:

1. Body dysmorphic disorder. The patient becomes preoccupied with a perceived physical defect that in reality is minimal or nonexistent. Such defects may include perceived ptosis, anisocoria, and other asymmetries (1).

417

2. Somatization disorder. This disorder is characterized by recurrent and multiple vague somatic complaints involving multiple organ systems. Anxiety and depression are usually present (1).
3. Hypochondriasis. In contrast to the vague complaints found in somatization disorder, the patient with hypochondriasis presents with more specific symptoms. As in somatization disorder, multiple organ systems are involved. The complaints are fueled by a strong fear of or belief in the presence of underlying disease. The patient typically practices excessive self-observation, reporting numerous signs and symptoms in support of the particular disease entity feared (1).
4. Conversion disorder. Typically characterized by the sudden and dramatic loss or alteration of a particular single physical function. Examples include blindness, paralysis, seizures, loss of speech, paresthesia of a body part, tunnel vision, etc (1).

Conversion symptoms are not under the voluntary control of the patient but are thought to represent the expression of a psychological conflict or need. The primary gain is relief from the conflict and reduction of anxiety (1).

The secondary gain, common to all psychogenic disorders, is found in the assumption of the sick role, which allows the patient to avoid unwanted responsibilities and receive support and sympathy from others (1).

Münchausen's Syndrome

In this syndrome, patients voluntarily produce physical symptoms and signs using a number of extraordinary methods, which include self-infliction of injury, self-administration of pharmacologic agents, and manipulation of laboratory tests. These patients appear to have an intense, pathological desire to assume the "sick" role. Such patients typically have an unusually extensive familiarity with medical terminology and procedures. Many are former health-care workers. A variant form of this syndrome, Münchausen's syndrome by proxy, has been described in which a parent, usually the mother, fabricates a history of illness in a child or actively induces illness in a child in the hope of generating extensive diagnostic evaluation and treatment (1,3).

General Considerations

When considering the diagnosis of nonorganic disease, the physician must first ensure that a complete and thorough ophthalmologic examination is performed. Once satisfied that no organic pathology is present on examination, the next objective is to make the patient see or do things that would be impossible in the face of a true organic disturbance. To meet this objective, it is critical to project a sincere and empathetic attitude toward the patient. A confrontational stance, although cathartic for the examiner, only serves to undermine patient trust and cooperation, essential elements in the unmasking of nonorganic disease (1,2).

DIAGNOSTIC TECHNIQUES

Evaluation of Decreased Visual Acuity

Patients Claiming Hand Motion to No Light Perception

1. Observe the patient during the history taking. In general, truly blind patients tend to look directly at the person to whom they are speaking. Patients with nonorganic disease often look in some other direction (1).

2. Ask the patient to touch the tips of the index fingers together. If the patient is claiming unilateral visual loss, the good eye is patched first. The patient with organic blindness will be able to bring the fingertips together easily, because this is a test of proprioception. The patient with nonorganic visual loss, especially the malingerer, will be unable to do this. A patient with organic disease will also be able to sign his or her name without difficulty, yet the patient with nonorganic visual loss may struggle (1,2).

3. Test for pupillary reactivity. A patient with true unilateral organic blindness will have a relative afferent pupillary defect. A patient with true bilateral blindness will have pupils that fail to react to light unless the lesion is in the postgeniculate pathways (i.e., cortical blindness). Magnetic resonance imaging (MRI) of the brain will demonstrate bilateral occipital lobe infarcts in most instances of cortical blindness (1,2).

4. Hold a large mirror in front of the patient's face and ask the patient to look directly ahead. If only unilateral visual loss is claimed, patch the seeing eye first. Rotate, twist, and tilt the mirror in various directions. A nystagmoid movement of the eye(s) will be elicited if the vision is better than light perception (1,2).

5. Place a loose prism with base down in front of the "blind" eye and ask the patient to view a distance target. A report of double vision upon questioning rules out monocular blindness (1,2).

6. Use a rotating optokinetic drum or horizontally moving tape to try to induce horizontal jerk nystagmus. If nystagmus is induced, vision is at least 20/400. For the patient claiming unilateral vision loss, the test begins with both eyes open. The examiner then suddenly covers the good eye and watches for the continuation of horizontal nystagmus. The patient with nonorganic visual loss will obviously show continued jerk nystagmus (1,2).

7. Perform a test of the patient's color vision, explaining that different "nerves" are used to sense color. Correct reading of color plates in one or both eyes indicates a visual acuity of at least 20/400.

8. Titmus Fly/Random Dot stereo plates: If the patient is able to perceive a three-dimensional effect, he or she must be using both eyes (1,2).

Patients Claiming 20/40 to Hand Motion Vision

1. Test the vision "from the bottom up." Begin visual acuity testing with the smallest line available, usually the 20/10 line. When the patient claims inabil-

ity to see the letters, feign amazement and explain that the patient should certainly be able to see the next line, which will be "double" the size of the preceding line. Show the 20/15 line next and give the patient several minutes to read it. This process is continued until the patient eventually is able to read a line. If the projector contains several 20/20 lines, each may be used sequentially as the patient is told that the lines are increasing in size. In this fashion, the patient may be tricked into admitting a better visual acuity than initially claimed (1).

2. Test near vision with a near card. A discrepancy between distance and near visual acuity not explained by refractive error or a disturbance of the media provides a good case for nonorganic disease (1).

3. Perform the reading bar test. Hold a tongue depressor blade vertically about 6 inches in front of the patient's face and place some reading material about 10 to 14 inches in front of the patient. If vision is good in both eyes, the patient will be able to read continuously. However, if one eye has poor vision, the patient will soon reach a point in the text when the good eye is blocked by the vertical blade. Reading will thus be impaired. The patient with nonorganic disease may not be sophisticated enough to appreciate this and continue to read without impairment (1,2).

4. Potential acuity meter (PAM) test. Determine best corrected visual acuity for each eye. Dilate each eye, then tell the patient that you are going to perform a test of "best potential vision." Explain that this test will bypass the current problem and allow you to know what the patient's vision would be if he or she did not have the current problem. The PAM is then used. A significant improvement in vision unassociated with any disturbance of the media or retina signals nonorganic visual loss (1).

5. Diagnostic "refraction." If the patient is claiming decreased vision in one eye, fog the normal eye with high plus power (+5.00 or higher sphere) and place a lens with minimal power (plus or minus 0.50 sphere or cylinder) over the affected eye. Ask the patient to read the chart with both eyes. In this fashion, the patient may be tricked into reading with the affected eye (1,2).

6. Paired cylinder "refraction." Plus and minus cylinders of the same power (2 to 6 diopters) are placed in a trial frame with their axes parallel in front of the good eye. Place the patient's usual correction, if any, in front of the bad eye. Ask the patient to use both eyes to read a line that has been read previously by the good eye but not by the affected eye. As the patient begins to read, blur the vision in the good eye by rotating the axis of one of the cylinders about 10 to 15 degrees. If the patient keeps reading or is able to read the line again when asked, the patient is obviously using the affected eye (1,2).

7. Red-green duochrome chart test. Place the red-green glasses on the patient so that the red lens covers the affected eye. Next, project the red-green duochrome letter chart and ask the patient to read with both eyes. The eye behind the red lens will see both sets of letters. The eye behind the green lens will only be able to see the green side of the chart. If the patient is able to read the

entire chart, he or she must be using the affected eye. If the patient is claiming monocular vision loss worse than 20/400, Ishihara color plates may be substituted for the duochrome slide. It must first be established that the patient has at least normal color vision in the unaffected eye. The red-green glasses are then placed on the patient with the red lens over the affected eye. The patient is then shown the Ishihara color plates. None of the plates, with the exception of 1 and 36, can be seen through a green lens. All plates can be seen through a red lens. If the patient is able to read the plates, the visual acuity must be at least 20/400 in the affected eye (1,2).

8. Tropicamide test. Instill tropicamide in the unaffected eye while putting in anesthetic drops for the intraocular pressure check. This is done after it has been established that the patient is able to read at distance and at near with both eyes. After about 30 minutes, test distance and near vision again. Because accommodation has been selectively paralyzed in the normal eye, successful reading at near signals use of the affected eye (1,2).

9. Prism dissociation test. Tell the patient you are going to perform a test of eye movement and alignment. Explain that the test will produce double vision. This test is performed only after confirming that the patient is not experiencing double vision in addition to the current visual loss. Place a loose prism (4 prism diopters) base down in front of the normal eye while a 1/2-prism diopter prism is placed over the affected eye (base in any direction). Dual prisms are used to allay any suspicion that the examiner is directing specific attention to one eye or the other. Project a 20/20 or larger Snellen letter in the distance, asking the patient if he or she has double vision. Assuming an affirmative response, ask the patient whether the two letters are of equal quality or sharpness. In this fashion, a reasonable assessment of true visual acuity can be made (1,2).

10. Titmus stereopsis test. Correct identification of nine of nine circles indicates 20 seconds of arc stereo acuity, which correlates with 20/20 vision in each eye. Based on the data obtained by Levy and Glick (4), there is an excellent correlation between Titmus score and Snellen visual acuity (Table 29-1) (1,2).

11. Size consistency test. Have the patient read the Snellen chart at half of the testing distance. At half the distance, the patient should be able to read letters at

TABLE 29–1. *Relationship of visual acuity and titmus stereopsis* (1,4)

Titmus score	Snellen acuity
9	20/20
8	20/30
7	20/40
6	20/50
5	20/70
4	20/100
3	20/200

Note: Poor stereoscopic acuity is inconclusive.

least half the size of the letters read at the full testing distance. (If the patient
reads 20/80 at 20 feet, he or she should be able to read 20/40 at 10 feet.) If the
vision is worse than expected, the visual loss is nonorganic. Organic processes
will result in similar Snellen acuities at varying distances with different test
objects with only a one- to two-line variation at maximum (1,2).

12. American Optical polarizing test. The projected letters are seen alternately by
each eye when special polarizing glasses are worn. One letter may be visible to
both eyes, the next by the left eye, the next by the right eye, etc. In this fashion,
the patient may be tricked into seeing with the affected eye (1,2).

If the examiner fails to demonstrate nonorganic visual loss in a patient with un-
explained, unilateral vision loss without any sign of a relative afferent pupillary
defect on examination, electrophysiologic testing is indicated (i.e., full-field and
macular ERG and pattern-reversal and flash-evoked visual evoked potentials
(VEP)). The absence of a relative afferent pupillary defect in a patient claiming
monocular vision loss does not clinch the diagnosis of nonorganic vision loss. The
patient may in fact have a bilateral optic neuropathy that is asymmetric. It is possible for a patient to have electrophysiologic evidence of bilateral optic neuropathy
with asymmetric visual acuity and no relative afferent pupillary defect (1).

Patients Claiming Visual Field Loss

1. Saccade test. Inform the patient that you want to test eye movements. Ask the
patient to pursue an object as it is moved in various directions. Next, have the
patient perform saccades from central gaze to eccentric target objects. Move the
target object from one area to another, asking the patient to look straight ahead
(usually at the examiner's nose) and then to the target object. Successful sac-
cadic movements into areas of claimed field loss indicates a nonorganic process. A complaint of not being able to see far enough into the periphery to complete the saccade may be countered with an explanation by the examiner that he
or she understands the patient's difficulty, and that is why the patient should try
to look directly at the object rather than try to see it in the peripheral vision (1).

2. Perform visual field testing monocularly and then binocularly. If the field defect
is present in only one eye on monocular testing but is still present in binocular
testing, the defect is assumed to be nonorganic. Obviously, this method is of no
use in patients claiming bilateral field defects (1).

3. Kinetic testing using Goldmann perimetry or a tangent screen may show a field
that becomes smaller and smaller as the test object is moved circumferentially
around the field. This "spiraling" field is a classic manifestation of nonorganic
disease (1).

4. A patient claiming nonorganic field loss may be coaxed into seeing a larger
field during perimetry testing. The examiner compliments the patient on a job
well done but explains that instead of waiting until he or she is completely cer-

tain of seeing the object, the patient should respond right at the moment when the light stimulus is just barely detected. The field test is repeated after this coaxing (1).

5. Perform tangent screen testing at different distances while maintaining the same ratio of the size of the test object and the distance of the patient from the screen. Accordingly, the size of a test object used at a distance of 1 m should be doubled when used at a distance of 2 m. A patient with organic field constriction will demonstrate an increase in the absolute size of the visual field when the test distance is moved from 1 to 2 m. In contrast, a patient with nonorganic field constriction will show no change in the size of the absolute field constriction (1).

Monocular Diplopia

Refractive error must be ruled out. Mild lens opacities and/or mild corneal epithelial dystrophies are among the possible refractive culprits. Diplopia caused by disturbances of the refractive media usually results in one image that is fairly clear and one image that is fuzzy, ghostlike, or shadowy. This usually resolves with a pinhole, better spectacle correction, or contact lens correction. True monocular diplopia where two separate and equal images are seen is almost never caused by an organic process. For the sake of completeness, it should be mentioned that there have been rare case reports of monocular diplopia and polyopia in patients with central nervous system disease located in the temporoparietal region. Such patients usually complain of multiple images of different sizes and shapes, yet these images are seen with equal clarity and tend not to overlap (1).

MANAGEMENT ISSUES

1. The diagnosis of nonorganic disease is most safely applied as a diagnosis of exclusion. Occult organic disease must be ruled out before the diagnosis on nonphysiologic visual loss can be made. A full ophthalmologic examination must be performed. Consider brain MRI/computed tomography if central lesions are suspected. ERG and VEP also should be considered.

2. Empathic reassurance is the rule for patients with documented nonorganic visual disturbance. The patient is told that there is no serious abnormality of the eye that could account for the patient's symptoms. In the patient with a psychogenic disturbance, the clinician should provide compassionate assurances that things will improve with time. Psychiatric referral may be helpful.

3. In cases of nonorganic visual disturbance in children, the physician should use reassurance and empathy. Some clinicians advocate a "tropicamide cure," where the child is told that he or she has an eye problem but that it will be cured by some very powerful eyedrops. Tropicamide is instilled and the child's distance acuity is retested 30 minutes later. It is important to remember that nonorganic visual loss may signal underlying emotional or psychological conflicts.

The astute clinician should ask the child without the parents present if there is anything else on the child's mind. Appropriate psychiatric and/or social work referrals may be indicated.

4. Cases of ocular Münchausen's syndrome are rare but present unique diagnostic and treatment problems. Because these particular patients are prone to self-infliction of injury in order to make their stories plausible, they tend to present with true ocular abnormalities and/or ocular emergencies requiring real management. Multiple presentations with similarly dramatic ocular problems to multiple hospitals in varied locations and a long list of physicians may tip the clinician toward suspecting the diagnosis of Münchausen's syndrome. Although patients afflicted with this rare syndrome are as varied and diverse as their illness presentations, the unifying characteristic appears to be an extensive and nomadic journey through various health-care institutions over time and space. A few well-placed phone calls to other institutions may help crack the case. If a diagnosis of Münchausen's syndrome is considered, psychiatric referral is indicated (3).

5. Münchausen's syndrome by proxy, a condition in which a parent simulates or produces illness in a child, is rare. No case reports of an ocular form of this syndrome currently exist in the literature. Nevertheless, consider this diagnosis if a child presents with persistent and recurrent ocular findings with no real explanation, the clinical findings and the history seem to make no sense, the child has seen multiple experienced clinicians who have never seen a case like it before, symptoms and signs disappear whenever the parent is absent, the parent is extremely attentive and refuses to leave the child alone, the parent has a previous medical background, and the parent seems to be less concerned about the child's condition than the medical staff is. Münchausen's syndrome by proxy is a form of child abuse; appropriate social work, protective services and psychiatric referrals are indicated if this diagnosis is seriously considered (5).

GENERAL MEDICAL/LEGAL CONSIDERATIONS

Although highly valuable in the unique clinical setting of the evaluation of nonorganic visual loss, the following points should be applied to all clinical situations:

1. Be sure to rigorously document all findings, tests, and verbal discussion with the patient. The medical chart is the only tangible and concrete record of what has transpired between you and your patient. If it was not written down, it did not happen.

2. Rigorously document the plans for both the acute management and later follow-up. Every chart should reflect a specific plan of action. Avoid general directives such as "return as required" and "follow up as needed."

3. Document all phone conversations between you and your patient. Be sure to include a specific and detailed record of what was discussed, along with the time and date of the conversation.

4. Maintain a polite and professional demeanor with all patients and families of patients, regardless of their attitude or behavior toward you.
5. Establish good communication and rapport with your patients. Let the patient know what to expect during and after all diagnostic interventions and procedures you perform.
6. Obtain informed consent before all invasive and surgical procedures. This includes an explanation of the procedure, the indications for the procedure, the risks involved, and the alternatives. Make sure all procedures are thoroughly documented with a procedure note.
7. If a patient refuses treatment or evaluation, make sure the patient is able to understand your rationale for the evaluation and/or treatment as well as the likely consequences of refusing the evaluation and/or treatment. This should be well documented in the chart.
8. Although the task may be difficult, strive to maintain patient confidentiality in the emergency room setting.
9. Have a chaperon present whenever examining a child.
10. If the examiner feels that a patient is making sexual overtures toward him or her, no matter how subtle or innocent, a chaperon should be in attendance for the entire clinical encounter.
11. Some experienced clinicians, male and female, prefer to have chaperons present during all clinical encounters in order to avoid the devastating consequences of unfounded claims of physical abuse and/or sexual harassment. Although having a chaperon present during every examination in the emergency room may be impractical, the emergency room physician will no doubt encounter specific situations, in addition to those noted above, where the attendance of a chaperon will serve him or her well.

REFERENCES

1. Miller NR. *Walsh and Hoyt's Clinical Neuro-Ophthalmology.* 4th ed. Part 2. Baltimore: Williams & Wilkins; 1995:4541–4563.
2. Kramer KK, La Piana FG, Appleton B. Ocular malingering and hysteria: diagnosis and management. *Surv Ophthalmol* 1979;24:89–96.
3. Leland DG. Münchausen's syndrome. A brief review. *S D J Med* 1993;April:109–112.
4. Sofinowski RE, Butler PM. Münchausen syndrome by proxy: a review. *Tex Med* 1991;87:66–69.
5. Levy NS, Glick EB. Stereoscopic perception and Snellen visual acuity. *Am J Ophthalmol* 1974;78:722–724.

Management of Ocular Injuries and Emergencies,
edited by Mathew W. MacCumber.
Lippincott–Raven Publishers, Philadelphia © 1998.

Appendix A: Pediatric Dosing of Commonly Used Medications

Sharon Fekrat

Department of Ophthalmology, Wilmer Eye Institute, The Johns Hopkins University School of Medicine, Baltimore, Maryland 21287

TABLE AA–1. *Pediatric dosing of commonly used medications*

Medication	Route	Dose
Ceftazidime	IV	100–150 mg/kg/day, every 8 h
Clindamycin	IV	25–40 mg/kg/day, every 6–8 h
Diamox	IV	20–40 mg/kg/day, every 6 h (not to exceed 1 g/day)
	PO	8–30 mg/kg/day, every 8 h
Compazine[a]	PO	0.4 mg/kg/day, every 8 h as needed
	PR	0.4 mg/kg/day, every 8 h as needed
	IM	0.1–0.15 mg/kg/dose, every 4–6 h as needed
Demerol	All	1.0–1.5 mg/kg/dose, every 4–6 h as needed (not to exceed 100 mg per dose)
Tylenol elixir	PO or PR	15 mg/kg/dose, every 4 h as needed
Codeine elixir	PO	0.5–1.0 mg/kg/dose, every 4–6 h as needed

Atropine drops for cycloplegia in children, if used, should be 0.5% twice daily. Do not use the 1% four times daily dose that is used in our adult patients.
IV, intravenously; PO, orally; PR, rectally; IM, intramuscularly.
[a]Not recommended in children <24 mo of age.

Management of Ocular Injuries and Emergencies,
edited by Mathew W. MacCumber.
Lippincott–Raven Publishers, Philadelphia © 1998.

Appendix B: Preparation of Antibiotics

Shannath L. Merbs and Peter A. Campochiaro

*Department of Ophthalmology, Wilmer Eye Institute, The Johns Hopkins University
School of Medicine, Baltimore, Maryland 21287*

Sterile techniques should be used in preparation of all antibiotics (1).

TOPICAL ANTIBIOTICS

Amphotericin B, topical 1.5 mg/ml

1. To the 50-mg amphotericin B injection vial, add 10 ml of sterile water for injection, USP (preservative free) (vial 1, 5 mg/ml).
2. Transfer 3 ml from vial 1 to sterile ophthalmic dropper bottle and add 7 ml of sterile water for injection, USP (preservative free), mix, and label (1.5 mg/ml). Refrigerate. Do not filter, as the drug is a colloidal suspension.

Cefazolin, 50 mg/ml

1. To the 500-mg cefazolin injection vial, add 10 ml of sodium chloride 0.9% for injection, USP (preservative free) (50 mg/ml).
2. Filter into a sterile empty vial. Refrigerate.

Tobramycin, 14 mg/ml (preserved)

1. To a 5-ml bottle of commercial ophthalmic tobramycin (3 mg/ml), add 2 ml parenteral tobramycin (40 mg/ml).
2. Cap the dropper bottle, shake to mix, and label (14 mg/ml). Filter into a sterile empty vial.

Vancomycin, 50 mg/ml

1. To the 500-mg vancomycin injection vial, add 10 ml of sterile water for injection, USP (preservative free), and shake to mix (50 mg/ml).
2. Filter into a sterile empty vial.

SUBCONJUNCTIVAL ANTIBIOTICS AND STEROID

Cefazolin, subconjunctival 100 mg/0.5 ml

1. To the 500-mg cefazolin injection vial, add 2.5 ml of sterile water for injection, USP (preservative free) (500 mg/2.5 ml or 100 mg/0.5 ml).
2. Filter into a sterile empty vial. Refrigerate.

Ceftazidime, subconjunctival 100 mg/0.5 ml

1. To the 1-g Ceftazidime injection vial, add 5 ml of sterile water for injection, USP (preservative free) (100 mg/0.5 ml).
2. Filter into a sterile empty vial. Refrigerate.

Vancomycin, subconjunctival 25 mg/0.5 ml

1. To the 500-mg vancomycin injection vial, add 10 ml of sodium chloride 0.9% for injection, USP (preservative free) (50 mg/ml).
2. Filter into a sterile empty vial.

Dexamethasone, subconjunctival 1 mg/0.25 ml

From the 4 mg/ml dexamethasone phosphate injection vial, withdraw desired dose.

INTRAVITREAL ANTIBIOTICS

Amphotericin B, intravitreal 0.005 mg/0.1 ml

1. To the 50-mg amphotericin B injection vial, add 10 ml of sterile water for injection, USP (preservative free) (vial 1, 5 mg/ml).
2. Transfer 0.1 ml from vial 1 to 10-ml empty sterile vial and add 9.9 ml sterile water for injection, USP (preservative free) (vial 2, 0.005 mg/0.1 ml).
3. Do not filter as the drug is a colloidal suspension. Refrigerate.

Ceftazidime, intravitreal 2 mg/0.1 ml

1. To the 1-g Ceftazidime injection vial, add 10 ml sterile water for injection, USP (preservative free) (vial 1, 100 mg/ml).
2. Transfer 2 ml from vial 1 to a 10-ml empty sterile vial and add 8 ml sodium chloride 0.9% for injection, USP (preservative free) (2 mg/0.1 ml).
3. Filter into a sterile empty vial. Refrigerate.

Clindamycin, intravitreal 0.5 mg/0.1 ml

1. From the 300 mg/2 ml clindamycin injection vial, withdraw 0.5 ml and transfer to a 20-ml empty sterile injection vial and add 14.5 ml of sodium chloride 0.9% for injection, USP (preservative free) (5 mg/ml).
2. Filter into a sterile empty vial

Vancomycin, intravitreal 1 mg/0.1 ml

1. To the 500-mg vancomycin injection vial, add 10 ml of sodium chloride 0.9% for injection, USP (preservative free) (vial 1, 50 mg/ml).
2. Transfer 2 ml from vial 1 to 10-ml sterile empty vial and add 8 ml of sodium chloride 0.9% for injection, USP (preservative free) (10 mg/ml).
3. Filter into a sterile empty vial.

REFERENCE

1. Reynolds LA, Closson RG. *Extemporaneous Ophthalmic Preparations.* Vancouver, WA: Applied Therapeutics, Inc.; 1993.

Management of Ocular Injuries and Emergencies,
edited by Mathew W. MacCumber.
Lippincott–Raven Publishers, Philadelphia ©1998.

Appendix C: Evaluation of Visual Disability

J. B. Harlan, Jr., and Neil R. Miller

*Department of Ophthalmology, Wilmer Eye Institute, The Johns Hopkins University
School of Medicine, Baltimore, Maryland 21287*

DEFINITION OF BLINDNESS (1)

In the United States, blindness is defined as central visual acuity equal to 20/200 or less in the better eye with best correction, or the widest diameter of visual field subtending an angle of no greater than 20 degrees.

The World Health Organization (WHO) defines five levels of visual impairment:

Level 1, 20/70
Level 2, 20/200
Level 3, 20/400
Level 4, 5/300
Level 5, no light perception

Patients with widest visual field radius no greater than 10 degrees but greater than 5 degrees around central fixation are considered level 3.

Patients with widest visual field radius no greater than 5 degrees around central fixation are considered level 4.

Blindness is defined by the WHO as an impairment level of 3 or worse.

DETERMINATION OF PERCENTAGE OF VISUAL IMPAIRMENT

In accordance with the standards set forth by the American Medical Association (2), the percentage of visual impairment is based on loss of function in each of the following three areas:

1. Central visual acuity
2. Visual fields
3. Ocular motility

The percentage loss of function is first determined in each of these three areas. These measurements are then translated into a final estimation of impairment of the entire visual system and of the person as a whole.

DETERMINATION OF IMPAIRMENT OF CENTRAL VISION (2)

1. Record best corrected visual acuity for distance and near for each eye. Distance acuity is measured in Snellen notation. Near acuity may be measured using revised Jaeger standard notation or American point type notation and then converting to near Snellen acuity using Table AC–1.

TABLE AC–1. *Visual acuity notations with corresponding percentages of loss of central vision*

For distance			
	Snellen notations		
English	Metric 6	Metric 4	% Loss
20/15	6/5	4/3	0
20/20	6/6	4/4	0
20/25	6/7.5	4/5	5
20/30	6/10	4/6	10
20/40	6/12	4/8	15
20/50	6/15	4/10	25
20/60	6/20	4/12	35
20/70	6/22	4/14	40
20/80	6/24	4/16	45
20/100	6/30	4/20	50
20/125	6/38	4/25	60
20/150	6/50	4/30	70
20/200	6/60	4/40	80
20/300	6/90	4/60	85
20/400	6/120	4/80	90
20/800	6/240	4/160	95

For near				
Near Snellen		Revised Jaeger Standard	American point-type	% Loss
Inches	Centimeters			
14/14	35/35	1	3	0
14/18	35/45	2	4	0
14/21	35/53	3	5	5
14/24	35/60	4	6	7
14/28	35/70	5	7	10
14/35	35/88	6	8	50
14/40	35/100	7	9	55
14/45	35/113	8	10	60
14/60	35/150	9	11	80
14/70	35/175	10	12	85
14/80	35/200	11	13	87
14/88	35/220	12	14	90
14/112	35/280	13	21	95
14/140	35/350	14	23	98

Reprinted with permission (1).

2. Table AC–2 is then used to find the central vision impairment for each eye. Locate the Snellen rating for near vision along the top row and then the Snellen rating for distance along the first column. Reading down from the near acuity value (top row) and across from the distance acuity value (first column), one locates the point of intersection. This point contains two impairment values. The top value is the percentage of visual loss without allowance for monocular aphakia or monocular pseudophakia. The bottom value is the percentage of visual loss allowing for monocular aphakia or monocular pseudophakia. Monocular aphakia or pseudophakia is considered to be an additional impairment due to greater light scatter, greater chance of glare, decreased contrast sensitivity, spherical aberration, loss of accommodation, increased likelihood of capsular opacification, chance of lens decentralization with visualization of the lens edge, and pupillary abnormalities. This is factored into the table by allowing a 50% impairment rating simply for aphakia/pseudophakia, and then adding half of the actual observed impairment to calculate the final total impairment.

DETERMINATION OF IMPAIRMENT OF VISUAL FIELD (2)

The Goldmann perimeter is used to evaluate the visual field for each eye. The standard stimulus is the III-4e kinetic stimulus for phakic and pseudophakic patients. The IV-4e kinetic stimulus is used for aphakic patients without a lens implant or contact lens.

Table AC–3 contains the accepted normal values for degrees of visual field in each of the eight principal meridians.

Record the maximum extent of the visual field in each of the eight principal meridians using the following rules:

1. If the border of the field coincides with a principal meridian (i.e., hemianopia or nasal step) the value recorded is the mid-point. In the example of a nasal step extending along the nasal meridian from 20 degrees to 60 degrees, the maximum extent of the field along that meridian would end at the mid-point between 20 degrees and 60 degrees, i.e., at 40 degrees. In the case of a hemianopia with its border at the vertical meridian (direct up) extending from 0 degrees to 40 degrees, the maximum extent of the field in the vertical meridian would be recorded as 20 degrees.
2. If a meridian passes through a scotoma, the width of the scotoma is subtracted from the maximum number of degrees for that meridian.
3. The maximum extent of a meridian cannot exceed the standard normal value for that particular meridian (Table AC–3).

Next, sum the measurements for all meridians to determine total degrees of visual field (maximum 500 degrees). The percentage of loss of monocular visual field is then read directly from Table AC–4.

TABLE AC–2. *Loss (%) of central vision in a single eye*

Snellen rating for distance in feet[a]	Approximate Snellen rating for near in inches[a]					
	$\frac{14}{14}$	$\frac{14}{18}$	$\frac{14}{21}$	$\frac{14}{24}$	$\frac{14}{28}$	$\frac{14}{35}$
$\frac{20}{15}$	0	0	3	4	5	25
	50	50	52	52	53	63
$\frac{20}{20}$	0	0	3	4	5	25
	50	50	52	52	53	63
$\frac{20}{25}$	3	3	5	6	8	28
	52	52	53	53	54	64
$\frac{20}{30}$	5	5	8	9	10	30
	53	53	54	54	55	65
$\frac{20}{40}$	8	8	10	11	13	33
	54	54	55	56	57	67
$\frac{20}{50}$	13	13	15	16	18	38
	57	57	58	58	59	69
$\frac{20}{60}$	16	16	18	20	22	41
	58	58	59	60	61	70
$\frac{20}{70}$	18	18	21	22	23	43
	59	59	61	61	62	72
$\frac{20}{80}$	20	20	23	24	25	45
	60	60	62	62	63	73
$\frac{20}{100}$	25	25	28	29	30	50
	63	63	64	64	65	75
$\frac{20}{125}$	30	30	33	34	35	55
	65	65	67	67	68	78
$\frac{20}{150}$	34	34	37	38	39	59
	67	67	68	69	70	80
$\frac{20}{200}$	40	40	43	44	45	65
	70	70	72	72	73	83
$\frac{20}{300}$	43	43	45	46	48	68
	72	72	73	73	74	84
$\frac{20}{400}$	45	45	48	49	50	70
	73	73	74	74	75	85
$\frac{20}{800}$	48	48	50	51	53	73
	74	74	75	76	77	87

[a]Upper number shows % loss of central vision without allowance for monocular aphakia or monocular pseudophakia; low number shows % loss of central vision with allowance for monocular aphakia or monocular pseudophakia.
Reprinted with permission (1).

TABLE AC–2. *Continued*

Approximate Snellen rating for near in inches[a]							
14/40	14/45	14/60	14/70	14/80	14/88	14/112	14/140
27/64	30/65	40/70	43/72	44/72	45/73	48/74	49/75
27/64	30/65	40/70	43/72	44/72	46/73	48/74	49/75
30/65	33/67	43/72	45/73	46/73	48/74	50/75	52/76
32/66	35/68	45/73	48/74	49/74	50/75	53/76	54/77
35/68	38/69	48/74	50/75	51/76	53/77	55/78	57/79
40/70	43/72	53/77	55/78	56/78	58/79	60/80	62/81
44/72	46/73	56/78	59/79	60/80	61/81	64/82	65/83
46/73	48/74	58/79	61/81	62/81	63/82	66/83	67/84
47/74	50/75	60/80	63/82	64/82	65/83	68/84	69/85
52/76	55/78	65/83	68/84	69/84	70/85	73/87	74/87
57/79	60/80	70/85	73/87	74/87	75/88	78/89	79/90
61/81	64/82	74/87	77/88	78/89	79/90	82/91	83/92
67/84	70/85	80/90	83/91	84/92	85/93	88/94	89/95
70/85	73/87	83/91	85/93	86/93	88/94	90/95	92/96
72/86	75/88	85/93	88/94	89/94	90/95	93/97	94/97
75/88	78/89	88/94	90/95	91/96	93/97	95/98	97/99

TABLE AC–3. *Normal visual fields for eight principal meridians*

Direction of vision	Degrees of field
Temporally	85
Down temporally	85
Direct down	65
Down nasally	50
Nasally	60
Up nasally	55
Direct up	45
Up temporally	55
Total	500

Reprinted with permission (1).

TABLE AC–4. *Loss of monocular visual field*

Total degrees		% of	Total degrees		% of	Total degrees		% of
Lost	Retained	Loss	Lost	Retained	Loss	Lost	Retained	Loss
0	500[a]	0	170	330	34	340	160	68
5	495	1	175	325	35	345	155	69
10	490	2	180	320	36	350	150	70
15	485	3	185	315	37	355	145	71
20	480	4	190	310	38	360	140	72
25	475	5	195	305	39	365	135	73
30	470	6	200	300	40	370	130	74
35	465	7	205	295	41	375	125	75
40	460	8	210	290	42	380	120	76
45	455	9	215	285	43	385	115	77
50	450	10	220	280	44	390	110	78
55	445	11	225	275	45	395	105	79
60	440	12	230	270	46	400	100	80
65	435	13	235	265	47	405	95	81
70	430	14	240	260	48	410	90	82
75	425	15	245	255	49	415	85	83
80	420	16	250	250	50	420	80	84
85	415	17	255	245	51	425	75	85
90	410	18	260	240	52	430	70	86
95	405	19	265	235	53	435	65	87
100	400	20	270	230	54	440	60	88
105	395	21	275	225	55	445	55	89
110	390	22	280	220	56	450	50	90
115	385	23	285	215	57	455	45	91
120	380	24	290	210	58	460	40	92
125	375	25	295	205	59	465	35	93
130	370	26	300	200	60	470	30	94
135	365	27	305	195	61	475	25	95
140	360	28	310	190	62	480	20	96
145	355	29	315	185	63	485	15	97
150	350	30	320	180	64	490	10	98
155	345	31	325	175	65	495	5	99
160	340	32	330	170	66	500	0	100
165	335	33	335	165	67			

[a]Or more.
Reprinted with permission (1).

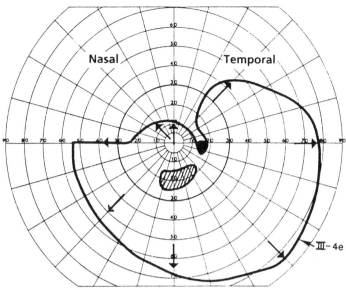

Direction of vision	Degrees of field	Comments
Temporally	77	
Down temporally	84	
Direct down	55	65° maximum from table, minus 10° of scotoma between 15° and 25°
Down nasally	50	Not 55°, because maximum from table is 50°
Nasally	37	Midway between 22° and 52°
Up nasally	15	
Direct up	10	
Up temporally	33	40° peripheral extent, minus 7° excluded by isopter between 10° and 17°
Total	361	361 divided by 5 = 72

Thus, the retained visual field is 72%, and the impairment is 28%.

FIG. AC–1. Sample field *(above)*, with sample calculations *(below)*. Reprinted with permission (1).

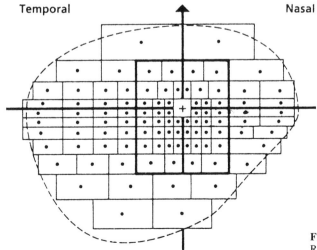

FIG. AC–2. Esterman grid. Reprinted with permission (1).

Consider the following example monocular field (Fig. AC–1):

If an inferior quadrant loss is present in an eye, 5% is added to the total percentage field loss in that eye. If an inferior hemianoptic loss is present in an eye (i.e., both inferior quadrants), 10% is added to the total percentage loss of field in that eye. This is done because major inferior visual field loss has more of a functional consequence than an equivalent loss above.

An alternate method of determining the percentage visual field loss is the use of the Esterman grid, which can be obtained from the American Academy of Ophthalmology, 655 Beech St., San Francisco, CA 94120-7424.

The recorded monocular kinetic field is transferred onto the Esterman 100 unit monocular grid. A count of the number of dots seen within the field among the 100 dots that are in the grid gives the percentage of retained field. A count of the number of dots outside the borders of the field gives the percentage field loss (Fig. AC-2).

DETERMINATION OF VISUAL IMPAIRMENT DUE TO ABNORMAL MOTILITY (2)

The amount of diplopia in different directions of gaze can be determined using an arc perimeter at 33 cm, a bowl perimeter, or a tangent screen. Diplopia usually

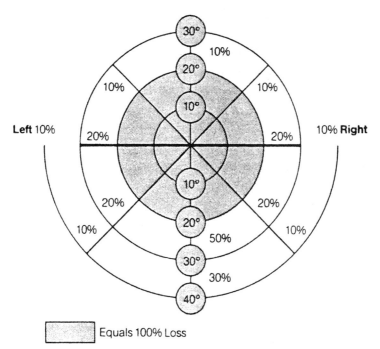

Equals 100% Loss

FIG. AC–3. Percentage loss of ocular motility of one eye in diplopia fields. Reprinted with permission (1).

causes significant visual impairment only if it exists within 30 degrees of the center of fixation.

The patient is tested with both eyes open and the chin supported in a chin rest. The face should be centered with the eyes equidistant from the sides of the central fixation target.

The presence or absence of double vision is noted as the patient follows the fixation target from the center of fixation outward to 30 degrees along each of the eight principal meridians. The percentage loss of motility is determined for each of the eight meridians using Fig. AC–3. Note that diplopia within the central 20 degrees of binocular field is scored as 100% loss. The percentage motility loss in the meridian with maximal impairment is recorded as the amount of motility loss for that patient.

DETERMINING TOTAL IMPAIRMENT OF THE VISUAL SYSTEM AND OF THE WHOLE PERSON (2)

1. The recorded percentage loss of central vision for a given eye and the recorded percentage loss of visual field for that eye are combined into a single percentage impairment using the combined values table (Table AC–5).
2. This process is repeated for the fellow eye.
3. The percentage impairment value of the eye with the greater impairment and the previously recorded ocular motility impairment are then combined into a single impairment value using the same combined values table (Table AC–5). Thus, the rating of ocular motility impairment is combined only with the impairment value of the worse eye to yield a total impairment value for that eye.
4. The examiner is allowed to estimate up to an additional 10% of impairment for an ocular abnormality that he or she feels is not adequately reflected in the central visual acuity, visual fields, or motility testing for a given eye. This additional percentage is simply combined with the existing percentage loss in the given eye to yield the total impairment for that eye. This is done using the combined values table (Table AC–5).
5. Once the total impairment of each eye has been determined using the above methods, Table AC–6 is then used to determine the percentage impairment of the entire visual system. If bilateral aphakia is present and corrected visual acuity has been used in the evaluation, the impairment of the visual system as a whole is increased by 25% of the value of the remaining corrected vision. For example, a 40% impairment of the visual system as a whole (60% remaining) would be increased to 40% + (0.25)(60%) = 40% + 15% = 55%.
6. The percentage impairment of the whole person resulting from a given level of visual system impairment may be read from Table AC–7.

APPENDIX C

TABLE AC–5. *Combined values chart*

	1	2	3	4	5	6	7	8	9	10	11	12	13	14	15	16	17	18	19	20	21	22	23	24	25
1	2																								
2	3	4																							
3	4	5	6																						
4	5	6	7	8																					
5	6	7	8	9	10																				
6	7	8	9	10	11	12																			
7	8	9	10	11	12	13	14																		
8	9	10	11	12	13	14	14	15																	
9	10	11	12	13	14	14	15	16	17																
10	11	12	13	14	15	15	16	17	18	19															
11	12	13	14	15	15	16	17	18	19	20	21														
12	13	14	15	16	16	17	18	19	20	21	22	23													
13	14	15	16	16	17	18	19	20	21	22	23	23	24												
14	15	16	17	17	18	19	20	21	22	23	23	24	25	26											
15	16	17	18	18	19	20	21	22	23	24	24	25	26	27	28										
16	17	18	19	19	20	21	22	23	24	24	25	26	27	28	29	29									
17	18	19	19	20	21	22	23	24	24	25	26	27	28	29	29	30	31								
18	19	20	20	21	22	23	24	25	25	26	27	28	29	29	30	31	32	33							
19	20	21	21	22	23	24	25	25	26	27	28	29	30	30	31	32	33	34	34						
20	21	22	22	23	24	25	26	26	27	28	29	30	30	31	32	33	34	34	35	36					
21	22	23	23	24	25	26	27	27	28	29	30	30	31	32	33	34	34	35	36	37	38				
22	23	24	24	25	26	27	27	28	29	30	31	31	32	33	34	34	35	36	37	38	38	39			
23	24	25	25	26	27	28	28	29	30	31	31	32	33	34	35	35	36	37	38	38	39	40	41		
24	25	26	26	27	28	29	29	30	31	32	32	33	34	35	35	36	37	38	38	39	40	41	41	42	
25	26	27	27	28	29	30	30	31	32	33	33	34	35	36	36	37	38	39	39	40	41	42	42	43	44
26	27	27	28	29	30	30	31	32	33	33	34	35	36	36	37	38	39	39	40	41	42	42	43	44	45
27	28	28	29	30	31	31	32	33	34	34	35	36	36	37	38	39	39	40	41	42	42	43	44	45	45
28	29	29	30	31	32	32	33	34	34	35	36	37	37	38	39	40	40	41	42	42	43	44	45	45	46
29	30	30	31	32	33	33	34	35	35	36	37	38	38	39	40	40	41	42	42	43	44	45	45	46	47
30	31	31	32	33	34	34	35	36	36	37	38	38	39	40	41	41	42	43	43	44	45	45	46	47	48
31	32	32	33	34	34	35	36	37	37	38	39	39	40	41	41	42	43	43	44	45	45	46	47	48	48
32	33	33	34	35	35	36	37	37	38	39	39	40	41	42	42	43	44	44	45	46	46	47	48	48	49
33	34	34	35	36	36	37	38	38	39	40	40	41	42	42	43	44	44	45	46	46	47	48	48	49	50
34	35	35	36	37	37	38	39	39	40	41	41	42	43	43	44	45	45	46	47	47	48	49	49	50	51
35	36	36	37	38	38	39	40	40	41	42	42	43	43	44	45	45	46	47	47	48	49	49	50	51	51
36	37	37	38	39	39	40	40	41	42	42	43	44	44	45	46	46	47	48	48	49	49	50	51	51	52
37	38	38	39	40	40	41	41	42	43	43	44	45	45	46	46	47	48	48	49	50	50	51	51	52	53
38	39	39	40	40	41	42	42	43	44	44	45	45	46	47	47	48	49	49	50	50	51	52	52	53	54
39	40	40	41	41	42	43	43	44	44	45	46	46	47	48	48	49	49	50	51	51	52	52	53	54	54
40	41	41	42	42	43	44	44	45	45	46	47	47	48	48	49	50	50	51	51	52	53	53	54	54	55
41	42	42	43	43	44	45	45	46	46	47	47	48	49	49	50	50	51	52	52	53	53	54	55	55	56
42	43	43	44	44	45	45	46	47	47	48	48	49	50	50	51	51	52	52	53	54	54	55	55	56	57
43	44	44	45	45	46	46	47	48	48	49	49	50	50	51	52	52	53	53	54	54	55	56	56	57	57
44	45	45	46	46	47	47	48	48	49	50	50	51	51	52	52	53	54	54	55	55	56	56	57	57	58
45	46	46	47	47	48	48	49	49	50	51	51	52	52	53	53	54	54	55	55	56	57	57	58	58	59
46	47	47	48	48	49	49	50	50	51	51	52	52	53	54	54	55	55	56	56	57	57	58	58	59	60
47	48	48	49	49	50	50	51	51	52	52	53	53	54	54	55	55	56	57	57	58	58	59	59	60	60
48	49	49	50	50	51	51	52	52	53	53	54	54	55	55	56	56	57	57	58	58	59	59	60	60	61
49	50	50	51	51	52	52	53	53	54	54	55	55	56	56	57	57	58	58	59	59	60	60	61	61	62
50	51	51	52	52	53	53	54	54	55	55	56	56	57	57	58	58	59	59	60	60	61	61	62	62	63
	1	2	3	4	5	6	7	8	9	10	11	12	13	14	15	16	17	18	19	20	21	22	23	24	25

TABLE AC–5. *Continued*

26	27	28	29	30	31	32	33	34	35	36	37	38	39	40	41	42	43	44	45	46	47	48	49	50
45																								
46	47																							
47	47	48																						
47	48	49	50																					
48	49	50	50	51																				
49	50	50	51	52	52																			
50	50	51	52	52	53	54																		
50	51	52	52	53	54	54	55																	
51	52	52	53	54	54	55	56	56																
52	53	53	54	55	55	56	56	57	58															
53	53	54	55	55	56	56	57	58	58	59														
53	54	55	55	56	57	57	58	58	59	60	60													
54	55	55	56	57	57	58	58	59	60	60	61	62												
55	55	56	57	57	58	59	59	60	60	61	62	62	63											
56	56	57	57	58	59	59	60	60	61	62	62	63	63	64										
56	57	58	58	59	59	60	60	61	62	62	63	63	64	65	65									
57	58	58	59	59	60	61	61	62	62	63	63	64	65	65	66	66								
58	58	59	60	60	61	61	62	62	63	64	64	65	65	66	66	67	68							
59	59	60	60	61	61	62	62	63	64	64	65	65	66	66	67	68	68	69						
59	60	60	61	62	62	63	63	64	64	65	65	66	66	67	68	68	69	69	70					
60	61	61	62	62	63	63	64	64	65	65	66	67	67	68	68	69	69	70	70	71				
61	61	62	62	63	63	64	64	65	66	66	67	67	68	68	69	69	70	70	71	71	72			
62	62	63	63	64	64	65	65	66	66	67	67	68	68	69	69	70	70	71	71	72	72	73		
62	63	63	64	64	65	65	66	66	67	67	68	68	69	69	70	70	71	71	72	72	73	73	74	
63	64	64	65	65	66	66	67	67	68	68	69	69	70	70	71	71	72	72	73	73	74	74	75	75

TABLE AC–5. *Continued*

	1	2	3	4	5	6	7	8	9	10	11	12	13	14	15	16	17	18	19	20	21	22	23	24	25
51	51	52	52	53	53	54	54	55	55	56	56	57	57	58	58	59	59	60	60	61	61	62	62	63	63
52	52	53	53	54	54	55	55	56	56	57	57	58	58	59	59	60	60	61	61	62	62	63	63	64	64
53	53	54	54	55	55	56	56	57	57	58	58	59	59	60	60	61	61	61	62	62	63	63	64	64	65
54	54	55	55	56	56	57	57	58	58	59	59	59	60	60	61	61	62	62	63	63	64	64	65	65	66
55	55	56	56	57	57	58	58	59	59	60	60	60	61	61	62	62	63	63	64	64	64	65	65	66	66
56	56	57	57	58	58	59	59	60	60	60	61	61	62	62	63	63	63	64	64	65	65	66	66	67	67
57	57	58	58	59	59	60	60	60	61	61	62	62	63	63	63	64	64	65	65	66	66	66	67	67	68
58	58	59	59	60	60	61	61	61	62	62	63	63	63	64	64	65	65	66	66	66	67	67	68	68	68
59	59	60	60	61	61	61	62	62	63	63	64	64	64	65	65	66	66	66	67	67	68	68	68	69	69
60	60	61	61	62	62	62	63	63	64	64	64	65	65	66	66	66	67	67	68	68	68	69	69	70	70
61	61	62	62	63	63	63	64	64	65	65	65	66	66	66	67	67	68	68	68	69	69	70	70	70	71
62	62	63	63	64	64	64	65	65	65	66	66	67	67	67	68	68	68	69	69	70	70	70	71	71	72
63	63	64	64	64	65	65	66	66	66	67	67	67	68	68	69	69	69	70	70	70	71	71	72	72	72
64	64	65	65	65	66	66	67	67	67	68	68	68	69	69	69	70	70	70	71	71	72	72	72	73	73
65	65	66	66	66	67	67	67	68	68	69	69	69	70	70	70	71	71	71	72	72	72	73	73	73	74
66	66	67	67	67	68	68	68	69	69	69	70	70	70	71	71	71	72	72	72	73	73	73	74	74	75
67	67	68	68	68	69	69	69	70	70	70	71	71	71	72	72	72	73	73	73	74	74	74	75	75	75
68	68	69	69	69	70	70	70	71	71	71	72	72	72	72	73	73	73	74	74	74	75	75	75	76	76
69	69	70	70	70	71	71	71	71	72	72	72	73	73	73	74	74	74	75	75	75	76	76	76	76	77
70	70	71	71	71	72	72	72	72	73	73	73	74	74	74	75	75	75	75	76	76	76	77	77	77	78
71	71	72	72	72	72	73	73	73	74	74	74	74	75	75	75	76	76	76	77	77	77	77	78	78	78
72	72	73	73	73	73	74	74	74	75	75	75	75	76	76	76	76	77	77	77	78	78	78	78	79	79
73	73	74	74	74	74	75	75	75	75	76	76	76	77	77	77	77	78	78	78	78	79	79	79	79	80
74	74	75	75	75	75	76	76	76	76	77	77	77	77	78	78	78	78	79	79	79	79	80	80	80	81
75	75	76	76	76	76	77	77	77	77	78	78	78	78	79	79	79	79	80	80	80	80	81	81	81	81
76	76	76	77	77	77	77	78	78	78	78	79	79	79	79	80	80	80	80	81	81	81	81	82	82	82
77	77	77	78	78	78	78	79	79	79	79	80	80	80	80	80	81	81	81	81	82	82	82	82	83	83
78	78	78	79	79	79	79	80	80	80	80	80	81	81	81	81	82	82	82	82	82	83	83	83	83	84
79	79	79	80	80	80	80	80	81	81	81	81	82	82	82	82	82	83	83	83	83	83	84	84	84	84
80	80	80	81	81	81	81	81	82	82	82	82	82	83	83	83	83	83	84	84	84	84	84	85	85	85
81	81	81	82	82	82	82	82	83	83	83	83	83	84	84	84	84	84	84	85	85	85	85	85	86	86
82	82	82	83	83	83	83	83	83	84	84	84	84	84	85	85	85	85	85	85	86	86	86	86	86	87
83	83	83	84	84	84	84	84	84	85	85	85	85	85	85	86	86	86	86	86	87	87	87	87	87	87
84	84	84	84	85	85	85	85	85	85	86	86	86	86	86	86	87	87	87	87	87	87	88	88	88	88
85	85	85	85	86	86	86	86	86	86	87	87	87	87	87	87	87	88	88	88	88	88	88	88	89	89
86	86	86	86	87	87	87	87	87	87	87	88	88	88	88	88	88	88	89	89	89	89	89	89	89	90
87	87	87	87	88	88	88	88	88	88	88	88	89	89	89	89	89	89	89	89	90	90	90	90	90	90
88	88	88	88	88	89	89	89	89	89	89	89	89	90	90	90	90	90	90	90	90	91	91	91	91	91
89	89	89	89	89	90	90	90	90	90	90	90	90	90	91	91	91	91	91	91	91	91	91	92	92	92
90	90	90	90	90	91	91	91	91	91	91	91	91	91	91	92	92	92	92	92	92	92	92	92	92	93
91	91	91	91	91	91	92	92	92	92	92	92	92	92	92	92	92	93	93	93	93	93	93	93	93	93
92	92	92	92	92	92	92	93	93	93	93	93	93	93	93	93	93	93	93	94	94	94	94	94	94	94
93	93	93	93	93	93	93	93	94	94	94	94	94	94	94	94	94	94	94	94	94	94	95	95	95	95
94	94	94	94	94	94	94	94	94	95	95	95	95	95	95	95	95	95	95	95	95	95	95	95	95	96
95	95	95	95	95	95	95	95	95	95	96	96	96	96	96	96	96	96	96	96	96	96	96	96	96	96
96	96	96	96	96	96	96	96	96	96	96	96	96	97	97	97	97	97	97	97	97	97	97	97	97	97
97	97	97	97	97	97	97	97	97	97	97	97	97	97	97	97	97	98	98	98	98	98	98	98	98	98
98	98	98	98	98	98	98	98	98	98	98	98	98	98	98	98	98	98	98	98	98	98	98	98	98	99
99	99	99	99	99	99	99	99	99	99	99	99	99	99	99	99	99	99	99	99	99	99	99	99	99	99
	1	2	3	4	5	6	7	8	9	10	11	12	13	14	15	16	17	18	19	20	21	22	23	24	25

TABLE AC–5. *Continued*

26	27	28	29	30	31	32	33	34	35	36	37	38	39	40	41	42	43	44	45	46	47	48	49	50
64	64	65	65	66	66	67	67	68	68	69	69	70	70	71	71	72	72	73	73	74	74	75	75	76
64	65	65	66	66	67	67	68	68	69	69	70	70	71	71	72	72	73	73	74	74	75	75	76	76
65	66	66	67	67	68	68	69	69	69	70	70	71	71	72	72	73	73	74	74	75	75	76	76	77
66	66	67	67	68	68	69	69	70	70	71	71	71	72	72	73	73	74	74	75	75	76	76	77	77
67	67	68	68	69	69	69	70	70	71	71	72	72	73	73	73	74	74	75	75	76	76	77	77	78
67	68	68	69	69	70	70	71	71	71	72	72	73	73	74	74	74	75	75	76	76	77	77	78	78
68	69	69	69	70	70	71	71	72	72	72	73	73	74	74	75	75	75	76	76	77	77	78	78	79
69	69	70	70	71	71	71	72	72	73	73	74	74	74	75	75	76	76	76	77	77	78	78	79	79
70	70	70	71	71	72	72	73	73	73	74	74	75	75	75	76	76	77	77	77	78	78	79	79	80
70	71	71	72	72	72	73	73	74	74	74	75	75	76	76	76	77	77	78	78	78	79	79	80	80
71	72	72	72	73	73	73	74	74	75	75	75	76	76	77	77	77	78	78	79	79	79	80	80	81
72	72	73	73	73	74	74	75	75	75	76	76	76	77	77	78	78	78	79	79	79	80	80	81	81
73	73	73	74	74	74	75	75	76	76	76	77	77	77	78	78	79	79	79	80	80	80	81	81	82
73	74	74	74	75	75	76	76	76	77	77	77	78	78	78	79	79	79	80	80	81	81	81	82	82
74	74	75	75	76	76	76	77	77	77	78	78	78	79	79	79	80	80	80	81	81	81	82	82	83
75	75	76	76	76	77	77	77	78	78	78	79	79	79	80	80	80	81	81	81	82	82	82	83	83
76	76	76	77	77	77	78	78	78	79	79	79	80	80	80	81	81	81	82	82	82	83	83	83	84
76	77	77	77	78	78	78	79	79	79	80	80	80	81	81	81	81	82	82	82	83	83	83	84	84
77	77	78	78	78	79	79	79	80	80	80	80	81	81	81	82	82	82	83	83	83	84	84	84	85
78	78	78	79	79	79	80	80	80	81	81	81	81	82	82	82	83	83	83	84	84	84	84	85	85
79	79	79	79	80	80	80	81	81	81	81	82	82	82	83	83	83	83	84	84	84	85	85	85	86
79	80	80	80	80	81	81	81	82	82	82	82	83	83	83	83	84	84	84	85	85	85	85	86	86
80	80	81	81	81	81	82	82	82	82	83	83	83	84	84	84	84	85	85	85	85	86	86	86	87
81	81	81	82	82	82	82	83	83	83	83	84	84	84	84	85	85	85	85	86	86	86	86	87	87
82	82	82	82	83	83	83	83	84	84	84	84	85	85	85	85	86	86	86	86	87	87	87	87	88
82	82	83	83	83	83	84	84	84	84	85	85	85	85	86	86	86	86	87	87	87	87	88	88	88
83	83	83	84	84	84	84	85	85	85	85	86	86	86	86	86	87	87	87	87	88	88	88	88	89
84	84	84	84	85	85	85	85	85	86	86	86	86	87	87	87	87	87	88	88	88	88	89	89	89
84	85	85	85	85	86	86	86	86	86	87	87	87	87	87	88	88	88	88	88	89	89	89	89	90
85	85	86	86	86	86	86	87	87	87	87	87	88	88	88	88	88	89	89	89	89	89	90	90	90
86	86	86	87	87	87	87	87	87	88	88	88	88	88	89	89	89	89	89	90	90	90	90	90	91
87	87	87	87	87	88	88	88	88	88	88	89	89	89	89	89	90	90	90	90	90	90	91	91	91
87	88	88	88	88	88	88	89	89	89	89	89	89	90	90	90	90	90	90	91	91	91	91	91	92
88	88	88	89	89	89	89	89	89	90	90	90	90	90	90	91	91	91	91	91	91	92	92	92	92
89	89	89	89	90	90	90	90	90	90	90	91	91	91	91	91	91	91	92	92	92	92	92	92	93
90	90	90	90	90	90	90	91	91	91	91	91	91	91	92	92	92	92	92	92	92	93	93	93	93
90	91	91	91	91	91	91	91	91	92	92	92	92	92	92	92	93	93	93	93	93	93	93	93	94
91	91	91	91	92	92	92	92	92	92	92	92	93	93	93	93	93	93	93	93	94	94	94	94	94
92	92	92	92	92	92	93	93	93	93	93	93	93	93	93	94	94	94	94	94	94	94	94	94	95
93	93	93	93	93	93	93	93	93	94	94	94	94	94	94	94	94	94	94	95	95	95	95	95	95
93	93	94	94	94	94	94	94	94	94	94	94	94	95	95	95	95	95	95	95	95	95	95	95	96
94	94	94	94	94	94	95	95	95	95	95	95	95	95	95	95	95	95	96	96	96	96	96	96	96
95	95	95	95	95	95	95	95	95	95	96	96	96	96	96	96	96	96	96	96	96	96	96	96	97
96	96	96	96	96	96	96	96	96	96	96	96	96	96	96	96	97	97	97	97	97	97	97	97	97
96	96	96	96	96	97	97	97	97	97	97	97	97	97	97	97	97	97	97	97	97	97	97	97	98
97	97	97	97	97	97	97	97	97	97	97	97	98	98	98	98	98	98	98	98	98	98	98	98	98
98	98	98	98	98	98	98	98	98	98	98	98	98	98	98	98	98	98	98	98	98	98	98	98	99
99	99	99	99	99	99	99	99	99	99	99	99	99	99	99	99	99	99	99	99	99	99	99	99	99
99	99	99	99	99	99	99	99	99	99	99	99	99	99	99	99	99	99	99	99	99	99	99	99	100
26	27	28	29	30	31	32	33	34	35	36	37	38	39	40	41	42	43	44	45	46	47	48	49	50

	51	52	53	54	55	56	57	58	59	60	61	62	63	64	65	66	67	68	69	70	71	72	73	74	75
51	76																								
52	76	77																							
53	77	77	78																						
54	77	78	78	79																					
55	78	78	79	79	80																				
56	78	79	79	80	80	81																			
57	79	79	80	80	81	81	82																		
58	79	80	80	81	81	82	82	82																	
59	80	80	81	81	82	82	82	83	83																
60	80	81	81	82	82	82	83	83	84	84															
61	81	81	82	82	82	83	83	84	84	84	85														
62	81	82	82	83	83	83	84	84	84	85	85	86													
63	82	82	83	83	83	84	84	84	85	85	86	86	86												
64	82	83	83	83	84	84	85	85	85	86	86	86	87	87											
65	83	83	84	84	84	85	85	85	86	86	86	87	87	87	88										
66	83	84	84	84	85	85	85	86	86	86	87	87	87	88	88	88									
67	84	84	84	85	85	85	86	86	86	87	87	87	88	88	88	89	89								
68	84	85	85	85	86	86	86	87	87	87	88	88	88	88	89	89	89	90							
69	85	85	85	86	86	86	87	87	87	88	88	88	89	89	89	89	90	90	90						
70	85	86	86	86	87	87	87	87	88	88	88	89	89	89	90	90	90	90	91	91					
71	86	86	86	87	87	87	88	88	88	88	89	89	89	90	90	90	90	91	91	91	92				
72	86	87	87	87	87	88	88	88	89	89	89	89	90	90	90	90	91	91	91	92	92	92			
73	87	87	87	88	88	88	88	89	89	89	89	90	90	90	91	91	91	91	92	92	92	92	93		
74	87	88	88	88	88	89	89	89	89	90	90	90	90	91	91	91	91	92	92	92	92	93	93	93	
75	88	88	88	89	89	89	89	90	90	90	90	91	91	91	91	92	92	92	92	93	93	93	93	94	94
76	88	88	89	89	89	89	90	90	90	90	91	91	91	91	92	92	92	92	93	93	93	93	94	94	94
77	89	89	89	89	90	90	90	90	91	91	91	91	91	92	92	92	92	93	93	93	93	94	94	94	94
78	89	89	90	90	90	90	91	91	91	91	91	92	92	92	92	93	93	93	93	93	94	94	94	94	95
79	90	90	90	90	91	91	91	91	91	92	92	92	92	92	93	93	93	93	93	94	94	94	94	95	95
80	90	90	91	91	91	91	91	92	92	92	92	92	93	93	93	93	93	94	94	94	94	94	95	95	95
81	91	91	91	91	91	92	92	92	92	92	93	93	93	93	93	94	94	94	94	94	94	95	95	95	95
82	91	91	92	92	92	92	92	92	93	93	93	93	93	94	94	94	94	94	94	95	95	95	95	95	96
83	92	92	92	92	92	93	93	93	93	93	93	94	94	94	94	94	94	95	95	95	95	95	95	96	96
84	92	92	92	93	93	93	93	93	93	94	94	94	94	94	94	95	95	95	95	95	95	96	96	96	96
85	93	93	93	93	93	93	94	94	94	94	94	94	94	95	95	95	95	95	95	96	96	96	96	96	96
86	93	93	93	94	94	94	94	94	94	94	95	95	95	95	95	95	95	96	96	96	96	96	96	96	97
87	94	94	94	94	94	94	94	95	95	95	95	95	95	95	95	96	96	96	96	96	96	96	96	97	97
88	94	94	94	94	95	95	95	95	95	95	95	95	96	96	96	96	96	96	96	96	97	97	97	97	97
89	95	95	95	95	95	95	95	95	95	96	96	96	96	96	96	96	96	96	97	97	97	97	97	97	97
90	95	95	95	95	96	96	96	96	96	96	96	96	96	96	97	97	97	97	97	97	97	97	97	97	98
91	96	96	96	96	96	96	96	96	96	96	96	97	97	97	97	97	97	97	97	97	97	97	98	98	98
92	96	96	96	96	96	96	97	97	97	97	97	97	97	97	97	97	97	97	98	98	98	98	98	98	98
93	97	97	97	97	97	97	97	97	97	97	97	97	97	97	98	98	98	98	98	98	98	98	98	98	98
94	97	97	97	97	97	97	97	97	98	98	98	98	98	98	98	98	98	98	98	98	98	98	98	98	99
95	98	98	98	98	98	98	98	98	98	98	98	98	98	98	98	98	98	98	98	99	99	99	99	99	99
96	98	98	98	98	98	98	98	98	98	98	98	98	99	99	99	99	99	99	99	99	99	99	99	99	99
97	99	99	99	99	99	99	99	99	99	99	99	99	99	99	99	99	99	99	99	99	99	99	99	99	99
98	99	99	99	99	99	99	99	99	99	99	99	99	99	99	99	99	99	99	99	99	99	99	99	99	100
99	100	100	100	100	100	100	100	100	100	100	100	100	100	100	100	100	100	100	100	100	100	100	100	100	100
	51	**52**	**53**	**54**	**55**	**56**	**57**	**58**	**59**	**60**	**61**	**62**	**63**	**64**	**65**	**66**	**67**	**68**	**69**	**70**	**71**	**72**	**73**	**74**	**75**

The values are derived from the formula A + B (1−A) = *combined* value of A and B, where A and B are the decimal equivalents of the impairment ratings. In the chart all values are expressed as percentages. To *combine* any two impairment values, locate the larger of the values on the side of the chart and read along that row until you come to the column indicated by the smaller value at the bottom of the chart. At the intersection of the row and the column is the combined value.

For example, to combine 35% and 20% read down the side of the chart until you come to the larger value, 35%. Then read across the 35% row until you come to the column indicated by 20% at the bottom of the chart. At the intersection of the row and column is the number 48. Therefore, 35% combined with 20% is 48%.

If three or more impairment values are to be combined, select any two and find their combined value as

76	77	78	79	80	81	82	83	84	85	86	87	88	89	90	91	92	93	94	95	96	97	98	99
94																							
94	95																						
95	95	95																					
95	95	95	96																				
95	95	96	96	96																			
95	96	96	96	96	96																		
96	96	96	96	96	97	97																	
96	96	96	96	97	97	97	97																
96	96	96	97	97	97	97	97	97															
96	97	97	97	97	97	97	97	98	98														
97	97	97	97	97	97	97	98	98	98	98													
97	97	97	97	97	98	98	98	98	98	98	98												
97	97	97	97	98	98	98	98	98	98	98	98	99											
97	97	98	98	98	98	98	98	98	98	98	99	99	99										
98	98	98	98	98	98	98	98	98	99	99	99	99	99	99									
98	98	98	98	98	98	98	98	99	99	99	99	99	99	99	99								
98	98	98	98	98	98	99	99	99	99	99	99	99	99	99	99	99							
98	98	98	99	99	99	99	99	99	99	99	99	99	99	99	99	99	100						
99	99	99	99	99	99	99	99	99	99	99	99	99	99	99	99	100	100	100					
99	99	99	99	99	99	99	99	99	99	99	99	99	99	100	100	100	100	100	100	100			
99	99	99	99	99	99	99	99	99	99	99	99	100	100	100	100	100	100	100	100	100	100		
99	99	99	99	99	99	99	99	100	100	100	100	100	100	100	100	100	100	100	100	100	100	100	
100	100	100	100	100	100	100	100	100	100	100	100	100	100	100	100	100	100	100	100	100	100	100	100
100	100	100	100	100	100	100	100	100	100	100	100	100	100	100	100	100	100	100	100				

above. Then use that value and the third value to locate the combined value of all. This process can be repeated indefinitely, the final value in each instance being the combination of all the previous values. In each step of this process the larger impairment value must be identified at the side of the chart.

Note: If impairment from two or more organ systems are to be *combined* to express a whole-person impairment, each must first be expressed as a whole-person impairment percent.

Reprinted with permission (1).

TABLE AC–6 *Visual system impairment for both eyes*

% Impairment worse eye	0	1	2	3	4	5	6	7	8	9	10	11	12	13	14	15	16	17	18	19	20	21	22	23	24
0	0																								
1	0	1																							
2	1	1	2																						
3	1	2	2	3																					
4	1	2	3	3	4																				
5	1	2	3	4	4	5																			
6	2	2	3	4	5	5	6																		
7	2	3	3	4	5	6	6	7																	
8	2	3	4	4	5	6	7	7	8																
9	2	3	4	5	5	6	7	8	8	9															
10	3	3	4	5	6	6	7	8	9	9	10														
11	3	4	4	5	6	7	7	8	9	10	10	11													
12	3	4	5	5	6	7	8	8	9	10	11	11	12												
13	3	4	5	6	6	7	8	9	9	10	11	12	12	13											
14	4	4	5	6	7	7	8	9	10	10	11	12	13	13	14										
15	4	5	5	6	7	8	8	9	10	11	11	12	13	14	14	15									
16	4	5	6	6	7	8	9	9	10	11	12	12	13	14	15	15	16								
17	4	5	6	7	7	8	9	10	10	11	12	13	13	14	15	16	16	17							
18	5	5	6	7	8	8	9	10	11	11	12	13	14	14	15	16	17	17	18						
19	5	6	6	7	8	9	9	10	11	12	12	13	14	15	15	16	17	18	18	19					
20	5	6	7	7	8	9	10	10	11	12	13	13	14	15	16	16	17	18	19	19	20				
21	5	6	7	8	8	9	10	11	11	12	13	14	14	15	16	17	17	18	19	20	20	21			
22	6	6	7	8	9	9	10	11	12	12	13	14	15	15	16	17	18	18	19	20	21	21	22		
23	6	7	7	8	9	10	10	11	12	13	13	14	15	16	16	17	18	19	19	20	21	22	22	23	
24	6	7	8	8	9	10	11	11	12	13	14	14	15	16	17	17	18	19	20	20	21	22	23	23	24
25	6	7	8	9	9	10	11	12	12	13	14	15	15	16	17	18	18	19	20	21	21	22	23	24	24
26	7	7	8	9	10	10	11	12	13	13	14	15	16	16	17	18	19	19	20	21	22	22	23	24	25
27	7	8	8	9	10	11	11	12	13	14	14	15	16	17	17	18	19	20	20	21	22	23	23	24	25
28	7	8	9	9	10	11	12	12	13	14	15	15	16	17	18	18	19	20	21	21	22	23	24	24	25
29	7	8	9	10	10	11	12	13	13	14	15	16	16	17	18	19	19	20	21	22	22	23	24	25	25
30	8	8	9	10	11	11	12	13	14	14	15	16	17	17	18	19	20	20	21	22	23	23	24	25	26
31	8	9	9	10	11	12	12	13	14	15	15	16	17	18	18	19	20	21	21	22	23	24	24	25	26
32	8	9	10	10	11	12	13	13	14	15	16	16	17	18	19	19	20	21	22	22	23	24	25	25	26
33	8	9	10	11	11	12	13	14	14	15	16	17	17	18	19	20	20	21	22	23	23	24	25	26	26
34	9	9	10	11	12	12	13	14	15	15	16	17	18	18	19	20	21	21	22	23	24	24	25	26	27
35	9	10	10	11	12	13	13	14	15	16	16	17	18	19	19	20	21	22	22	23	24	25	25	26	27
36	9	10	11	11	12	13	14	14	15	16	17	17	18	19	20	20	21	22	23	23	24	25	26	26	27
37	9	10	11	12	12	13	14	15	15	16	17	18	18	19	20	21	21	22	23	24	24	25	26	27	27
38	10	10	11	12	13	13	14	15	16	16	17	18	19	19	20	21	22	22	23	24	25	25	26	27	28
39	10	11	11	12	13	14	14	15	16	17	17	18	19	20	20	21	22	23	23	24	25	26	26	27	28
40	10	11	12	12	13	14	15	15	16	17	18	18	19	20	21	21	22	23	24	24	25	26	27	27	28
41	10	11	12	13	13	14	15	16	16	17	18	19	19	20	21	22	22	23	24	25	25	26	27	28	28
42	11	11	12	13	14	14	15	16	17	17	18	19	20	20	21	22	23	23	24	25	26	26	27	28	29
43	11	12	12	13	14	15	15	16	17	18	18	19	20	21	21	22	23	24	24	25	26	27	27	28	29
44	11	12	13	13	14	15	16	16	17	18	19	19	20	21	22	22	23	24	25	25	26	27	28	28	29
45	11	12	13	14	14	15	16	17	17	18	19	20	20	21	22	23	23	24	25	26	26	27	28	29	29
46	12	12	13	14	15	15	16	17	18	18	19	20	21	21	22	23	24	24	25	26	27	27	28	29	30
47	12	13	13	14	15	16	16	17	18	19	19	20	21	22	22	23	24	25	25	26	27	28	28	29	30
48	12	13	14	14	15	16	17	17	18	19	20	20	21	22	23	23	24	25	26	26	27	28	29	29	30
49	12	13	14	15	15	16	17	18	18	19	20	21	21	22	23	24	24	25	26	27	27	28	29	30	30

% Impairment better eye

TABLE AC–6. *Continued*

25	26	27	28	29	30	31	32	33	34	35	36	37	38	39	40	41	42	43	44	45	46	47	48	49
25																								
25	26																							
26	26	27																						
26	27	27	28																					
26	27	28	28	29																				
26	27	28	29	29	30																			
27	27	28	29	30	30	31																		
27	28	28	29	30	31	31	32																	
27	28	29	29	30	31	32	32	33																
27	28	29	30	30	31	32	33	33	34															
28	28	29	30	31	31	32	33	34	34	35														
28	29	29	30	31	32	32	33	34	35	35	36													
28	29	30	30	31	32	33	33	34	35	36	36	37												
28	29	30	31	31	32	33	34	34	35	36	37	37	38											
29	29	30	31	32	32	33	34	35	35	36	37	38	38	39										
29	30	30	31	32	33	33	34	35	36	36	37	38	39	39	40									
29	30	31	31	32	33	34	34	35	36	37	37	38	39	40	40	41								
29	30	31	32	32	33	34	35	35	36	37	38	38	39	40	41	41	42							
30	30	31	32	33	33	34	35	36	36	37	38	39	39	40	41	42	42	43						
30	31	31	32	33	34	34	35	36	37	37	38	39	40	40	41	42	43	43	44					
30	31	32	32	33	34	35	35	36	37	38	38	39	40	41	41	42	43	44	44	45				
30	31	32	33	33	34	35	36	36	37	38	39	39	40	41	42	42	43	44	45	45	46			
31	31	32	33	34	34	35	36	37	37	38	39	40	40	41	42	43	43	44	45	46	46	47		
31	32	32	33	34	35	35	36	37	38	38	39	40	41	41	42	43	44	44	45	46	47	47	48	
31	32	33	33	34	35	36	36	37	38	39	39	40	41	42	42	43	44	45	45	46	47	48	48	49
25	26	27	28	29	30	31	32	33	34	35	36	37	38	39	40	41	42	43	44	45	46	47	48	49

TABLE AC–6 *Continued*

% Impairment worse eye

	0	1	2	3	4	5	6	7	8	9	10	11	12	13	14	15	16	17	18	19	20	21	22	23	24
50	13	13	14	15	16	16	17	18	19	19	20	21	22	22	23	24	25	25	26	27	28	28	29	30	31
51	13	14	14	15	16	17	17	18	19	20	20	21	22	23	23	24	25	26	26	27	28	29	29	30	31
52	13	14	15	15	16	17	18	18	19	20	21	21	22	23	24	24	25	26	27	27	28	29	30	30	31
53	13	14	15	16	16	17	18	19	19	20	21	22	22	23	24	25	25	26	27	28	28	29	30	31	31
54	14	14	15	16	17	17	18	19	20	20	21	22	23	23	24	25	26	26	27	28	29	29	30	31	32
55	14	15	15	16	17	18	18	19	20	21	21	22	23	24	24	25	26	27	27	28	29	30	30	31	32
56	14	15	16	16	17	18	19	19	20	21	22	22	23	24	25	25	26	27	28	28	29	30	31	31	32
57	14	15	16	17	17	18	19	20	20	21	22	23	23	24	25	26	26	27	28	29	29	30	31	32	32
58	15	15	16	17	18	18	19	20	21	21	22	23	24	24	25	26	27	27	28	29	30	30	31	32	33
59	15	16	16	17	18	19	19	20	21	22	22	23	24	25	25	26	27	28	28	29	30	31	31	32	33
60	15	16	17	17	18	19	20	20	21	22	23	23	24	25	26	26	27	28	29	29	30	31	32	32	33
61	15	16	17	18	18	19	20	21	21	22	23	24	24	25	26	27	27	28	29	30	30	31	32	33	33
62	16	16	17	18	19	19	20	21	22	22	23	24	25	25	26	27	28	28	29	30	31	31	32	33	34
63	16	17	17	18	19	20	20	21	22	23	23	24	25	26	26	27	28	29	29	30	31	32	32	33	34
64	16	17	18	18	19	20	21	21	22	23	24	24	25	26	27	27	28	29	30	30	31	32	33	33	34
65	16	17	18	19	19	20	21	22	22	23	24	25	25	26	27	28	28	29	30	31	31	32	33	34	34
66	17	17	18	19	20	20	21	22	23	23	24	25	26	26	27	28	29	29	30	31	32	32	33	34	35
67	17	18	18	19	20	21	21	22	23	24	24	25	26	27	27	28	29	30	30	31	32	33	33	34	35
68	17	18	19	19	20	21	22	22	23	24	25	25	26	27	28	28	29	30	31	31	32	33	34	34	35
69	17	18	19	20	20	21	22	23	23	24	25	26	26	27	28	29	29	30	31	32	32	33	34	35	35
70	18	18	19	20	21	21	22	23	24	24	25	26	27	27	28	29	30	30	31	32	33	33	34	35	36
71	18	19	19	20	21	22	22	23	24	25	25	26	27	28	28	29	30	31	31	32	33	34	34	35	36
72	18	19	20	20	21	22	23	23	24	25	26	26	27	28	29	29	30	31	32	32	33	34	35	35	36
73	18	19	20	21	21	22	23	24	24	25	26	27	27	28	29	30	30	31	32	33	33	34	35	36	36
74	19	19	20	21	22	22	23	24	25	25	26	27	28	28	29	30	31	31	32	33	34	34	35	36	37
75	19	20	20	21	22	23	23	24	25	26	26	27	28	29	29	30	31	32	32	33	34	35	35	36	37
76	19	20	21	21	22	23	24	24	25	26	27	27	28	29	30	30	31	32	33	33	34	35	36	36	37
77	19	20	21	22	22	23	24	25	25	26	27	28	28	29	30	31	31	32	33	34	34	35	36	37	37
78	20	20	21	22	23	23	24	25	26	26	27	28	29	29	30	31	32	32	33	34	35	35	36	37	38
79	20	21	21	22	23	24	24	25	26	27	27	28	29	30	30	31	32	33	33	34	35	36	36	37	38
80	20	21	22	22	23	24	25	25	26	27	28	28	29	30	31	31	32	33	34	34	35	36	37	37	38
81	20	21	22	23	23	24	25	26	26	27	28	29	29	30	31	32	32	33	34	35	35	36	37	38	38
82	21	21	22	23	24	24	25	26	27	27	28	29	30	30	31	32	33	33	34	35	36	36	37	38	39
83	21	22	22	23	24	25	25	26	27	28	28	29	30	31	31	32	33	34	34	35	36	37	37	38	39
84	21	22	23	23	24	25	26	26	27	28	29	29	30	31	32	32	33	34	35	35	36	37	38	38	39
85	21	22	23	24	24	25	26	27	27	28	29	30	30	31	32	33	33	34	35	36	36	37	38	39	39
86	22	22	23	24	25	25	26	27	28	28	29	30	31	31	32	33	34	34	35	36	37	37	38	39	40
87	22	23	23	24	25	26	26	27	28	29	29	30	31	32	32	33	34	35	35	36	37	38	38	39	40
88	22	23	24	24	25	26	27	27	28	29	30	30	31	32	33	33	34	35	36	36	37	38	39	39	40
89	22	23	24	25	25	26	27	28	28	29	30	31	31	32	33	34	34	35	·36	37	37	38	39	40	40
90	23	23	24	25	26	26	27	28	29	29	30	31	32	32	33	34	35	35	36	37	38	38	39	40	41
91	23	24	24	25	26	27	27	28	29	30	30	31	32	33	33	34	35	36	36	37	38	39	39	40	41
92	23	24	25	25	26	27	28	28	29	30	31	31	32	33	34	34	35	36	37	37	38	39	40	40	41
93	23	24	25	26	26	27	28	29	29	30	31	32	32	33	34	35	35	36	37	38	38	39	40	41	41
94	24	24	25	26	27	27	28	29	30	30	31	32	33	33	34	35	36	36	37	38	39	39	40	41	42
95	24	25	25	26	27	28	28	29	30	31	31	32	33	34	34	35	36	37	37	38	39	40	40	41	42
96	24	25	26	26	27	28	29	29	30	31	32	32	33	34	35	35	36	37	38	38	39	40	41	41	42
97	24	25	26	27	27	28	29	30	30	31	32	33	33	34	35	36	36	37	38	39	39	40	41	42	42
98	25	25	26	27	28	28	29	30	31	31	32	33	34	34	35	36	37	37	38	39	40	40	41	42	43
99	25	26	26	27	28	29	29	30	31	32	32	33	34	35	35	36	37	38	38	39	40	41	41	42	43
100	25	26	27	27	28	29	30	30	31	32	33	33	34	35	36	36	37	38	39	39	40	41	42	42	43
	0	1	2	3	4	5	6	7	8	9	10	11	12	13	14	15	16	17	18	19	20	21	22	23	24

% Impairment better eye

TABLE AC–6 *Continued*

25	26	27	28	29	30	31	32	33	34	35	36	37	38	39	40	41	42	43	44	45	46	47	48	49	
31	32	33	34	34	35	36	37	37	38	39	40	40	41	42	43	43	44	45	46	46	47	48	49	49	50
32	32	33	34	35	35	36	37	38	38	39	40	41	41	42	43	44	44	45	46	47	47	48	49	50	51
32	33	33	34	35	36	36	37	38	39	39	40	41	42	42	43	44	45	45	46	47	48	48	49	50	52
32	33	34	34	35	36	37	37	38	39	40	40	41	42	43	43	44	45	46	46	47	48	49	49	50	53
32	33	34	35	35	36	37	38	38	39	40	41	41	42	43	44	44	45	46	47	47	48	49	50	50	54
33	33	34	35	36	36	37	38	39	39	40	41	42	42	43	44	45	45	46	47	48	48	49	50	51	55
33	34	34	35	36	37	37	38	39	40	40	41	42	43	43	44	45	46	46	47	48	49	49	50	51	56
33	34	35	35	36	37	38	38	39	40	41	41	42	43	44	44	45	46	47	47	48	49	50	50	51	57
33	34	35	36	36	37	38	39	39	40	41	42	42	43	44	45	45	46	47	48	48	49	50	51	51	58
34	34	35	36	37	37	38	39	40	40	41	42	43	43	44	45	46	46	47	48	49	49	50	51	52	59
34	35	35	36	37	38	38	39	40	41	41	42	43	44	44	45	46	47	47	48	49	50	50	51	52	60
34	35	36	36	37	38	39	39	40	41	42	42	43	44	45	45	46	47	48	48	49	50	51	51	52	61
34	35	36	37	37	38	39	40	40	41	42	43	43	44	45	46	46	47	48	49	49	50	51	52	52	62
35	35	36	37	38	38	39	40	41	41	42	43	44	44	45	46	47	47	48	49	50	50	51	52	53	63
35	36	36	37	38	39	39	40	41	42	42	43	44	45	45	46	47	48	48	49	50	51	51	52	53	64
35	36	37	37	38	39	40	40	41	42	43	43	44	45	46	46	47	48	49	49	50	51	52	52	53	65
35	36	37	38	38	39	40	41	41	42	43	44	44	45	46	47	47	48	49	50	50	51	52	53	53	66
36	36	37	38	39	39	40	41	42	42	43	44	45	45	46	47	48	48	49	50	51	51	52	53	54	67
36	37	37	38	39	40	40	41	42	43	43	44	45	46	46	47	48	49	49	50	51	52	52	53	54	68
36	37	38	38	39	40	41	41	42	43	44	44	45	46	47	47	48	49	50	50	51	52	53	53	54	69
36	37	38	39	39	40	41	42	42	43	44	45	45	46	47	48	48	49	50	51	51	52	53	54	54	70
37	37	38	39	40	40	41	42	43	43	44	45	46	46	47	48	49	49	50	51	52	52	53	54	55	71
37	38	38	39	40	41	41	42	43	44	44	45	46	47	47	48	49	50	50	51	52	53	53	54	55	72
37	38	39	39	40	41	42	42	43	44	45	45	46	47	48	48	49	50	51	51	52	53	54	54	55	73
37	38	39	40	40	41	42	43	43	44	45	46	46	47	48	49	49	50	51	52	52	53	54	55	55	74
38	38	39	40	41	41	42	43	44	44	45	46	47	47	48	49	50	50	51	52	53	53	54	55	56	75
38	39	39	40	41	42	42	43	44	45	45	46	47	48	48	49	50	51	51	52	53	54	54	55	56	76
38	39	40	40	41	42	43	43	44	45	46	46	47	48	49	49	50	51	52	52	53	54	55	55	56	77
38	39	40	41	41	42	43	44	44	45	46	47	47	48	49	50	50	51	52	53	53	54	55	56	56	78
39	39	40	41	42	42	43	44	45	45	46	47	48	48	49	50	51	51	52	53	54	54	55	56	57	79
39	40	40	41	42	43	43	44	45	46	46	47	48	49	49	50	51	52	52	53	54	55	55	56	57	80
39	40	41	41	42	43	44	44	45	46	47	47	48	49	50	50	51	52	53	53	54	55	56	56	57	81
39	40	41	42	42	43	44	45	45	46	47	48	48	49	50	51	51	52	53	54	54	55	56	57	57	82
40	40	41	42	43	43	44	45	46	46	47	48	49	49	50	51	52	52	53	54	55	55	56	57	58	83
40	41	41	42	43	44	44	45	46	47	47	48	49	50	50	51	52	53	53	54	55	56	56	57	58	84
40	41	42	42	43	44	45	45	46	47	48	48	49	50	51	51	52	53	54	54	55	56	57	57	58	85
40	41	42	43	43	44	45	46	46	47	48	49	49	50	51	52	52	53	54	55	55	56	57	58	58	86
41	41	42	43	44	44	45	46	47	47	48	49	50	50	51	52	53	53	54	55	56	56	57	58	59	87
41	42	42	43	44	45	45	46	47	48	48	49	50	51	51	52	53	54	54	55	56	57	57	58	59	88
41	42	43	43	44	45	46	46	47	48	49	49	50	51	52	52	53	54	55	55	56	57	58	58	59	89
41	42	43	44	44	45	46	47	47	48	49	50	50	51	52	53	53	54	55	56	56	57	58	59	59	90
42	42	43	44	45	45	46	47	48	48	49	50	51	51	52	53	54	54	55	56	57	57	58	59	60	91
42	43	43	44	45	46	46	47	48	49	49	50	51	52	52	53	54	55	55	56	57	58	58	59	60	92
42	43	44	44	45	46	47	47	48	49	50	50	51	52	53	53	54	55	56	56	57	58	59	59	60	93
42	43	44	45	45	46	47	48	48	49	50	51	51	52	53	54	54	55	56	57	57	58	59	60	60	94
43	43	44	45	46	46	47	48	49	49	50	51	52	52	53	54	55	55	56	57	58	58	59	60	61	95
43	44	44	45	46	47	47	48	49	50	50	51	52	53	53	54	55	56	56	57	58	59	59	60	61	96
43	44	45	45	46	47	48	48	49	50	51	51	52	53	54	54	55	56	57	57	58	59	60	60	61	97
43	44	45	46	46	47	48	49	49	50	51	52	52	53	54	55	55	56	57	58	58	59	60	61	61	98
44	44	45	46	47	47	48	49	50	50	51	52	53	53	54	55	56	56	57	58	59	59	60	61	62	99
44	45	45	46	47	48	48	49	50	51	51	52	53	54	54	55	56	57	57	58	59	60	60	61	62	100
25	26	27	28	29	30	31	32	33	34	35	36	37	38	39	40	41	42	43	44	45	46	47	48	49	

Worse	50	51	52	53	54	55	56	57	58	59	60	61	62	63	64	65	66	67	68	69	70	71	72	73	74
50	50																								
51	50	51																							
52	51	51	52																						
53	51	52	52	53																					
54	51	52	53	53	54																				
55	51	52	53	54	54	55																			
56	52	52	53	54	55	55	56																		
57	52	53	53	54	55	56	56	57																	
58	52	53	54	54	55	56	57	57	58																
59	52	53	54	55	55	56	57	58	58	59															
60	53	53	54	55	56	56	57	58	59	59	60														
61	53	54	54	55	56	57	57	58	59	60	60	61													
62	53	54	55	55	56	57	58	58	59	60	61	61	62												
63	53	54	55	56	56	57	58	59	59	60	61	62	62	63											
64	54	54	55	56	57	57	58	59	60	60	61	62	63	63	64										
65	54	55	55	56	57	58	58	59	60	61	61	62	63	64	64	65									
66	54	55	56	56	57	58	59	59	60	61	62	62	63	64	65	65	66								
67	54	55	56	57	57	58	59	60	60	61	62	63	63	64	65	66	66	67							
68	55	55	56	57	58	58	59	60	61	61	62	63	64	64	65	66	67	67	68						
69	55	56	56	57	58	59	59	60	61	62	62	63	64	65	65	66	67	68	68	69					
70	55	56	57	57	58	59	60	60	61	62	63	63	64	65	66	66	67	68	69	69	70				
71	55	56	57	58	58	59	60	61	61	62	63	64	64	65	66	67	67	68	69	70	70	71			
72	56	56	57	58	59	59	60	61	62	62	63	64	65	65	66	67	68	68	69	70	71	71	72		
73	56	57	57	58	59	60	60	61	62	63	63	64	65	66	66	67	68	69	69	70	71	72	72	73	
74	56	57	58	58	59	60	61	61	62	63	64	64	65	66	67	67	68	69	70	70	71	72	73	73	74
75	56	57	58	59	59	60	61	62	62	63	64	65	65	66	67	68	68	69	70	71	71	72	73	74	74
76	57	57	58	59	60	60	61	62	63	63	64	65	66	66	67	68	69	69	70	71	72	72	73	74	75
77	57	58	58	59	60	61	61	62	63	64	64	65	66	67	67	68	69	70	70	71	72	73	73	74	75
78	57	58	59	59	60	61	62	62	63	64	65	65	66	67	68	68	69	70	71	71	72	73	74	74	75
79	57	58	59	60	60	61	62	63	63	64	65	66	66	67	68	69	69	70	71	72	72	73	74	75	75
80	58	58	59	60	61	61	62	63	64	64	65	66	67	67	68	69	70	70	71	72	73	73	74	75	76
81	58	59	59	60	61	62	62	63	64	65	65	66	67	68	68	69	70	71	71	72	73	74	74	75	76
82	58	59	60	60	61	62	63	63	64	65	66	66	67	68	69	69	70	71	72	72	73	74	75	75	76
83	58	59	60	61	61	62	63	64	64	65	66	67	67	68	69	70	70	71	72	73	73	74	75	75	76
84	59	59	60	61	62	62	63	64	65	65	66	67	68	68	69	70	71	71	72	73	74	74	75	76	77
85	59	60	60	61	62	63	63	64	65	66	66	67	68	69	69	70	71	72	72	73	74	75	75	76	77
86	59	60	61	61	62	63	64	64	65	66	67	67	68	69	70	70	71	72	73	73	74	75	76	76	77
87	59	60	61	62	62	63	64	65	65	66	67	68	68	69	70	71	71	72	73	74	74	75	76	77	77
88	60	60	61	62	63	63	64	65	66	66	67	68	69	69	70	71	72	72	73	74	75	75	76	77	78
89	60	61	61	62	63	64	64	65	66	67	67	68	69	70	70	71	72	73	73	74	75	76	76	77	78
90	60	61	62	62	63	64	65	65	66	67	68	68	69	70	71	71	72	73	74	74	75	76	77	77	78
91	60	61	62	63	63	64	65	66	66	67	68	69	69	70	71	72	72	73	74	75	75	76	77	78	78
92	61	61	62	63	64	64	65	66	67	67	68	69	70	70	71	72	73	73	74	75	76	76	77	78	79
93	61	62	62	63	64	65	65	66	67	68	68	69	70	71	71	72	73	74	74	75	76	77	77	78	79
94	61	62	63	63	64	65	66	66	67	68	69	69	70	71	72	72	73	74	75	75	76	77	78	78	79
95	61	62	63	64	64	65	66	67	67	68	69	70	70	71	72	73	73	74	75	76	76	77	78	79	79
96	62	62	63	64	65	65	66	67	68	68	69	70	71	71	72	73	74	74	75	76	77	77	78	79	80
97	62	63	63	64	65	66	66	67	68	69	69	70	71	72	72	73	74	75	75	76	77	78	78	79	80
98	62	63	64	64	65	66	67	67	68	69	70	70	71	72	73	73	74	75	76	76	77	78	79	79	80
99	62	63	64	65	65	66	67	68	68	69	70	71	71	72	73	74	74	75	76	77	77	78	79	80	80
100	63	63	64	65	66	66	67	68	69	69	70	71	72	72	73	74	75	75	76	77	78	78	79	80	81

% Impairment better eye

The values in this table are based on the following formula:

$$\frac{3 \times \text{impairment value of better eye} + \text{impairment value of worse eye}}{4} = \text{impairment of visual system}$$

The guides to the table are percentage impairment values for each eye. The percentage for the worse eye is read at the side of the table. The percentage for the better eye is read at the bottom of the table. At the intersection of the column for the worse eye and the column for the better eye is the impairment of visual system value.

75	76	77	78	79	80	81	82	83	84	85	86	87	88	89	90	91	92	93	94	95	96	97	98	99	100
75																									
75	76																								
76	76	77																							
76	77	77	78																						
76	77	78	78	79																					
76	77	78	79	79	80																				
77	77	78	79	80	80	81																			
77	78	78	79	80	81	81	82																		
77	78	79	79	80	81	82	82	83																	
77	78	79	80	80	81	82	83	83	84																
78	78	79	80	81	81	82	83	84	84	85															
78	79	79	80	81	82	82	83	84	85	85	86														
78	79	80	80	81	82	83	83	84	85	86	86	87													
78	79	80	81	81	82	83	84	84	85	86	87	87	88												
79	79	80	81	82	82	83	84	85	85	86	87	88	88	89											
79	80	80	81	82	83	83	84	85	86	86	87	88	89	89	90										
79	80	81	81	82	83	84	84	85	86	87	87	88	89	90	90	91									
79	80	81	82	82	83	84	85	85	86	87	88	88	89	90	91	91	92								
80	80	81	82	83	83	84	85	86	86	87	88	89	89	90	91	92	92	93							
80	81	81	82	83	84	84	85	86	87	87	88	89	90	90	91	92	93	93	94						
80	81	82	82	83	84	85	85	86	87	88	88	89	90	91	91	92	93	94	94	95					
80	81	82	83	83	84	85	86	86	87	88	89	89	90	91	92	92	93	94	95	95	96				
81	81	82	83	84	84	85	86	87	87	88	89	90	90	91	92	93	93	94	95	96	96	97			
81	82	82	83	84	85	85	86	87	88	88	89	90	91	91	92	93	94	94	95	96	97	97	98		
81	82	83	83	84	85	86	86	87	88	89	89	90	91	92	92	93	94	95	95	96	97	98	98	99	
81	82	83	84	84	85	86	87	87	88	89	90	90	91	92	93	93	94	95	96	96	97	98	99	99	100

For example, when there is 60% impairment of one eye and 30% impairment of the other eye, read down the side of the table until you come to the larger value (60%). The follow across the row until it is intersected by the column designated by 30% at the bottom of the page. At the intersection of these two columns is printed the number 38. This number (38) represents the percentage impairment of the visual system when there is 60% impairment of one eye and 30% impairment of the other eye.

If bilateral aphakia is present and corrected central vision has been used in evaluation, impairment of the visual system is weighted by an additional 25% decrease in the value of the remaining corrected vision. For example, a 38% impairment (62% remaining) would be increased to 38% + (25%)(62%) = 54%.

Reprinted with permission (1).

TABLE AC–7. *Impairment of the visual system as it relates to impairment of the whole person*

% Impairment of the											
Visual system	Whole person	Visual system	Whole person	Visual system	Whole person	Visual system	Whole person	Visual system	Whole person	Visual system	Whole person
0	0	15	14	30	28	45	42	60	57	75	71
1	1	16	15	31	29	46	43	61	58	76	72
2	2	17	16	32	30	47	44	62	59	77	73
3	3	18	17	33	31	48	45	63	59	78	74
4	4	19	18	34	32	49	46	64	60	79	75
5	5	20	19	35	33	50	47	65	61	80	76
6	6	21	20	36	34	51	48	66	62	81	76
7	7	22	21	37	35	52	49	67	63	82	77
8	8	23	22	38	36	53	50	68	64	83	78
9	8	24	23	39	37	54	51	69	65	84	79
10	9	25	24	40	38	55	52	70	66	85	80
11	10	26	25	41	39	56	53	71	67	86	81
12	11	27	25	42	40	57	54	72	68	87	82
13	12	28	26	43	41	58	55	73	69	88	83
14	13	29	27	44	42	59	56	74	70	89	84
										90–100	85

	% Impairment of the	
	Visual system	Whole person
Total loss of vision of one eye	25	24
Total loss of vision of both eyes	100	85

Reprinted with permission (1).

REVIEW

1. Impairment of central visual acuity is determined for each eye.
2. Impairment of visual field is determined for each eye. Remember to adjust for inferior quadrant or inferior hemianopic loss.
3. For each eye, the acuity and field impairment values are then combined to yield a single impairment value using the special combined values table.
4. Impairment of ocular motility is determined (a binocular test).
5. This single value is combined with the impairment value of the worse eye to yield a final impairment value for that eye using the combined values table. At this stage, the examiner now has a percentage impairment for each eye that reflects central acuity, visual field, and motility.
6. Remember that an additional 10% impairment may be combined with the total impairment value in a given eye (using the combined values table) for any other abnormality not reflected adequately in the testing.
7. The impairment of the visual system as a whole is determined using Table AC–6. Remember to adjust for bilateral aphakia.
8. The impairment rating for the person as a whole due to impairment of the visual system as a whole is then read from Table AC–7.

REFERENCES

1. Riordan-Eva P. Blindness. In: Vaughan DG, Asbury T, Riordan-Eva P, eds. *General Ophthalmology.* 13th ed. Norwalk, CT: Appleton & Lange; 1992.
2. *Guides to the Evaluation of Permanent Impairment.* 4th ed. Chicago: American Medical Association; June 1993:209–222,322–324.

Subject Index

Page references followed by t or f indicate tables or figures, respectively.

A

Abducens nerve palsy, 375–376
Abrasion, corneal, 179–180
Abscess
  subperiosteal
    diagnostic imaging, 71
    management, 134
    radiologic findings, 71
    secondary to ethmoiditis, orbital
      cellulitis with, 131, 132f
  surgical drainage of, 128f, 129
Abuse, child, 50–52
  Münchausen's syndrome by proxy, 424
Acanthamoeba, 202–205
  diagnosis, 203
  management, 203–205
  risk factors, 203
Accidents, motor vehicle, 24
  ocular trauma secondary to, 24, 25t
Accommodation insufficiency, 381–382
  diagnosis, 381–382
  management, 382
ACIOL. *See* Anterior chamber intraocular
    lens implantation
Acute posterior multifocal placoid
    pigment epitheliopathy, 146
Adenovirus conjunctivitis, 191–192
  diagnosis, 191–192
  management, 192
Adenovirus syndromes, 191–192
Adult chlamydial keratoconjunctivitis,
    193
Afferent visual system disorders,
    351–367
  basic considerations, 351–352
Age
  common etiologic organisms related to,
    188, 188t
  and ocular trauma, 11–13
AION. *See* Anterior ischemic optic
    neuropathy

Airguns/BB guns, 20–21
Alkali burn, severe
  with corneal perforation, 168, 169f
  keratoprosthesis after, 170, 170f
  stromal ulceration with, 168, 168f
Allen cards, 30, 45, 45f
Allergic conjunctivitis, 177–178
  diagnosis, 177
  management, 177–178
Amaurosis fugax, 334–335
  diagnosis, 334
  management, 334
Amblyopia, 52–53
  deprivation, 53
  management, 53
  refractive, 53
  strabismic, 53
American Academy of Ophthalmology,
    208
American National Standards Institute
    Z87 specifications, 26
American Optical polarizing test,
    422
American Society for Testing and
    Materials F803 specifications,
    26
American Society of Anesthesiologists
    (ASA) Physical Status
    Classification, 93, 93t
Ammonia burn, penetrating keratoplasty
    after, 169f, 169–170
Amphotericin B
  intravitreal preparation, 430
  topical preparation, 429
Ancillary testing
  of corneoscleral lacerations and
    ruptures, 210
  of posterior segment, 37
Anesthesia, 91–96
Anesthesia plan, 94–96
Aneurysm, 390–391

Aneurysm (*contd.*)
  diagnosis, 390
  diagnostic imaging of, 62
  management, 390–391
  radiologic findings, 62
Angiography
  cerebral, 60
  magnetic resonance, 59
  of traumatic carotid-cavernous fistula,
    74
Angle closure, lens-induced, 259
Angle recession, 229–230
  diagnosis, 229, 230f
  management, 229
Angle width, classification system for
    grading, 236, 236f
Angle-closure glaucoma
  acute
    diagnosis, 239t, 239–240
    management, 240
    signs and symptoms of, 239t
  general characteristics of, 186, 186t
  management, 240
  Nd-YAG laser peripheral iridectomy
    for, 240
  neovascular, secondary to retinal
    diseases, 250, 251t
  primary, 237–241
Anisocoria, 32, 382–383
  diagnosis, 382–383
  emergent clinical scenario, 8
  management, 383
Anterior chamber
  examination of, 35
  flat, 401f, 401–403
    Grade 1, 401, 401f
    Grade 2, 401, 401f
    Grade 3, 401, 401f
  paracentesis procedure, 337, 337f
  washout for hyphema, 233–234
Anterior chamber angle foreign bodies,
    312–313
  management, 312–313, 313f
  removal through corneoscleral shelved
    incision, 312, 313f
Anterior chamber intraocular lens
  implantation, 262–263

Anterior chamber tap, 279
Anterior hordeolum, 125
Anterior ischemic optic neuropathy, 355
  arteritic, 357, 357f
  diagnosis, 355, 356
  emergent surgery for, 85
Anterior orbital inflammation, 157–158
Anterior scleritis
  diffuse, 153
  necrotizing, with inflammation, 153
  nodular, 153
Anterior segment
  examination of, 34–35
    pediatric, 48
  foreign bodies, 311–314
    basic considerations, 309
    removal through corneoscleral
      shelved incision, 312, 313f
  injuries of, 227–234
    basic considerations, 227–228
    mechanical damage, 227
    vascular damage, 227
  reconstruction of, 257–273
Anterior uveitis, 137–141
  description, 137–138
  diagnosis, 139–141
  etiology, 138–139
  herpes simplex virus, 138
  idiopathic, 138
  management, 141
  traumatic, 138
  varicella-zoster virus, 138
Antibiotics
  intravitreal, 430–431
  preparation of, 429–431
  subjunctival, 429–430
  topical, 429
Aphakic/pseudophakic pupillary block,
    253–254
  definition, 253
  diagnosis, 253
  management, 254
APMPPE. *See* Acute posterior multifocal
    placoid pigment epitheliopathy
Aponeurosis trauma management,
    103–106
Arteriography. *See also* Angiography

of aneurysm, 62
Arteritis, giant cell (temporal), 356–358
 emergent surgery for, 83
Arthritis, juvenile rheumatoid arthritis,
 138–139
ASA. *See* American Society of
 Anesthesiologists
Aspiration, lenticular, bimanual technique
 for, 261–262, 262f
Assault, 21–22
Astigmatism, postoperative, corneal
 suture placement to reduce, 214f,
 215–216, 217f
Atrophy, "bow tie" or "band," 365
Atropine drops, 427t
Avulsion of vitreous base, 290

B

Bacillus endophthalmitis, 277, 277t
Bacterial conjunctivitis, 190
 diagnosis, 190
 management, 190
Bacterial endophthalmitis
 acute and delayed postoperative and
  endogenous, 281
 panuveitis involvement, 149
Bacterial keratitis, 195–198, 196f
 agents that cause, 195, 196t
 clinical features, 195
 determinants, 195
 diagnosis, 195–197
 gram-negative, 195–197
 gram-positive, 195
 management, 197f, 197–198
 pathogenesis, 195
 ulcerative, 195, 197f
Baltimore Eye Survey, 10
"Band" atrophy, 365
Bandage contact lens, 211
Bard-Parker blades, 107
Battered child syndrome, 50–51
 diagnosis, 50–51
BB gun injuries, 20–21, 25f
Behcet's disease, 144–145
Bell's phenomenon, 43
Berlin's edema, 290, 323–324, 324f

Bilateral granulomatous panuveitis, 407
Bilateral internuclear ophthalmoplegia,
 380
 wall-eyed, 380
Bimanual technique for lenticular
 aspiration, limbal approach,
 261–262, 262f
Biomicroscopy, slit-lamp, 352
Biopsy, corneal punch, 201, 202f
Birdshot chorioretinopathy, 146
Birth trauma, 48–52
Blepharitis, 124–125
 diagnosis, 124–125
 etiology/microbiology, 124
 signs, 125
 symptoms, 124
 treatment, 125
Blindness
 cortical, retrogeniculate trauma and,
  365–366
 definition of, 433
 fleeting, 334–335
Blowout fractures. *See* Orbital floor
 (blowout) fractures
Blunt injuries
 conjunctival, 175
 corneal, 178–179
 direct, 320
 emergent clinical scenario, 3
 traumatic retinopathy after, 324,
  324f
"Blurred" optic nerve head, 8
Body dysmorphic disorder, 417
Bonn iris hooks, 269, 270f, 271f, 272
"Bow tie" atrophy, 365
Branch retinal artery occlusion, 335
Branch retinal vein occlusion, 339
 diagnosis, 339, 339f
 management, 339
BRAO. *See* Branch retinal artery
 occlusion
Brightness
 relative, 352
 testing, 33
Burns
 chemical, 163–170
 ocular, 163–171

Burns (*contd.*)
    retinal, 320, 328–330
    thermal, 170–171

C

Caldwell projection, 61
Canal fracture
    diagnostic imaging, 74
    radiologic findings, 74
Canaliculitis, 119–121
    diagnosis, 120
    etiology, 120
    management, 121
    signs, 120, 120f
"Candle wax dripping," 146
Cantholysis
    for full-thickness eyelid defects, 102,
        102f
    for traumatic orbital hemorrhage, 109,
        109f
Canthotomy
    for full-thickness eyelid defects, 102,
        102f
    lateral, for traumatic orbital
        hemorrhage, 109, 109f
Capsular integrity, 259
Capsular rupture, traumatic cataracts
    with, 261–263
Capsular support, IOL placement in eyes
    without, 266–267
Carotid-cavernous fistula, 387–389
    diagnosis, 388
    management, 388–389
    traumatic
        diagnostic imaging, 74
        radiologic findings, 74
Cataractous lens, traumatically subluxed
    or dislocated, 263–269
Cataracts, 40t
    extraction of, dropped cortical and
        nuclear lens material during, 400
    ruptured wounds, 219–220
    traumatic, with minimal or no zonular
        dehiscence and/or capsular
        rupture, 261–263
Cavernous sinus thrombosis, 389
    diagnosis, 389
    management, 389

CC fistula. *See* Carotid-cavernous fistula
Cefazolin
    subconjunctival preparation, 429–430
    topical preparation, 429
Ceftazidime
    intravitreal preparation, 430
    pediatric dosing, 427t
    subconjunctival preparation, 430
Cellulitis
    orbital, 130–134
        diagnostic imaging, 68–69
        radiologic findings, 68–69
        secondary to sinusitis, 85–86
    preseptal, 126–130
Central retinal artery occlusion, 323,
        335
    diagnosis, 323, 335–336, 336f
    management, 323
Central retinal vein occlusion, 338–339
    diagnosis, 338
    management, 338–339
Central serous chorioretinopathy,
        341–342
    diagnosis, 341–342, 342f
    management, 342
Central vision impairment
    corresponding visual acuity notations,
        434, 434t
    determination of, 434t, 434–435
    in single eye, Snellen ratings for, 435,
        436t–437t
Cerebral angiography, 60
Chalazion, 126
    excision, 126, 127f
Chemical burns, 163–170
    basic considerations, 163
    common causes of, 163, 164t
    diagnosis, 163–165
    initial management, 165–167,
        166f
    options, 167–168
    intermediate treatment, 168, 169f
    rehabilitation, 169–170
    Thoft's classification of, 164, 165t,
        166f
Chemosis, subconjunctival hemorrhagic,
        175, 175f
Chiasm, optic, trauma to, 363–364
Child abuse, 50–52

Münchausen's syndrome by proxy, 424
  ophthalmic manifestations of, 51, 51t
  suspected, 52
  systemic signs of, 49, 49t
Children. *See under* Pediatric
Chlamydia conjunctivitis, 193–194
  diagnosis, 193–194
  management, 194
Chlamydia keratoconjunctivitis, adult,
    193
Chloral hydrate hypnotic, 43, 44t
Chorioretinitis sclopeteria, 290–291
  diagnosis, 290–291
  medical management, 291
  surgical management, 291
Chorioretinopathy
  birdshot, 146
  central serous, 341–342, 342f
Choroid
  examination of, 36
  injuries and emergencies, 290–295
  visual disorders affecting, 334–347
Choroidal detachment, 291–295
  diagnosis, 292
  diagnostic imaging of, 62–63
  hemorrhagic, 293, 293t
  "kissing," 293
  management, 292–295
  medical management, 292–293
    indications for, 292, 292t
  radiologic findings, 62–63, 63f, 64f
  serous, 293, 293t
  surgical management, 293–295, 294f
    indications for, 293, 293t
Choroidal hemorrhage, expulsive, 397
Choroidal neovascularization, 339–341
  diagnosis, 340, 341f
  management, 340–341, 341f
  photocoagulation procedure, 326–327,
    340–341
  secondary to choroidal rupture, 325,
    325f
Choroidal rupture, 325–327
  choroidal neovascularization secondary
    to, 325, 325f
  diagnosis, 325, 325f
  management, 325f, 325–326, 326f
  submacular hemorrhage secondary to,
    326, 326f

Choroiditis, multifocal, 146
Choroidopathy
  punctate inner, 147
  serpiginous, 145–146
Clarity, 258–259
Clindamycin
  intravitreal preparation, 430
  pediatric dosing, 427t
Closed globe injury, 208
Clot, expression of, 233
Cloudy cornea, in infancy, 46, 46t
CMV. *See* Cytomegalovirus
CNDO. *See* Congenital nasolacrimal duct
    obstruction
CNV. *See* Choroidal neovascularization
Codeine elixir, 427t
Color vision testing, 33, 419
  in neuro-ophthalmic evaluation,
    352
Coma, ocular movements in, 381
Commotio retinae (Berlin's edema),
    323–324, 324f
  diagnosis, 324, 324f
  management, 324
Compazine, 427t
Compressive optic neuropathy, 363
  diagnosis, 363
  management, 363
  orbital bone fractures with, 85
Computed tomography, 55, 56–57
  of aneurysm, 62
  of choroidal detachments, 62–63, 64f
  of endophthalmitis, 63, 65f
  of foreign bodies, 65, 66f
  of inflammatory disorders, 66–67
  of optic neuritis, 69
  of orbital cellulitis, 68–69
  of orbital fractures, 68, 68f
  of orbital hemorrhage or hematoma,
    69
  of retinal detachment, 69
  of ruptured or lacerated globes, 70, 72f
  of subperiosteal abscess, 71
  of subperiosteal hematoma, 71–73
  of thyroid orbitopathy, 74
  of traumatic carotid-cavernous fistula,
    74
  of traumatic optic neuropathy and
    canal fracture, 74

Computed tomography (contd.)
of vitreous hemorrhage, 75
Concept Guibor stents, 103
Congenital glaucoma, 252–253
diagnosis, 252
management, 253
Shaffer-Weiss classification of, 252,
252t
Congenital nasolacrimal duct obstruction,
123
Conjunctiva
examination of, 35
noninfectious disorders of, 173–183
basic considerations, 174
ocular examination, 174–175
patient evaluation, 174
Conjunctival bleb, infected with
endophthalmitis, 277, 278f
Conjunctival blunt injury, 175
Conjunctival foreign body, 176
diagnosis, 176
management, 176
Conjunctival lacerations, 176–177
diagnosis, 176
management, 176–177, 177f
Conjunctival peritomy, 411, 412f
Conjunctivitis
acute follicular, 191
adenovirus, 191–192
allergic, 177–178
bacterial, 190
basic considerations, 185
chlamydia, 193–194
differential diagnosis based on clinical
signs, 186–187
general characteristics of, 186, 186t
gonorrheal, 187–190
hemorrhagic, 192
herpes simplex, 192
hyperacute, 187, 189f
infectious, 185–206
microbial, 187
signs and symptoms of, 186–187
toxic, 178
viral, 190–194
Conscious sedation
drugs for, 43, 44t
in pediatric patients, 43

Contact lenses after corneoscleral
laceration repair, 218–219
Contusion injuries, 257
lens, 258–269
associated complications, 259–261
diagnosis, 258–259
management, 261–269
retinal pigment epithelial, 324
Conversion disorder, 418
Cornea
damage to, 49–50
diagnosis, 49
management, 50
examination of, 35
foreign bodies, 181–182, 311–312
diagnosis, 181, 182f
examination, 311
management, 182, 182f, 311–312
foreign body sensation, sudden, 6
noninfectious disorders of, 173–183
basic considerations, 174
ocular examination, 174–175
patient evaluation, 174
perforation
infectious keratitis with, 83
with severe chemical burn, 168, 169f
red eye, 186, 186t
Corneal abrasion, 179–180
diagnosis, 179, 180f
management, 179–180
semi-pressure patch for, 180, 180f
Corneal blunt trauma, 178–179
diagnosis, 178, 179f
management, 178–179
Corneal culture, 196f, 197
Corneal lacerations
emergent surgery for, 81
stellate, 215, 217f
surgical management of, 212–218
Corneal punch biopsy, 201, 202f
Corneal recurrent erosion, 180–181
diagnosis, 180–181, 181f
management, 181
Corneal scrapings, 197, 197f
Corneal sutures, placement to reduce
postoperative astigmatism, 214f,
215–216, 217f
Corneal swabbing, 196f, 196–197

Corneoscleral lacerations, 207–225
  ancillary testing, 210
  bandage contact lens for, 211
  basic considerations, 207–208
  definitions, 208–209
  emergent surgery for, 81–82
  examination, 209–210
  history, 209
  initial management, 210
  isolated, 211
  medical management, 211
  patching for, 211
  patient evaluation, 209–210
  postoperative management, 218
  prognostic factors, 210–211
  surgical management of, 212–218, 213,
    214f, 215, 215f
  visual rehabilitation, 218–219
Corneoscleral ruptures, 207–225
  ancillary testing, 210
  basic considerations, 207–208
  definitions, 208–209
  examination, 209–210
  history, 209
  initial management, 210
  patient evaluation, 209–210
  postoperative management, 218
  prognostic factors, 210–211
  surgical management of, 212–218, 215f
  visual rehabilitation, 218–219
Corneoscleral sutures, 215, 216f
Corneoscleral tunnels, self-sealing, 271f,
  272
Cortical blindness, retrogeniculate trauma
  and, 365–366
Cortical material, dropped into vitreous
  during cataract extraction, 400
Corticosteroids, oral, 143–144
CRAO. *See* Central retinal artery
  occlusion
Cryotherapy, 298–299, 299f
Crystallin lens examination, 35
CSR. *See* Central serous
  chorioretinopathy
CT. *See* Computed tomography
Culture
  corneal, 196f, 197
  endophthalmitis, 279–280

Cyclodialysis, 230–231
  diagnosis, 230
  management, 230–231
Cyclodialysis clefts, 269
  repair procedure, 272
Cytomegalovirus retinitis, 145
  fulminant, 145, 145f
  indolent, 145, 145f
  treatment, 140t

D

Dacryoadenitis, 117–119, 158–159
  acute suppurative, 117–118
    diagnosis, 118
    etiology, 117
    management, 118
  chronic, 118–119
    diagnosis, 119
    etiology, 118–119
    management, 119
Dacryocystitis, 121–124
  acute, 122, 122f
  causes of obstruction, 121
  diagnosis, 122
  etiology/microbiology, 121–122
  management, 122–123
  neonatal, 123–124
  signs, 122, 122f
Dacryocystography, 61
Dalen-Fuch's nodules, 408, 408f
Databases, 9–10
Dehiscence
  wound, 220, 220f
  zonular
    signs of, 259, 259t
    traumatic cataracts with minimal or
      no, 261–263
Demerol
  for conscious sedation, 43, 44t
  pediatric dosing, 427t
Deprivation amblyopia, 53
Descemet's membrane
  breaks in, 49–50
  vertical breaks in, 178, 179f
Desert Shield, 22
Desert Storm, 22
Dexamethasone, 430

Diabetic retinopathy, proliferative, 349
Dialysis
    cyclodialysis, 230–231
    cyclodialysis clefts, 269
        repair procedure, 272
    iridodialysis, 228–229
        repair procedure, 271f, 272
    retinal, 295
Diamox, 427t
Diffuse anterior scleritis, 153
Diffuse orbital inflammation, 157
Dilated fundus examination, pediatric,
    48
Diplopia, monocular, 423
Disability
    visual
        evaluation of, 433–455
        nonorganic, 417–425
        sudden nontraumatic, 333–350
    of whole person, visual system
        impairment and, 441, 454t
Dislocated cataractous lens, management,
    263–269
    anterior techniques for, 263
    extracapsular techniques for, 264
    intracapsular technique for, 263f,
        263–264
    pars plana retrieval, 265f, 266
    posterior techniques for, 264
Dislocated lens
    and glaucoma, 248–249
    pars plana recovery of, 266
Dislocated lens-associated ocular
    injuries, 260–261
Disorders
    of afferent visual system, 351–
        367
    neurovascular, 387–391
    optic nerve, 351–367
    vitreous, 347–349
Double vision
    atraumatic, 3–4
    traumatic, 4
Droop, eyelid, acute, 8
Drugs. *See also* Antibiotics; *specific*
    drugs
    for conscious sedation, 43, 44t
    lens trauma due to, 257

muscle relaxants, 95
    pediatric dosing, 427t

E
E charts, 30, 46
"E game," 30
Echography, 59–60. *See also* Ultrasound
Ectopia lentis
    conditions associated with, 248, 249t
    glaucoma secondary to, 248t, 248–249
Edema, Berlin's, 290, 323–324, 324f
Electrical injury, 182–183
Emergencies
    choroid, 290–295
    clinical scenarios, 1–8
    glaucomatous, 235–255
    posterior segment, 285–307
    preventable, 9–28
    retinal, 295–306
    vitreous, 286–290
Emergent surgery
    for corneal laceration, 81
    for corneoscleral laceration, 81–82
    for endophthalmitis, 82–83
    for giant cell arteritis, 83
    indications for, 80, 80t
    for intraocular foreign body, 83–84
    intraoperative, 393–405
    for lid lacerations, 84–85
    for nonarteritic anterior ischemic optic
        neuropathy, 85
    for orbital bone fracture with and
        without muscle entrapment, 85
    for orbital bone fracture with optic
        nerve compression, 85
    for orbital cellulitis secondary to
        sinusitis, 85–86
    for orbital foreign body, 86
    overview, 80–81
    for perforating injury, 86–87
    for posterior perforating injury, 87
    postoperative, 393–405
    for retinal detachment, 87
    for sickle cell hyphema and elevated
        IOP, 88
    timing
        basic considerations, 79–80

guidelines for, 79–89
for traumatic retrobulbar hemorrhage,
87–88
Encircling scleral buckle procedure,
301–305, 305f
Endophthalmitis, 275–283
bacterial
acute and delayed postoperative and
endogenous, 281
panuveitis involvement, 149
basic considerations, 275–282
culture sites and methods, 279–280
diagnosis, 277–280
diagnostic imaging, 63
differential diagnosis, 278–279
emergent surgery for, 82–83
endogenous, 275, 276
differential diagnosis, 279
onset, 278
endogenous bacterial, 281
endogenous fungal, 281
epidemiology, 276
follow-up treatment, 282
fungal, endogenous, 281
imaging studies, 278
infected conjunctival bleb with, 277,
278f
onset, 277–278
organisms isolated from, 276–277,
277t
postoperative, 275, 276
differential diagnosis, 278–279
onset, 278
postoperative bacterial, 281
postoperative fungal, 281
prophylaxis for penetrating trauma,
280–281
radiologic findings, 63, 64f, 65f
signs and symptoms of, 277, 278f
traumatic, 275, 276
differential diagnosis, 278
onset, 277
treatment, 280–282
follow-up, 282
types of, 275
Endophthalmitis-Vitrectomy Study
(EVS), 82
Enucleation, 409–413

complications of, 412–413
indications for, 410
with insertion of plastic sphere or
Medpor implant, 411, 412f–413f
postoperative management, 411–412
procedure, 411, 412f–413f
Epidemic keratoconjunctivitis, 192
Epidemiology, 9–28
Episcleritis, 150–151
basic considerations, 150
diagnosis/workup, 151
etiology, 150
management, 151
Epithelial contusion, retinal pigment, 324
Epithelial keratophy, punctate, 125
Epitheliopathy, acute posterior multifocal
placoid pigment, 146
Erosion, corneal recurrent, 180–181
Erythropsia, 346–347
diagnosis, 347
management, 347
Esterman grid, 439f, 440
ETDRS charts, 30
Ethmoiditis, orbital cellulitis with SPA
secondary to, 131, 132f
Evaluation, 29–37
recommended guidelines for timing of,
1–8
Evisceration, 413–414
indications for, 414
postoperative management, 414
procedure summary, 414
EVS. *See* Endophthalmitis-Vitrectomy
Study
Examination, 30
anterior segment, 34–35
pediatric, 48
with corneoscleral lacerations and
ruptures, 209–210
dilated fundus, pediatric, 48
external, 31
pediatric, 46
with glaucomatous emergencies, 237
neuro-ophthalmic, 351
for noninfectious disorders of
conjunctiva and cornea, 174–
175
with occult scleral ruptures, 220–221

Examination (*contd.*)
  pediatric, 41–48
  posterior segment, 36–37
  pupillary, 31
Explants, 302, 302f
  suture placement to secure, 302–304, 303f
Expulsive choroidal hemorrhage, 397
Expulsive suprachoroidal hemorrhage, 397
External examination, 31
  pediatric, 46
External hordeolum, 125
Extracapsular techniques for subluxed or dislocated cataractous lens, 264
Extraocular motility assessment, 33–34
Eye injuries. *See* Injuries; Ocular trauma
Eye movements
  acute disorders of, 369–385
  in coma, 381
  traumatic disorders of, 369–385
Eyelid closure, neonatal, 49
Eyelid droop (ptosis), acute, 8
Eyelid infections, 124–130
Eyelid injuries, 97–106
  basic considerations, 97
  diagnosis, 98
  management, 98–106
Eyelid lacerations
  canthotomy and cantholysis for, 102, 102f
  emergent surgery for, 84–85
  full-thickness defects, 102, 102f
  involving deeper structures, 103–106
  involving eyelid margin, 101f, 101–102, 102f
  involving lateral canthus, 103
  involving medial canthus and lacrimal system, 102–103, 104f–105f
  simple, skin alone or skin and orbicularis, 100, 100f
Eyelid margin
  lacerations involving, 101f, 101–102, 102f
  repair of, 101, 101f
Eyelid speculum, 41, 42f
Eyelid twitching, acute, 7
Eyewall, 208

F
Facial nerve function testing, 352
Fentanyl citrate (Sublimaze), 43, 44t
Fever, pharyngoconjunctival, 192
Fistula, carotid-cavernous, 387–389
  traumatic
    diagnostic imaging, 74
    radiologic findings, 74
Flashes of light (photopsia), 5
Flashing lights, 347–348
Fleeting blindness, 334–335
Floaters, 347–348
  emergent clinical scenario, 5
Fluid drainage, subretinal, during scleral buckling retinal reattachment surgery, 293–294, 294t
Follicular conjunctivitis, acute, 191
Forced duction testing, 34, 34f
Foreign bodies
  anterior chamber angle, 312–313
  conjunctival, 176
  corneal, 181–182, 311–312
  diagnostic imaging, 65–66
  identifying, 209, 210f
  intraocular
    definition, 209
    emergent surgery for, 83–84
    management of, 309–318
  intravitreal, 314–315
  iris, 312–313
  lenticular, 313–314
  orbital, 114–115
    emergent surgery for, 86
  radiologic findings, 65–66, 66f, 67f
  retained intraocular, 149
  retinal, 315–317
Foreign body sensation, sudden corneal, 6
Fourth (trochlear) nerve palsy, 372–375
  diagnosis, 372–374
    three-step test, 373f, 373–374
  management, 374–375
Fractures
  canal
    diagnostic imaging, 74
    radiologic findings, 74
  LeFort I, 113, 113f
  LeFort II, 113, 113f

LeFort III, 113f, 114
medial orbital wall, 111
naso-orbital-ethmoid, 114
orbital, 110
   complex, 113–114
   diagnostic imaging, 68
   radiologic findings, 68, 68f
orbital bone
   with optic nerve compression, 85
   with and without muscle entrapment,
     85
orbital floor (blowout), 110–111
   repair procedure, 111–113, 112f
orbital roof, 111–113
Fuchs' heterochromic iridocyclitis, 139
Fulminant keratitis, 196, 197f
Fungal endophthalmitis, 277, 277t
   endogenous, 281
   postoperative, delayed-onset, 281
Fungal keratitis, 201–202
   diagnosis, 201
   management, 201–202, 202f
Fungal orbital cellulitis, 133

G
Gaze palsy, 379
Gender, 10
Geniculate body, lateral, 365
Ghost cell glaucoma, 245–246
   diagnosis, 245
   management, 246
Giant cell arteritis, 356–358
   diagnosis, 357–358
   emergent surgery for, 83
   management, 358
Glaucoma
   angle-closure
     diagnosis, 239t, 239–240
     general characteristics of, 186, 186t
     primary, 237–241
   associated with phacoanaphylactic
     uveitis, 248t
   classification system for, 236, 236f
   congenital, 252–253
   ghost cell, 245–246
   inflammatory disorders associated
     with, 242, 243t

lens particle, 247–248, 248t
   after lens injury, 259
lens-induced, 247, 248t
malignant, 241–242
neovascular, 250
phacolytic (lens protein), 247, 248t
   after lens injury, 260
phacomorphic, 248t
pseudoexfoliative, 246
pupillary block, 237, 238f
secondary to ectopia lentis, 248t,
   248–249
steroid-response, 253
subluxed or dislocated lens and,
   248–249
Glaucomatocyclitic crisis, 244–245
Glaucomatous emergencies, 235–255
   basic considerations, 236–237
   examination, 237
Globe injuries
   closed, 208
   open, 257
     definition, 208
     occult, 219, 219t
     penetration
       diagnosis, 394
       management, 394–395
       precautions to prevent, 394
       during retrobulbar injection,
         393–395
       during strabismus surgery, 395
     rupture or laceration
       diagnostic imaging, 70
       radiologic findings, 70, 72f,
         73f
Goldmann lens, 237
Goldmann perimetry testing, 422
Goldmann visual field testing, 33
Gonioscopy, 35, 237
   Goldmann lens, 237
   for identifying foreign bodies, 209,
     210f
   Zeiss lens, 237
Gonorrheal conjunctivitis, 187–190
   diagnosis, 187, 189f
   management, 188–190
Gram-negative bacterial keratitis,
   195–197

Gram-negative endophthalmitis, 277, 277t
Gram-positive bacterial keratitis, 195
Granulomatous panuveitis, bilateral, 407
Guibor stents (Concept), 103

H

Hand motion vision
  patient claiming 20/40 to, 419–422
  patient claiming, to no light perception, 419
Hardy-Rand-Rittle plates, 33
Hematoma
  orbital
    diagnostic imaging, 69
    radiologic findings, 69, 70f
  subperiosteal
    diagnostic imaging, 71–73
    radiologic findings, 71–73
Hemophilus influenzae conjunctivitis, 190, 191f
  management, 190
Hemorrhage
  expulsive choroidal, 397
  orbital
    diagnostic imaging, 69
    radiologic findings, 69, 70f
    traumatic, 108–109
  preretinal, 51, 52f
  retinal, 50
  retrobulbar
    during retrobulbar injection, 395–397
    traumatic, 87–88
  subconjunctival, 175–176
  submacular, 326, 326f
  suprachoroidal
    drainage of, 293, 294f
    expulsive, 397
    intraoperative, 397–398
    risk factors for, 397
  traumatic orbital, 108–109
  traumatic retrobulbar, 87–88
  vitreous, 40t, 286–289
    diagnostic imaging, 74–75
    radiologic findings, 74–75, 75f
    spontaneous, 348–349

Hemorrhagic choroidal detachment, 293, 293t
Hemorrhagic conjunctivitis, 192
Hereditary optic neuropathy, 360–361
Herpes simplex virus infection
  anterior uveitis involvement, 138
  conjunctivitis, 192
  keratitis, 198–200, 199f
    diagnosis, 198–199, 199f
    management, 199–200
    signs and symptoms of, 199
Herpes zoster ophthalmicus, 200–201
  diagnosis, 200
  management, 200–201
Hertel measurements, 31f, 31–32
Histoplasmosis, 145
History, 29–30
  corneoscleral lacerations and ruptures, 209
  in neuro-ophthalmic evaluation, 351
  for noninfectious disorders of conjunctiva and cornea, 174
  with occult scleral ruptures, 220
  pediatric, 40–41
HLA-B27
  anterior uveitis involvement, 138
  -associated panuveitis, 149
Hordeolum, 125–126
  chalazion excision procedure, 126, 127f
  diagnosis, 126
  etiology, 126
  external or anterior, 125
  internal or posterior, 125
  management, 126, 127f
Horner's syndrome, 383–385
  diagnosis, 384–385
  management, 385
HOTV, 30
HSV. *See* Herpes simplex virus
Humphrey visual field testing, 33
Hyperacute conjunctivitis, 187, 189f
Hyphema, 231–234
  automated removal of, 233, 234f
  diagnosis, 231
  management, 231–233
  surgical management of
    indications for, 233
    procedures for, 233–234

Hypochondriasis, 418
HZO. *See* Herpes zoster ophthalmicus

I

Imaging, 55–77. *See also specific modalities*
  basic considerations, 55–56
  diagnostic, 62–75
  ordering, 56
  studies, 56–61
Immunocompromised individuals, acute visual disturbance in, 4
Impairment
  visual
    evaluation of, 433–455
    nonorganic, 417–425
    sudden nontraumatic, 333–350
  of whole person, visual system impairment and, 441, 454t
Implants
  Medpor, 411, 412f–413f
  selection of, 410–411
Incarceration, retinal, 305–306
Incidence, 10–13
Infants. *See also under* Pediatric
  cloudy cornea in, 46, 46t
  visual acuity testing, 45
Infections. *See also specific infections*
  conjunctival bleb, 277, 278f
  herpes simplex virus, 138
  lacrimal system, 117–124
  of lids, 124–130
  precautions to prevent spread in office setting, 191
  varicella-zoster virus, 138
Infectious conjunctivitis, 185–206
  etiologic agents, 188, 188t
Infectious inflammatory disorders
  diagnostic imaging of, 66–67
  radiologic findings, 66–67
Infectious keratitis with corneal perforation, 83
Infectious uveitis, 140t, 141
Inflammation
  necrotizing anterior scleritis with, 153
  orbital inflammatory syndrome, 155–160

Inflammatory disorders
  associated with glaucoma, 242, 243t
  infectious and noninfectious
    diagnostic imaging of, 66–67
    radiologic findings, 66–67
Inflammatory syndromes
  ocular, 137–161
  periocular, 137–161
Inflammatory uveitis, 242–244
  diagnosis, 242–243
  management, 244
Injection, retrobulbar
  penetration of globe during, 393–395
  retrobulbar hemorrhage during, 395–397
Injuries. *See also* Ocular trauma; Trauma
  anterior segment, 227–234
  assault-related, 21t, 21–22
  blunt
    conjunctival, 175
    direct, 320
    emergent clinical scenario, 3
    traumatic retinopathy after, 324, 324f
  chemical, 163–170
    common causes of, 163, 164t
    Thoft's classification of, 164, 165t, 166f
  in children, 11, 12t
  choroid, 290–295
  classification system, 208, 208f
  closed globe, 208
  contusion, 257
  dislocated lens-associated, 260–261
  electrical, 182–183
  intraocular foreign body, 209
  lacrimal system, 97–106
  lens
    contusion and lacerating, 258–269
    dislocated, 260–261
    management of, 257–273
  lid, 97–106
  occupational, 13–18
    key findings of reports on, 13, 14t–17t
  open globe, 208, 257
  penetrating

Induries, penetrating (*contd.*)
  definition, 209
  emergent clinical scenario, 3
  perforating
    definition, 209
    emergent surgery for, 86–87
    posterior, 87
  photic, 320
  posterior perforating, 87
  posterior segment, 285–307
  retinal, 295–306
  retinal vascular, 320
  splash, 1–2
  sports-related, 18–20, 19t
  thermal burns, 170–171
  vitreous, 286–290
  of war, 22, 22t
Injury databases, 9–10
Injury potential, determination of, 24, 25f
Inner choroidopathy, punctate, 147
INO. *See* Internuclear ophthalmoplegia
Intermediate uveitis, 141–144
  description, 141–142
  diagnosis, 142–143
  etiology, 142
  idiopathic, 142
  management, 143
  periocular therapy, 143
Internal hordeolum, 125
International Society of Ocular Trauma,
    208
Internuclear ophthalmoplegia, 380
  bilateral, 380
  wall-eyed bilateral, 380
Interstitial keratitis, 205
  diagnosis, 205
  management, 205
Intracapsular technique for traumatically
    dislocated cataractous lens, 263f,
    263–264
Intraocular foreign bodies
  anterior segment, 309, 311–314
  basic considerations, 309–311
  composition and size, 310
  emergent surgery for, 83–84
  initial management, 310–311
  injury due to, 209
  management of, 309–318

posterior segment, 310, 314–317
  retained, 149
Intraocular laser photocoagulation with
    endoprobe, 298
Intraocular lens, posterior chamber
  fixation in ciliary sulcus, 268f, 269
  insertion of, 268, 268f
  iris fixation procedure, 267
  scleral fixation procedure, 267–269
Intraocular lens implantation, 262–263
  anterior chamber, 262–263
  in eyes without capsular support,
      266–267
  posterior chamber, 262
    support alternatives for, 267
Intraocular lens-associated uveitis, 139
Intraocular magnets, 314–315, 315f
Intraocular pressure
  elevated, sickle cell hyphema and, 88
  evaluation of, 36
    pediatric, 47
Intraocular tumors, 344–345
  diagnosis, 344–345
  management, 345
Intraoperative emergencies, 393–405
Intravitreal antibiotics, 430–431
Intravitreal foreign bodies, 314–315
  examination, 314
  management, 314–315, 315f
  removal via vitrectomy and forceps,
      316, 317f
IOP. *See* Intraocular pressure
Iridectomy, Nd-YAG laser peripheral,
    241
Iridocyclitis, 137
  Fuchs' heterochromic, 139
Iridodialysis, 228–229
  diagnosis, 228, 228f
  management, 229
  repair procedure, 271f, 272
Iris
  configuration in pupillary block
      glaucoma, 237, 238f
  examination of, 35
Iris defects
  radial, 269–272
  traumatic, 269–272
Iris fixation of posterior chamber IOL, 267

Iris foreign bodies, 312–313
  management, 312–313
Iris plateau syndrome, 237, 238f
Iris sphincter tears, 228–229
  diagnosis, 228
  management, 229
Iritis, 137
  traumatic, 228
Irrigation, ocular
  Mediflow lens for, 165, 166f
  with neutral solution, 165, 166f
Ischemic optic neuropathy
  anterior, 355
  arteritic, 356–358
    diagnosis, 357f, 357–358
    management, 358
  nonarteritic, 355–356
    diagnosis, 355–356
    management, 356
  posterior, 355
Ishihara plates, 33
Itchiness, acute periocular, 6

J
JRA. *See* Juvenile rheumatoid arthritis
Juvenile rheumatoid arthritis, 138–139

K
Keratitis, 194–205
  bacterial, 195–198
  basic considerations, 185
  diagnostic stains for, 195, 196t
  differential diagnosis based on clinical
    signs, 186–187
  fulminant, 196, 197f
  fungal, 201–202
  herpes simplex, 198–200
  infectious, 194–205
    with corneal perforation, 83
  infectious agents that cause, 195, 196t
  interstitial (stromal), 205
  noninfectious, 185
    causes, 185
  parasitic, 202–205
  risk factors for, 194–195
  signs and symptoms of, 186–187
  superficial punctate, 182, 183f

ulcerative, 195, 197f
viral, 198–201
Keratoconjunctivitis
  adult chlamydial, 193
  epidemic, 192
Keratophy, punctate epithelial, 125
Keratoplasty, penetrating
  after chemical burn, 169f, 169–170
  after corneoscleral laceration repair,
    219
Keratoprostheses, 170, 170f
Ketamine hydrochloride, 43, 44t
Kimura spatulas, 107
"Kissing" choroidal detachments, 293

L
Laboratory testing, preoperative, 93–94,
    94t
Lacerations
  conjunctival, 176–177
  corneal
    emergent surgery for, 81
    stellate, 215, 217f
  corneoscleral, 207–225
    emergent surgery for, 81–82
    surgical management of, 213, 214f
  definition, 209
  globe
    diagnostic imaging, 70
    radiologic findings, 70, 72f, 73f
  lens, 258–269
    associated complications, 259–261
    diagnosis, 258–259
    management, 261–269
  lid
    emergent surgery for, 84–85
    involving deeper structures,
      103–106
    involving eyelid margin, 101f,
      101–102, 102f
    involving lacrimal system, 102–103,
      104f–105f
    involving lateral canthus, 103
    involving medial canthus, 102–103,
      104f–105f
    simple, skin alone or skin and
      orbicularis, 100, 100f

Lacerations (*contd.*)
  scleral
    partial-thickness, 212
    posterior full-thickness, 221–224, 222f
Lacrimal gland infection, 117–119
Lacrimal system infections, 117–124
  basic considerations, 117
  risk factors, 117
Lacrimal system injuries, 97–106
  basic considerations, 97
  diagnosis, 98
  management, 98–106
    general considerations, 98–100
Lacrimal system lacerations, 102–103, 104f–105f
Landholt C charts, 30
Laser
  indirect ophthalmoscope delivery system, 297–298
  slit-lamp delivery system, 297
  transscleral diode delivery system, 298
Laser photocoagulation
  intraocular, with endoprobe, 298
  of retinal breaks without retinal detachment, 297, 297f
Lateral canthus lacerations, 103
Lateral geniculate body trauma, 365
  diagnosis, 365
  management, 365
Leber hereditary optic neuropathy, 360–361
  diagnosis, 360–361
  management, 361
LeFort I fracture, 113, 113f
LeFort II fracture, 113, 113f
LeFort III fractures, 113f, 114
Left superior oblique palsy, 373f, 373–374
Legal considerations, 424–425
Lens
  cataractous, 263–269
  clarity, 258–259
  contusion, 258–269
  crystallin, 35
  injuries, 257–273
  lacerating injuries, 258–269

  nuclear material dropped into vitreous, 400
  position and stability, 259
  subluxed or dislocated, 248–249
  subluxed or dislocated cataractous, 263–269
  trauma mechanisms, 257
Lens particle glaucoma, 247–248, 248t
  diagnosis, 247
  after lens injury, 259
  management, 248
Lens protein glaucoma, 247
Lens stability, 259
Lensectomy, pars plana, 264–266, 265f
Lenses, contact, 218–219
Lens-induced angle closure, 259
Lens-induced glaucomas, 247, 248t
Lens-induced uveitis, 260
Lenticular aspiration, bimanual technique for, 261–262, 262f
Lenticular foreign bodies, 313–314
  examination, 313–314
Lesions, supranuclear, 379–381
Letters (for visual testing), 30
Leukocoria, 39, 40t
Levator muscle trauma, 103–106
LHON. *See* Leber hereditary optic neuropathy
Lids. *See under* Eyelid
Limbal approach to bimanual lenticular aspiration, 261–262, 262f
Limbal paracentesis, 269, 270f
Loss of vision. *See also* Visual impairment
  nonorganic, 417–425
  nontraumatic
    sudden, 333–350
    sudden painless, 2
    transient, 2
  sudden nontraumatic, 333–350
    basic considerations, 333–334
    painless, 2
  sudden painful, 3
  sudden painless nontraumatic, 2
  transient nontraumatic, 2
  traumatic, three-part strategy for preventing, 24–26

Lyme disease
  treatment of, 140t
  uveitis involvement, 142

M

Macular hole
  idiopathic, 343–345
    diagnosis, 344
    management, 344
  traumatic, 327f, 327–328
Maculopathy
  photic
    mild-to-moderate, 328–329, 329f
    severe, 329, 330f
  traumatic, 319–331
Magnetic resonance angiography, 59
Magnetic resonance imaging, 55, 57–59
  of aneurysm, 62
  of choroidal detachments, 62
  of optic neuritis, 69
  of orbital hemorrhage or hematoma, 69
  of retinal detachment, 69
  of thyroid orbitopathy, 74
  of traumatic carotid-cavernous fistula, 74
  of vitreous hemorrhage, 75
Magnets, intraocular, 314–315, 315f
"Malar rash," 125
Malignant glaucoma, 241–242
  diagnosis, 241–242
  management, 242
Malingering, 417
Maryland State Health Services Cost Review Commission, 10
Massachusetts Eye and Ear Infirmary, 11
Medial canthus lacerations, 102–103, 104f–105f
Medial orbital wall fractures, 111
Medical history interview, 92, 92t
Medical management
  of avulsion of vitreous base, 290
  of chorioretinitis sclopeteria, 291
  of choroidal detachment, 292–293
    indications for, 292, 292t
  of isolated corneoscleral lacerations, 211

of partial-thickness scleral lacerations, 212
  of vitreous hemorrhage, 287
Medical/legal considerations, 424–425
Medications. *See* Drugs
Mediflow lens, 165, 166f
Medpor implant, 411, 412f–413f
Meperidine hydrochloride (Demerol)
  for conscious sedation, 43, 44t
  pediatric dosing, 427t
Metabolic optic neuropathy, 362–363
Metal shields, 1, 2f
MEWDS. *See* Multiple evanescent white dot syndrome
Microbial conjunctivitis, 187
  etiologic agents, 188, 188t
Midazolam hydrochloride (Versed), 43, 44t
Migraine, 345–346
  common, 345
  diagnosis, 345–346
  management, 346
  ophthalmoplegic, 345
  retinal, 345
Monocular diplopia, 423
Monocular visual field
  loss of, 438, 438t
  sample, 439f
Moraxella conjunctivitis, 190
Morphine sulfate, 43, 44t
Motility, abnormal, visual impairment due to, 440f, 440–441
Motility evaluation
  extraocular, 33–34
  in neuro-ophthalmic evaluation, 351
  pediatric, 47
Motor vehicle accidents, 24
  ocular trauma secondary to, 24, 25t
MRI. *See* Magnetic resonance imaging
Mucormycosis
  diagnostic imaging of, 66–67
  radiologic findings, 66–67
Multifocal choroiditis, 146
Multifocal placoid pigment epitheliopathy, acute posterior, 146
Multiple evanescent white dot syndrome, 147

Multiple ocular motor nerve palsies,
376–377
diagnosis, 376–377
management, 377
Multiple sclerosis, 142
Münchausen's syndrome, 418
ocular, 424
Münchausen's syndrome by proxy, 424
Muscle entrapment, orbital bone fracture
with and without, 85
Muscle relaxants, 95
Myasthenia gravis, 377–379
diagnosis, 377–378
management, 378–379
Myopathy, traumatic, 114
Myositis, 158

N
Nasolacrimal duct obstruction,
congenital, 123
Nasolacrimal sac infection, 121
Naso-orbital-ethmoid fractures, 114
National Athletic Injury/Illness Reporting
System, 10
National Electronic Injury Surveillance
System (NEISS), 9–10
National Eye Trauma System (NETS)
Registry, 9, 10
National Hospital Discharge Survey, 10
National Institute for Occupational Safety
and Health (NIOSH), 9, 13
Nd-YAG laser peripheral iridectomy, 241
Near cards, 420
Near vision tests, 420
Necrotizing anterior scleritis, 153
NEISS. *See* National Electronic Injury
Surveillance System
Neisseria gonorrhoeae
hyperacute conjunctivitis due to, 187,
189f
ophthalmia neonatorum due to, 187,
189f
Nembutal. *See* Pentobarbital
Neonatal dacryocystitis, 123–124
diagnosis, 123
etiology, 123
management, 123–124

Neonatal eyelid closure, 49
diagnosis, 49
management, 49
Neonatorum, ophthalmia, 187, 189f
Neovascular glaucoma, 250
diagnosis, 250
management, 250
secondary to retinal diseases, 250, 251t
Neovascularization, choroidal, 339–341
photocoagulation procedure, 326–327
secondary to choroidal rupture, 325, 325f
NETS Registry. *See* National Eye Trauma
System Registry
Neuritis, optic, 358–360
diagnostic imaging, 69
radiologic findings, 69
Neuro-ophthalmic evaluation, 351
examination, 351
history, 351
Neuropathy, optic
arteritic ischemic, 356–358
compressive, 363
orbital bone fractures with, 85
Leber hereditary, 360–361
nonarteritic ischemic, 355–356
emergent surgery for, 85
toxic/metabolic, 362–363
traumatic
diagnosis, 354
diagnostic imaging, 74
direct, 353f, 353–355
indirect, 353–355
management, 354–355
radiologic findings, 74
Neurovascular disorders, 387–391
NIOSH. *See* National Institute for
Occupational Safety and Health
Nodular anterior scleritis, 153
Nonorganic visual loss, 417–425
definitions and terminology, 417–418
diagnostic techniques, 419–423
general considerations, 418
management issues, 423–424
medical/legal considerations, 424–425
Nuclear lens material dropped into
vitreous, 400
Nystagmus, 380
horizontal jerk, 419

O

Occupational injuries, 13–18
Ocular burns, 163–171
Ocular emergencies. *See* Emergencies
Ocular evaluation, 29–37
Ocular examination. *See also*
    Examination
  for noninfectious disorders of
      conjunctiva and cornea, 174–175
Ocular histoplasmosis, 145
Ocular history, 29–37
Ocular inflammatory syndromes,
    137–161
Ocular injuries. *See* Injuries; Ocular
    trauma
Ocular irrigation
  Mediflow lens for, 165, 166f
  with neutral solution, 165, 166f
Ocular motor nerve palsies, 369–377
  multiple, 376–377
Ocular movements in coma, 381
Ocular pulse amplitude, 388
Ocular trauma. *See also* Injuries
  classification system, 208, 208f
  costs of, 24
  epidemiology of, 9–28
  etiology, 13–24
  incidence, 10–13
  pediatric evaluation, 39–54
  prevention of, 24–26
  risk factors, 10–13
  secondary to motor vehicle accidents,
      24, 25t
Oculomotor nerve palsy, 369–372
One-eye patients, functional, 24, 25f
ONTT. *See* Optic neuritis treatment trial
OPA. *See* Ocular pulse amplitude
Open globe, occult, 219, 219t
Open globe injuries, 257
  definition, 208
Ophthalmia, sympathetic, 149, 407–409
Ophthalmia neonatorum, 187, 189f
Ophthalmologic emergencies requiring
    operative procedure, 80, 80t
Ophthalmologic evaluation, 1–8
Ophthalmoplegia, internuclear, 380
Ophthalmoplegic migraine, 345
Ophthalmoscopy, 352

Optic chiasm trauma, 363–364
  diagnosis, 364
  management, 364
Optic disk swelling
  in optic neuritis, 359, 359f
  in papilledema, 361, 362f
Optic nerve
  avulsion of, 353, 353f
  compression of, 85
  disorders of, 351–367
    basic considerations, 351–352
Optic nerve head
  "blurred," 8
  examination of, 37
Optic neuritis, 358–360
  diagnosis, 358–360
  diagnostic imaging, 69
  management, 360
  optic disk swelling in, 359, 359f
  radiologic findings, 69
Optic neuritis treatment trial (ONTT),
    358
Optic neuropathy
  arteritic ischemic, 356–358
  compressive, 363
    orbital bone fractures with, 85
  Leber hereditary, 360–361
  nonarteritic ischemic, 355–356
    emergent surgery for, 85
  toxic/metabolic, 362–363
  traumatic
    diagnosis, 354
    diagnostic imaging, 74
    direct, 353f, 353–355
    indirect, 353–355
    management, 354–355
    radiologic findings, 74
Optic tract trauma, 364–365
  diagnosis, 364–365
  management, 365
Oral corticosteroids, 143–144
Orbicularis, lid lacerations involving skin
    and, 100, 100f
Orbital bone fractures
  with optic nerve compression, 85
  with and without muscle entrapment,
    85
Orbital cellulitis, 130–134

Orbital cellulitis (*contd.*)
  diagnosis, 131–132
  diagnostic imaging, 68–69
  etiology/microbiology, 131
  fungal, 133
  management, 132–134
  radiologic findings, 68–69
  secondary to sinusitis, 85–86
  signs, 131, 132f
  with SPA secondary to ethmoiditis,
    131, 132f
Orbital floor (blowout) fractures,
    110–111
  diagnosis, 110
  management, 110–111
  repair procedure, 111–113, 112f
Orbital foreign bodies, 114–115
  diagnosis, 115
  emergent surgery for, 86
  management, 115
Orbital fractures, 110
  complex, 113–114
  diagnostic imaging, 68
  radiologic findings, 68, 68f
Orbital hemorrhage or hematoma
  diagnostic imaging, 69
  radiologic findings, 69
  traumatic, 108–109
Orbital inflammation
  anterior, 157–158
  diffuse form, 157
  idiopathic, 157
  posterior, 159
Orbital inflammatory syndrome, 155–160
  basic considerations, 155
  diagnosis, 157–159
  differential diagnosis, 155–156, 156t
  diffuse form, 157
  laboratory testing, 156–157
  management, 159–160
Orbital pseudotumor, 155–160. *See also*
    Orbital inflammatory syndrome
  differential diagnosis, 155–156, 156t
Orbital roof fractures, 111–113
Orbital teratoma, 40t
Orbital trauma, 107–116
  basic considerations, 107–108
Orbital wall fractures, medial, 111

Orbitopathy, thyroid
  diagnostic imaging, 74
  radiologic findings, 74

P

Pain, acute atraumatic periocular, 7
Painful loss of vision, sudden, 3
Painless atraumatic loss of vision,
    sudden, 2
Palsy
  fourth (trochlear) nerve, 372–375
  gaze, 379
  left superior oblique, 373f, 373–374
  ocular motor nerve, 369–377
    multiple, 376–377
  sixth (abducens) nerve, 375–376
  third (oculomotor) nerve, 369–372
PAM test. *See* Potential acuity meter test
Pan-retinal photocoagulation, 349
Panuveitis, 148–150
  bilateral granulomatous, 407
  description, 148
  diagnosis, 149–150
  etiology, 148–149
  idiopathic, 148
  management, 150
Paper cups, stiff, 1, 2f
Papilledema, 361, 362f
Papoose board, 41, 41f
Paracentesis
  anterior chamber, 337, 337f
  for hyphema, 233
  limbal, 269, 270f
Parasitic keratitis, 202–205
Pars plana lensectomy, 264–266, 265f
Pars plana recovery of posteriorly
    dislocated lens, 266
Pars plana retrieval of dislocated lens,
    265f, 266
Pars plana vitrectomy, 265f, 266
  for vitreous hemorrhage, 287–289,
    288f
Partial-thickness scleral lacerations, 212
  diagnosis, 212
  management, 212
    medical, 212
    surgical, 212

Patching
  for corneal abrasion, 180, 180f
  for corneoscleral lacerations, 211
  with metal shields, 1, 2f
  semi-pressure, 180, 180f
  with stiff paper cups, 1, 2f
Patient evaluation
  corneoscleral lacerations and ruptures,
    209–210
  for noninfectious disorders of
    conjunctiva and cornea, 174
  pediatric examination, 41–48
  preoperative assessment, 91–94
PCIOL. *See* Posterior chamber
    intraocular lens implantation
Pediatric examination, 41–48
  external, 46
  methods to restrain toddlers for, 42f,
    42–43
  pupillary, 47
Pediatric eye injuries, 11, 12t
Pediatric history, 40–41
  key information to be gathered, 40–41
Pediatric ocular trauma
  conscious sedation, 43
  dosing of medicines, 427t
  evaluation of, 39–54
    basic considerations, 39–40
PEK. *See* Punctate epithelial keratophy
Penetrating injury
  definition, 209
  emergent clinical scenario, 3
  endophthalmitis prophylaxis for,
    280–281
Penetrating keratoplasty
  after chemical burn, 169f, 169–170
  after corneoscleral laceration repair,
    219
Pentobarbital (Nembutal), 43, 44t
Perforating injury
  corneal, infectious keratitis with, 83
  definition, 209
  emergent surgery for, 86–87
  posterior, 87
Perimetry testing, 422
Perineuritis, 159
Periocular inflammatory syndromes,
    137–161

Periocular itchiness, acute, 6
Periocular pain, acute atraumatic, 7
Periocular swelling, atraumatic, 7
Peripheral iridectomy, Nd-YAG laser, 241
Periscleritis, 157–158
Peritomy, conjunctival, 411, 412f
Phacoanaphylactic uveitis, 260
  glaucoma associated with, 248t
Phacoantigenic uveitis, 260
Phacolytic glaucoma, 247, 248t
  diagnosis, 247
  after lens injury, 260
  management, 247
Phacomorphic glaucoma, 248t
Pharmacologic agents. *See* Drugs
Pharyngoconjunctival fever, 192
Photic injury, 320
Photic maculopathy
  mild-to-moderate, 328–329, 329f
  severe, 329, 330f
Photocoagulation
  of choroidal neovascularization,
    326–327
    procedure, 340–341
  laser
    intraocular, with endoprobe, 298
    of retinal breaks without retinal
      detachment, 297, 297f, 298
  pan-retinal, 349
  for proliferative diabetic retinopathy,
    349
Photopsia, 5
Physical examination, 92, 93t
Physical forces, lens trauma due to, 257
Physical status classification, 93, 93t
PION. *See* Posterior ischemic optic
    neuropathy
Placoid pigment epitheliopathy, acute
    posterior multifocal, 146
Plain radiography, 60–61
  Caldwell projection, 61
  of foreign bodies, 66
  Waters projection, 61
Plastic spheres, 411, 412f–413f
POHS. *See* Presumed ocular
    histoplasmosis syndrome
Polymicrobial endophthalmitis, 277, 277t
Posner-Schlossman syndrome, 244–245

Posner-Schlossman syndrome (*contd.*)
  diagnosis, 244–245
  management, 245
Posner-Schlossman/glaucomatocyclitic
    crisis, 139
Posterior chamber intraocular lens
  fixation in ciliary sulcus, 268f, 269
  insertion of, 268, 268f
  iris fixation procedure, 267
  scleral fixation procedure, 267–269
Posterior chamber intraocular lens
    implantation, 262
  support alternatives for, 267
Posterior full-thickness scleral lacerations
    and ruptures, 221–224, 222f, 223f
Posterior hordeolum, 125
Posterior ischemic optic neuropathy, 355
Posterior multifocal placoid pigment
    epitheliopathy, acute, 146
Posterior orbital inflammation, 159
Posterior perforating injury, 87
Posterior scleritis, 153
Posterior segment
  ancillary testing of, 37
  examination of, 36–37
    general principles for, 36
  foreign bodies, 314–317
    basic considerations, 310
  injuries and emergencies
    acute management of, 285–307
    basic considerations, 285–286
Posterior uveitis, 144–148
  description, 144
  diagnosis, 147–148
  etiology, 144–147
  idiopathic, 144
  management, 148
Posterior vitreous detachment, 347–348
  diagnosis, 347
  management, 348
Posteriorly dislocated lens, pars plana
    recovery of, 266
Postoperative acute visual disturbance,
    4–5
Postoperative emergencies, 393–405
Potential acuity meter test, 420
PPV. *See* Pars plana vitrectomy
Prematurity, retinopathy of, 40t

Preretinal hemorrhages, 51, 52f
Preschool children. *See also under*
    Pediatric
  visual acuity testing, 45–46
Preseptal cellulitis, 126–130
  diagnosis, 128–129
  etiology/microbiology, 127–128
  management, 128f, 129–130
  signs and symptoms, 128, 128f
Presumed ocular histoplasmosis
    syndrome, 145
Preventable ocular emergency, 9–28
Prevention, three-part strategy for, 24–26
Prism dissociation test, 421
Proptosis
  acute, 5
  differential diagnosis, 39, 40t
Prostheses
  eyes, 25f
  implants, 410–411
  keratoprosthesis, 170, 170f
Protective devices, 25f, 26
  suppliers, 26
Pseudoexfoliative glaucoma, 246
  diagnosis, 246
  management, 246
Pseudomonas aeruginosa fulminant
    keratitis, 196, 197f
Pseudophakic pupillary block, 253–254
  definition, 253
Pseudotumor
  diagnostic imaging of, 66–67
  orbital, 155–160
  radiologic findings, 66–67
Pseudotumor cerebri, 361–362
  diagnosis, 361, 362f
  management, 362
Psychogenic illness, 417–418
  categories, 417–418
Ptosis. *See* Eyelid droop
Punctate epithelial keratophy, 125
Punctate inner choroidopathy, 147
Punctate keratitis, superficial, 182, 183f
Pupillary block, aphakic/pseudophakic,
    253–254
Pupillary block glaucoma, 237, 238f
Pupillary defects, relative afferent,
    31–32, 32f

Pupillary examination, 31–33
  in evaluation of decreased visual
    acuity, 419
  important points, 32–33
  in neuro-ophthalmic evaluation, 351
  pediatric, 47
Pupils
  acute disorders of, 369–385
  traumatic disorders of, 369–385
Purtscher's retinopathy, 320–321, 321f
  diagnosis, 321
  management, 321

R
Race, 11
Radial iris defects, 269–272
  repair procedure, 269–272, 270f
Radiation, ultraviolet, 182–183
Radiography, plain film, 60–61
  of foreign bodies, 66
Radiology. *See also specific modalities*
  diagnostic findings, 62–75
RAO. *See* Retinal artery occlusion
RAPD. *See* Relative afferent pupillary
    defect
Rash, "malar," 125
Reconstruction, anterior segment,
    257–273
Red, seeing, 346–347
Red desaturation testing, 33
  in neuro-ophthalmic evaluation, 352
Red eye
  acute, 5–6
  general characteristics of, 186, 186t
Red reflex, 348
Red-green duochrome chart test, 420–421
Refraction
  diagnostic, 420
  paired cylinder, 420
Refractive amblyopia, 53
Rehabilitation
  after chemical burn, 169–170
  after corneoscleral laceration repair,
    218–219
Relative afferent pupillary defect
  examination for, 31, 33
  swinging flashlight test for, 31–32, 32f

Retained intraocular foreign bodies, 149
Retina
  diseases of, neovascular angle-closure
    glaucomas secondary to, 250, 251t
  examination of, 36
  injuries and emergencies, 295–306
  visual disorders affecting, 334–347
Retina Society, 208
Retinal artery occlusion, 335–337
  branch, 335
  central, 323, 335
    diagnosis, 335–336, 336f
  diagnosis, 335–336, 336f
  management, 336–337
Retinal breaks
  fishmouthing of, 304, 305f
  without retinal detachment, 295–299
    diagnosis, 296
    management, 296–299
    surgical management, 297–299
Retinal burns, 328–330
  basic considerations, 320
  diagnosis, 328–330
  management, 330
  mechanisms, 328
  prevention during ocular surgery,
    329–330
Retinal detachment, 40t
  diagnostic imaging, 69
  emergent surgery for, 87
  radiologic findings, 69, 71f
  retinal breaks without, 295–299
  rhegmatogenous
    nontraumatic, 342–343
    traumatic, 300–305
Retinal dialysis, 295
  diagnosis, 295, 296f
  surgical management, 295, 296f
Retinal foreign bodies, 315–317
  examination, 316
  management, 316–317
Retinal hemorrhages, 50
  diagnosis, 50
  management, 50
Retinal incarceration, 305–306
  diagnosis, 306, 306f
  mechanisms of, 305
  surgical management, 306

Retinal migraine, 345
Retinal necrosis
  acute, 146
    treatment of, 140t
  progressive outer, 146, 147f
    treatment of, 140t
Retinal pigment epithelial contusion, 324
  diagnosis, 324
  management, 324
Retinal reattachment surgery, scleral
    buckling
  encircling procedure, 301–305, 305f
  subretinal fluid drainage during,
    293–294, 294t
Retinal tears, vitreous hemorrhage
    secondary to, 74–75, 75f
Retinal vascular injuries, 320
Retinal vein occlusion
  branch, 339, 339f
  central, 338–339
Retinitis, cytomegalovirus, 145
  treatment, 140t
Retinoblastoma, 40t
Retinopathy
  of prematurity, 40t
  proliferative diabetic, 349
  Purtscher's, 320–321, 321f
  traumatic, 324, 324f
  Valsalva, 321–322
Retrobulbar hemorrhage
  during retrobulbar injection, 395–397
    diagnosis, 396
    management, 396–397
  traumatic, 87–88
Retrobulbar injection
  penetration of globe during, 393–395
    precautions to prevent, 394
  retrobulbar hemorrhage during,
    395–397
Retrogeniculate trauma, 365–366
  diagnosis, 366
  management, 366
Rhabdomyosarcoma, 40t
Rhegmatogenous retinal detachment
  diagnosis, 300, 342–343, 343f
  management, 300–305, 343
  nontraumatic, 342–343
  surgical management, 301–305
  traumatic, 300–305

Rheumatoid arthritis, juvenile, 138–139
Risk factors, 10–13
Rosacea, 125
RRD. *See* Rhegmatogenous retinal
    detachment
Ruptures
  capsular, traumatic cataracts with,
    261–263
  cataract wounds, 219–220
  choroidal, 325–327
  corneoscleral, 207–225
  definition, 209
  globe
    diagnostic imaging, 70
    radiologic findings, 70, 72f, 73f
  scleral
    posterior full-thickness, 221–224,
      222f
    signs of, 220, 220f

S

Saccade test, 422
Sarcoidosis
  anterior uveitis involvement, 139
  diagnostic imaging of, 66–67
  posterior uveitis involvement, 146
  radiologic findings, 66–67
School-age children. *See also under*
    Pediatric
  visual acuity testing, 46
Scleral buckle procedure
  encircling, 301–305, 305f
  indications for subretinal fluid drainage
    during, 293–294, 294t
Scleral fixation of posterior chamber
    IOL, 267–269
Scleral lacerations
  partial-thickness, 212
  posterior full-thickness, 221–224, 222f,
    223f
Scleral ruptures
  occult, 219–221
    diagnosis, 220–221
    management, 221
    signs of, 219, 219t
  posterior full-thickness, 221–224,
    222f
  signs of, 220, 220f

Scleral sutures, 214f, 216–217
Scleritis, 152–155
  basic considerations, 152
  diagnosis/workup, 152–154
  diffuse anterior, 153
  episcleritis, 150–151
  etiology, 152
  management, 154–155
  necrotizing anterior, 153
  nodular anterior, 153
  posterior, 153
  with secondary uveitis, 139
Scleromalacia perforans, 153
Sedation, conscious
  drugs for, 43, 44t
  in pediatric patients, 43
Seeing red, 346–347
Semi-pressure patches, 180, 180f
Serous chorioretinopathy, central,
  341–342, 342f
Serous choroidal detachment, 293,
  293t
Serpiginous choroidopathy, 145–146
Shaffer-Weiss classification, 252, 252t
Shaken baby syndrome, 51–52, 322–323
  diagnosis, 51–52, 322–323
  management, 323
  ophthalmic findings in, 322
  preretinal hemorrhages in, 51, 52f
Sickle cell hyphema and elevated IOP,
  88
Sinskey hooks, 269, 272
Sinusitis, orbital cellulitis secondary to,
  85–86
Sixth (abducens) nerve palsy, 375–376
  diagnosis, 375–376
  management, 376
Size consistency test, 421–422
Skew deviation, 379–380
Skin
  lid lacerations involving, 100, 100f
  lid lacerations involving orbicularis
    and, 100, 100f
Skin-muscle flap, 100, 100f
Slit-lamp biomicroscopy, 352
Slit-lamp laser delivery system, 297
Snellen charts, 30
Snellen visual acuity test, 421, 421t
  notations and corresponding

percentages of loss of central
  vision, 434, 434t
  ratings for central vision impairment in
    single eye, 435, 436t–437t
SO. *See* Sympathetic ophthalmia
Socioeconomic status, 11
Somatization disorder, 418
SPA. *See* Subperiosteal abscess
Speculum, eyelid, 41, 42f
Splash injury, 1–2
Spondyloarthropathy, 138
Spondyloarthropathy-associated
  panuveitis, 149
Sports-related injuries, 18–20, 19t
Staphylococcus aureus
  conjunctivitis due to, 190
  ulcerative keratitis due to, 195, 197f
Staphylococcus endophthalmitis,
  276–277, 277t
Steroid-response glaucoma, 253
  diagnosis, 253
  management, 253
Steroids, 429–430
Strabismic amblyopia, 53
Strabismus, 39, 40t
Strabismus surgery, 395
Streptococcus endophthalmitis, 277,
  277t
Streptococcus pneumoniae conjunctivitis,
  190
Stromal keratitis, 205
  algorithm for, 204f, 205
Stromal ulceration, 168, 168f
Stye. *See* Hordeolum
Subconjunctival hemorrhage, 175–176
  diagnosis, 175, 175f
  management, 175–176
Subjunctival antibiotics, 429–430
Sublimaze. *See* Fentanyl citrate
Subluxed or dislocated cataractous lens,
  management, 263–269
  anterior techniques for, 263
  extracapsular techniques for, 264
  intracapsular technique for, 263f,
    263–264
  posterior techniques for, 264
Subluxed or dislocated lens and
  glaucoma, 248–249
  diagnosis, 248–249

Subluxed or dislocated lens and glaucoma
        (*contd.*)
    management, 249
Submacular hemorrhage, 326, 326f
Subperiosteal abscess
    diagnostic imaging, 71
    management, 134
    radiologic findings, 71
    secondary to ethmoiditis, 131, 132f
Subperiosteal hematoma
    diagnostic imaging, 71–73
    radiologic findings, 71–73
Subretinal fluid drainage, 293–294,
        294t
Sungazing, moderate photic maculopathy
        secondary to, 329, 329f
Superficial punctate keratitis, 182, 183f
Superior oblique palsy, left, three-step
        test, 373f, 373–374
Suppurative dacryoadenitis, acute,
        117–118
    diagnosis, 118
    etiology, 117
    management, 118
Suprachoroidal hemorrhage
    delayed-onset, 398–399
        diagnosis, 398–399
        management, 399
    drainage of, 293, 294f
    expulsive, 397
    intraoperative, 397–398
        diagnosis, 397
        management, 397–398
    risk factors for, 397
Supranuclear lesions, 379–381
Surface culture, 279
Surgery. *See also specific procedures*
    anterior segment reconstruction,
        257–273
    for avulsion of vitreous base, 290
    bimanual lenticular aspiration
        technique, 261–262, 262f
    cataract extraction, 400
    for chorioretinitis sclopeteria, 291
    for choroidal detachment, 293–295,
        294f
        indications for, 293, 293t
    for corneal and corneoscleral

lacerations and ruptures, 212–218,
        215f
    preparations for, 213
    for corneoscleral lacerations, 213,
        214f, 215
    elective, 81
    emergent. *see* Emergent surgery
    immediate, 80
    intraocular lens implantation, 262–263
    intraoperative suprachoroidal
        hemorrhage, 397–398
    ophthalmologic emergencies requiring,
        80, 80t
    for partial-thickness scleral lacerations,
        212
    patient management for, 91
    patient preparation for, 94
    for posterior full-thickness scleral
        lacerations and ruptures, 221–224,
        222f, 223f
    preoperative preparation, 91–96
    repair of stellate corneal lacerations,
        215, 217f
    for retinal breaks without retinal
        detachment, 297f, 297–299
    retinal burn prevention during,
        329–330
    for retinal dialysis, 295, 296f
    for retinal incarceration, 306
    for rhegmatogenous retinal
        detachment, 301–305
    scleral buckling retinal reattachment,
        293–294, 294t
    semielective, 81
    strabismus, 395
    urgent, 80–81
    for vitreous hemorrhage, 287
Surgical blades, 197, 197f
Sutures
    corneal, 214f, 215–216, 217f
    corneoscleral, 215, 216f
    placement to secure explants, 302–304,
        303f
    scleral, 214f, 216–217
Swabbing, corneal, 196f, 196–197
Swelling
    atraumatic periocular, 7
    optic disk

in optic neuritis, 359, 359f
in papilledema, 361, 362f
Sympathetic ophthalmia, 149, 407–409
diagnosis, 408, 408f
differential diagnosis, 409
management, 409
Syphilis
posterior uveitis involvement, 147
treatment of, 139, 140t
uveitis involvement, 139
Systemic culture, 279

T

Tangent screen testing, 422, 423
Tears
acute, 6–7
iris sphincter, 228–229
retinal, 74–75, 75f
Temporal arteritis. *See* Giant cell arteritis
Teratoma, orbital, 40t
Terminology, 417–418
Terson's syndrome, 322
diagnosis, 322
management, 322
Testing. *See also specific tests*
ancillary
corneoscleral lacerations and
ruptures, 210
of posterior segment, 37
brightness, 33
color vision, 33, 419
in neuro-ophthalmic evaluation, 352
facial nerve function, 352
forced duction, 34, 34f
near vision, 420
perimetry, 422
preoperative laboratory, 93–94, 94t
red desaturation, 33
in neuro-ophthalmic evaluation, 352
size consistency, 421–422
tangent screen, 422, 423
vision, "bottom up," 419–420
visual acuity, 30–31
in neuro-ophthalmic evaluation, 351
pediatric, 43–46
with Titmus stereopsis and Snellen
tests, 421, 421t

visual field, 33
in neuro-ophthalmic evaluation, 351
with nonorganic visual loss, 422
pediatric, 47–48
Tetanus prophylaxis, 40t, 41, 129, 132
Thermal burns, 170–171
basic considerations, 170
diagnosis, 170–171
management, 171
Third (oculomotor) nerve palsy, 369–372
diagnosis, 371–372
management, 372
Thoft's classification of chemical injury,
164, 165t, 166f
Thrombosis, cavernous sinus, 389
Thyroid orbitopathy
diagnostic imaging, 74
radiologic findings, 74
Titmus stereopsis test, 421, 421t
TNO stereo test, 419
Tobramycin, 429
Toddlers. *See also under* Pediatric
methods to restrain, 42f, 42–43
visual acuity testing, 45
Topical antibiotics, 429
Toxic conjunctivitis, 178
diagnosis, 178
iatrogenic, 178
management, 178
Toxic/metabolic optic neuropathy,
362–363
diagnosis, 362
management, 363
Toxocariasis, 40t, 146
Toxoplasmosis
treatment of, 140t
uveitis involvement, 144
Transient atraumatic loss of vision, 2
Transscleral diode laser delivery system,
298
Trauma
to aponeurosis, 103–106
birth, 48–52
blunt corneal, 178–179
differential diagnosis, 39, 40t
to lateral geniculate body, 365
lens, 257
to levator muscle, 103–106

Trauma (*contd.*)
    ocular. *see also* Injuries
        classification system, 208, 208f
        epidemiology of, 9–28
        pediatric evaluation, 39–54
    to optic chiasm, 363–364
    optic tract, 364–365
    orbital, 107–116
    penetrating, 280–281
    retrogeniculate, 365–366
    supranuclear lesions after, 379–381
Traumatic carotid-cavernous fistula
    diagnostic imaging, 74
    radiologic findings, 74
Traumatic cataracts
    with minimal or no zonular dehiscence
        and/or capsular rupture, 261–
        263
    subluxed or dislocated lens, 263–269
Traumatic disorders
    of eye movements, 369–385
    of pupils, 369–385
Traumatic double vision, emergent
    clinical scenario, 4
Traumatic endophthalmitis, 275, 276
    differential diagnosis, 278
    onset, 277
Traumatic iris defects, 269–272
Traumatic iritis, 228
    diagnosis, 228
    management, 228
Traumatic loss of vision, 24–26
Traumatic macular hole, 327f, 327–
    328
    diagnosis, 327
    management, 327–328
Traumatic maculopathies, 319–331
    basic considerations, 319
Traumatic myopathy, 114
    diagnosis, 114
    management, 114
Traumatic optic neuropathy
    diagnostic imaging, 74
    direct, 353f, 353–355
    indirect, 353–355
    radiologic findings, 74
Traumatic orbital hemorrhage, 108–109
    diagnosis, 108
    management, 108–109

lateral canthotomy and cantholysis
    procedure, 109, 109f
Traumatic retinopathy, 324, 324f
Traumatic retrobulbar hemorrhage, 87–88
Trigeminal nerve function testing, 352
Trochlear nerve palsy, 372–375
Tropicamide cure, 423
Tropicamide test, 421
Tuberculosis
    diagnostic imaging of, 66–67
    radiologic findings, 66–67
Tumbling E, 30, 46
Tumors
    intraocular, 344–345
    orbital pseudotumor, 155–160
    pseudotumor cerebri, 361–362
Twitching, acute eyelid, 7
Tylenol elixir, 427t

U
Ulceration, stromal, 168, 168f
Ulcerative keratitis, 195, 197f
Ultrasonography. *See* Ultrasound
Ultrasound, 55, 59–60
    of choroidal detachments, 62, 63f
    of endophthalmitis, 63, 64f
    of foreign bodies, 65–66, 67f
    of inflammatory disorders, 66–67
    of orbital cellulitis, 69
    of orbital fractures, 68, 68f
    of orbital hemorrhage or hematoma,
        69, 70f
    of retinal detachment, 69, 71f
    of ruptured or lacerated globes, 70, 72f,
        73f
    of thyroid orbitopathy, 74
    of traumatic carotid-cavernous fistula,
        74
    of traumatic optic neuropathy and
        canal fracture, 74
    of vitreous hemorrhage, 74–75, 75f
Ultraviolet radiation, 182–183
    diagnosis, 182, 183f
    management, 183
United States Eye Injury Registry
    (USEIR), 9, 10
USEIR. *See* United States Eye Injury
    Registry

Uveitis, 137–150
anterior, 137–141
basic considerations, 137
general characteristics of, 186, 186t
infectious, 140t, 141
inflammatory, 242–244
intermediate, 141–144
intraocular lens-associated, 139
lens-induced, 260
panuveitis, 148–150
bilateral granulomatous, 407
phacoanaphylactic, 260
glaucoma associated with, 248t
phacoantigenic, 260
posterior, 144–148
secondary, 139

V

Valsalva retinopathy, 321–322
diagnosis, 321–322
management, 322
Vancomycin
intravitreal preparation, 430–431
subconjunctival preparation, 430
topical preparation, 429
Varicella-zoster virus infection, 138
Vascular injuries, retinal, 320
Versed. *See* Midazolam hydrochloride
Viral conjunctivitis, 190–194
Viral keratitis, 198–201
Virus. *See also specific viruses*
precautions to prevent spread in office
setting, 191
Vision testing. *See also* Testing
"bottom up," 419–420
Visual acuity
corresponding percentages of loss of
central vision, 434, 434t
decreased
evaluation of, 419–423
patient claiming hand motion to no
light perception, 419
normal optotype, 45
Visual acuity testing, 30–31
in neuro-ophthalmic evaluation, 351
pediatric, 43–46
with Titmus stereopsis and Snellen
tests, 421, 421t

Visual disability. *See* Visual impairment
Visual disorders
affecting retina and choroid, 334–347
affecting vitreous, 347–349
of afferent visual system, 351–367
of optic nerve, 351–367
Visual distortion, acute, 4
Visual disturbances
acute
in immunocompromised individual,
4
in postoperative patient, 4–5
nonorganic, 417
sudden nontraumatic, 333–350
basic considerations, 333–334
Visual field
monocular
loss of, 438, 438t
sample, 439f
normal values, 435, 438t
Visual field impairment
determination of, 435–440, 438t,
439f
patients claiming, 422–423
Visual field testing, 33
in neuro-ophthalmic evaluation, 351
with nonorganic visual loss, 422
pediatric, 47–48
Visual impairment
for both eyes, 441, 448t–453t
central, 434t, 434–435, 436t–437t
combined values chart, 441, 442t–
447t
definition of, 433
due to abnormal motility, 440f,
440–441
evaluation of, 433–455
review, 441–455
and impairment of whole person, 441,
454t
nonorganic, 417–425
nontraumatic
sudden, 333–350
sudden painless, 2
transient, 2
percentage of, 433
sudden nontraumatic, 333–350
sudden painful, 3
sudden painless nontraumatic, 2

Visual impairment (*contd.*)
  total, 441, 442t–447t, 448t–453t, 454t
  transient nontraumatic, 2
  traumatic, 24–26
Visual loss. *See* Loss of vision
Visual rehabilitation
  after chemical burn, 169–170
  after corneoscleral laceration repair,
    218–219
Vitrectomy
  intravitreal foreign body removal via,
    316, 317f
  pars plana, 265f, 266
    for vitreous hemorrhage, 287–289,
      288f
Vitreous
  disorders affecting, 347–349
  dropped cortical and nuclear lens
    material into, 400
  examination of, 36
  foreign bodies in, 314–315
  injuries and emergencies, 286–290
  posterior detachment, 347–348
Vitreous base avulsion, 290
  diagnosis, 290
  medical management, 290
  surgical management, 290
Vitreous biopsy, 279–280
Vitreous hemorrhage, 40t, 286–289
  diagnosis, 286
  diagnostic imaging, 74–75
  management, 286–289
    medical, 287
    pars plana vitrectomy, 287–289,
      288f
    surgical, 287

  radiologic findings, 74–75, 75f
  spontaneous, 348–349
    diagnosis, 348
    management, 348–349
Vitreous loss, 399–400
Vitreous Society, 208
Vitreous tap, 279
VKH syndrome. *See* Vogt-Koyanagi-
  Harada syndrome
Vogt-Koyanagi-Harada syndrome, 149
VZV. *See* Varicella-zoster virus

W
Wall-eyed bilateral internuclear
  ophthalmoplegia, 380
War injuries, 22, 22t
Waters projection, 61
WEBINO. *See* Wall-eyed bilateral
  internuclear ophthalmoplegia
Wegener's granulomatosis
  diagnostic imaging of, 66–67
  radiologic findings, 66–67
White dots, 147
WHO. *See* World Health Organization
Work-related eye injuries, 13, 14t–17t
World Health Organization (WHO), 433
Wound dehiscence, 220, 220f
Wounds, cataract, 219–220

Z
Zeiss lens, 237
Zonular dehiscence
  signs of, 259, 259t
    traumatic cataracts with minimal or no,
      261–263